Application of Nanotechnology in Drug Delivery

Application of Nanotechnology in Drug Delivery

Editor: Miranda Cowan

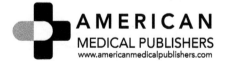

AMERICAN
MEDICAL PUBLISHERS
www.americanmedicalpublishers.com

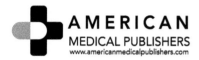

Cataloging-in-Publication Data

Application of nanotechnology in drug delivery / edited by Miranda Cowan.
    p. cm.
Includes bibliographical references and index.
ISBN 978-1-63927-894-7
1. Drug delivery systems. 2. Nanoparticles. 3. Nanotechnology. 4. Pharmaceutical technology.
5. Pharmaceutical biotechnology. I. Cowan, Miranda.
RS199.5 .A67 2023
615.6--dc23

American Medical Publishers,
41 Flatbush Avenue,
1st Floor, New York,
NY 11217, USA

ISBN 978-1-63927-894-7 (Hardback)

Contents

Preface...VII

Chapter 1   **Buspirone Nanovesicular Nasal System for Non-Hormonal Hot Flushes Treatment**...1
Elka Touitou, Hiba Natsheh and Shaher Duchi

Chapter 2   **Dual pH/Redox-Responsive Mixed Polymeric Micelles for Anticancer Drug Delivery and Controlled Release**..14
Yongle Luo, Xujun Yin, Xi Yin, Anqi Chen, Lili Zhao, Gang Zhang, Wenbo Liao, Xiangxuan Huang, Juan Li and Can Yang Zhang

Chapter 3   **Photo-Magnetic Irradiation-Mediated Multimodal Therapy of Neuroblastoma Cells Using a Cluster of Multifunctional Nanostructures**.................27
Rohini Atluri, Rahul Atmaramani, Gamage Tharaka, Thomas McCallister, Jian Peng, David Diercks, Somesree GhoshMitra and Santaneel Ghosh

Chapter 4   **Development of Parvifloron D-Loaded Smart Nanoparticles to Target Pancreatic Cancer**...44
Ana Santos-Rebelo, Catarina Garcia, Carla Eleutério, Ana Bastos, Sílvia Castro Coelho, Manuel A. N. Coelho, Jesús Molpeceres, Ana S. Viana, Lia Ascensão, João F. Pinto, Maria M. Gaspar, Patrícia Rijo and Catarina P. Reis

Chapter 5   **Nanolipid-Trehalose Conjugates and Nano-Assemblies as Putative Autophagy Inducers**...59
Eleonora Colombo, Michele Biocotino, Giulia Frapporti, Pietro Randazzo, Michael S. Christodoulou, Giovanni Piccoli, Laura Polito, Pierfausto Seneci and Daniele Passarella

Chapter 6   **Fluorescence and Cytotoxicity of Cadmium Sulfide Quantum Dots Stabilized on Clay Nanotubes**...76
Anna V. Stavitskaya, Andrei A. Novikov, Mikhail S. Kotelev, Dmitry S. Kopitsyn, Elvira V. Rozhina, Ilnur R. Ishmukhametov, Rawil F. Fakhrullin, Evgenii V. Ivanov, Yuri M. Lvov and Vladimir A. Vinokurov

Chapter 7   **Protein Corona Fingerprints of Liposomes: New Opportunities for Targeted Drug Delivery and Early Detection in Pancreatic Cancer**...............87
Sara Palchetti, Damiano Caputo, Luca Digiacomo, Anna Laura Capriotti, Roberto Coppola, Daniela Pozzi and Giulio Caracciolo

Chapter 8   **Chitosan-Based Polyelectrolyte Complexes for Doxorubicin and Zoledronic Acid Combined Therapy to Overcome Multidrug Resistance**............99
Simona Giarra, Silvia Zappavigna, Virginia Campani, Marianna Abate, Alessia Maria Cossu, Carlo Leonetti, Manuela Porru, Laura Mayol, Michele Caraglia and Giuseppe De Rosa

Chapter 9   **MIL-100(Al) Gels as an Excellent Platform Loaded with Doxorubicin
Hydrochloride for pH-Triggered Drug Release and Anticancer Effect**.......................111
Yuge Feng, Chengliang Wang, Fei Ke, Jianye Zang and Junfa Zhu

Chapter 10   **Development of Multifunctional Liposomes Containing Magnetic/Plasmonic
MnFe$_2$O$_4$/Au Core/Shell Nanoparticles** 122
Ana Rita O. Rodrigues, Joana O. G. Matos, Armando M. Nova Dias,
Bernardo G. Almeida, Ana Pires, André M. Pereira, João P. Araújo,
Maria-João R. P. Queiroz, Elisabete M. S. Castanheira and Paulo J. G. Coutinho

Chapter 11   **Systemic Administration of Polyelectrolyte Microcapsules: Where do they
Accumulate and When? In Vivo and Ex Vivo Study**.......................................140
Nikita A. Navolokin, Sergei V. German, Alla B. Bucharskaya, Olga S. Godage,
Viktor V. Zuev, Galina N. Maslyakova, Nikolaiy A. Pyataev, Pavel S. Zamyshliaev,
Mikhail N. Zharkov, Georgy S. Terentyuk, Dmitry A. Gorin and Gleb B. Sukhorukov

Chapter 12   **Intratumoral Delivery of Doxorubicin on Folate-Conjugated Graphene Oxide by
In-Situ Forming Thermo-Sensitive Hydrogel for Breast Cancer Therapy**...........154
Yi Teng Fong, Chih-Hao Chen and Jyh-Ping Chen

Chapter 13   **Trends towards Biomimicry in Theranostics**...178
Michael Evangelopoulos, Alessandro Parodi, Jonathan O. Martinez and
Ennio Tasciotti

Chapter 14   **Inhibition of Glycolysis by Using a Micro/Nano-Lipid Bromopyruvic Chitosan
Carrier as a Promising Tool to Improve Treatment of Hepatocellular Carcinoma**.....197
Nemany A. Hanafy, Luciana Dini, Cinzia Citti, Giuseppe Cannazza and
Stefano Leporatti

Chapter 15   **Magnetic Graphene Oxide for Dual Targeted Delivery of Doxorubicin and
Photothermal Therapy**...209
Yu-Jen Lu, Pin-Yi Lin, Pei-Han Huang, Chang-Yi Kuo, K.T. Shalumon,
Mao-Yu Chen and Jyh-Ping Chen

Permissions

List of Contributors

Index

Preface

Every book is initially just a concept; it takes months of research and hard work to give it the final shape in which the readers receive it. In its early stages, this book also went through rigorous reviewing. The notable contributions made by experts from across the globe were first molded into patterned chapters and then arranged in a sensibly sequential manner to bring out the best results.

Drug delivery is an area of research concerned with the development of novel materials or carrier systems for the effective therapeutic delivery of drugs. One of the emerging technologies for drug delivery is nanotechnology. It enables enhanced treatments with lesser side effects and targeted delivery of drugs. Nanotechnology involves the characterization, production, design and application of nanoscale materials in different key areas, which helps in providing site specific treatment, which in turn decreases the accumulation of drugs in the healthy tissues. Furthermore, it helps in retention of drugs in the body for efficient treatment and helps in transfer of drugs across the endothelial and epithelial barriers. This leads to fewer plasma fluctuations, thereby reducing the side effects. This book provides significant information on the application of nanotechnology for drug delivery. Scientists and students actively engaged in the study of drug delivery systems will find this book full of crucial and unexplored concepts.

It has been my immense pleasure to be a part of this project and to contribute my years of learning in such a meaningful form. I would like to take this opportunity to thank all the people who have been associated with the completion of this book at any step.

Editor

Buspirone Nanovesicular Nasal System for Non-Hormonal Hot Flushes Treatment

Elka Touitou *, Hiba Natsheh and Shaher Duchi

The Institute for Drug Research, School of Pharmacy, Faculty of Medicine, The Hebrew University of Jerusalem, P.O. Box 12065, Jerusalem 91120, Israel; hiba.natsheh@mail.huji.ac.il (H.N.); shaherd75@gmail.com (S.D.)
* Correspondence: elka.touitou@mail.huji.ac.il;

Abstract: The aim of this work was to design and characterize a new nanovesicular nasal delivery system (NDS) containing buspirone, and investigate its efficiency in an animal model for the treatment of hot flushes. The presence of multilamellar vesicles with a mean size distribution of 370 nm was evidenced by transition electron microscopy (TEM), cryo-scanning electron microscopy (Cryo-SEM), and dynamic light scattering (DLS) tests. Pharmacodynamic evaluation of the nasal treatment efficacy with the new system was carried out in ovariectomized (OVX) rat—an animal model for hot flushes—and compared with other treatments. We found that the nasal administration of a buspirone NDS resulted in a significant reduction in tail skin temperature (TST). This effect was not observed in the control buspirone-treated groups. Buspirone levels in the plasma and brain of nasally-treated normal rats were quantified and compared with those of rats that had received oral administration by a LC-MS/MS assay. A significantly higher bioavailability was achieved with the new treatment relative to an oral administration of the same drug dose. No pathological changes in the nasal cavity were observed following sub-chronic nasal administration of buspirone NDS. In conclusion, the data of our investigation show that buspirone in the new nanovesicular nasal carrier could be considered for further studies for the development of a treatment for the hot flushes ailment.

Keywords: nanovesicular nasal carrier; nasal delivery system; buspirone; hot flushes; ovariectomized rat

1. Introduction

Currently, most of therapeutic products for hot flushes are based on hormone therapy (HT), involving the administration of estrogen alone or in combination with progesterone. There is a growing demand for a safer treatment alternative to HT for hot flushes [1].

Drugs affecting serotonin levels were investigated for non-hormonal therapies for hot flushes. In a previous study, we reported that buspirone administrated in a transdermal system has efficiently treated hot flushes in an animal model [2]. Buspirone—a 5-HT1A agonist—is currently administered orally and indicated for the treatment of generalized anxiety disorder (GAD). Buspirone HCl belongs to biopharmaceutics classification system (BCS) class I, being highly soluble and highly permeable. However, oral administration of this drug is associated with low bioavailability: ~4% due to an extensive first-pass metabolism [3]. In addition, this centrally acting drug lacks the ability to penetrate the blood–brain barrier (BBB).

Nasal administration, being able to circumvent the first pass metabolism and bypass the BBB, could be a promising alternative for the oral administration of buspirone. Despite this, the nasal delivery of many molecules is poor, due to the low permeability of the nasal mucosa [4,5].

Touitou and Illum emphasized the role of the carrier in the design of an efficient nasal product [4]. To overcome the above drawbacks, we propose here the nasal administration of buspirone incorporated in a new nanovesicular delivery system (NDS) to be tested in a hot flushes animal model. We have shown that the new vesicular nasal carrier enhanced the pharmacodynamic effect of a number of other drugs [6–8].

Various aspects of nasal delivery of buspirone were previously studied [9–12]. Khan et al. investigated the nasal clearance, bioavailability, and delivery to brain of buspirone in chitosan mucoadhesive nasal formulation in vivo [9–11]. Mathure et al. studied the ex vivo permeation of buspirone niosomes gel through sheep nasal mucosa [12].

In this work, we designed and characterized buspirone NDS, tested its pharmacodynamic effect in an ovariectomized (OVX) animal model for hot flushes, and measured the drug levels in brain and plasma. The safety of the local application of the nanovesicular system on the animal nasal cavity was also examined.

To our knowledge, this pharmacodynamic effect of nasally administrated buspirone in a nanovesicular carrier has not been previously investigated.

2. Materials and Methods

2.1. Materials

Buspirone HCl was a gift from Unipharm, Israel. Ethinylestradiol (EE) was purchased from Sigma (Jerusalem, Israel). Phosphatidylcholine phospholipid, Phospholipon 90 G, was bought from Lipoid GmbH (Berlin, Germany). Propylene glycol and Vitamin E (Tocopheryl acetate) were acquired from Tamar (Rishon Lezion, Israel). Ethanol absolute (Gadot, Netanya, Israel) was acquired from the Hebrew University warehouse. All of the other materials used in this work were of analytical or pharmaceutical grade.

2.2. Animals

All of the procedures performed on animals were conducted according to The National Institutes of Health regulations and approved by the Committee for Animal Care and Experimental Use of the Hebrew University of Jerusalem, Ethics No. MD-11-12833-3 (2011–2015).

Sprague–Dawley female rats (weighing 250–360 g) were purchased from Harlan (Rehovot, Israel). The rats were housed in separate cages and were maintained on a 12 h light, 12 h dark cycle, with lights on from 07:00 to 19:00 daily with free access to food and water.

The administration of buspirone from all of the systems was carried out under short anesthesia with isoflurane, including the animals in the control groups. This was sufficient to keep the rats sedated for a short period of 1–2 min during the instillation of nasal formulations to prevent sneezing.

2.3. Preparation and Characterization of Buspirone NDS

The new carrier was composed of phospholipid: propylene glycol: ethanol at the ratio 1:4:3 per weight. Additional components were vitamin E and water [6].

Buspirone NDS was prepared by a simple mixing method using an overhead Heidolph® stirrer (Heidolph Digital 200 RZR-2000, Schwabach, Germany). Briefly, phospholipid was dissolved in ethanol; then, propylene glycol and vitamin E were added. Buspirone HCl aqueous solution was then added slowly with continuous mixing; the nanovesicles were generated at this stage.

In this work, we present the results obtained with 3% w/w buspirone NDS. The system was tested for drug chemical content, the presence of nanovesicles, the size distribution of vesicles, viscosity, pH, and three months' stability.

2.3.1. Drug Chemical Content

The concentration of buspirone in the system was quantified by HPLC (Merck-Hitachi D-7000 equipped with an L-7400 variable UV detector, L-7300 column oven, L-7200 auto-sampler, L-7100 pump, and an Hardware Security Module (HSM) computerized analysis program, Tokyo, Japan). The drug concertation in the samples was determined using a modified method described by

Foroutan et al. [13]. The chromatographic conditions were set as follows: UV detection 240 nm, a Nucleosil C18 125 mm × 4 mm 5 micron column with a mobile phase of acetonitrile: phosphate buffer 0.01 M pH 3.5 (40:60, v/v) at a flow of 1 mL/min.

2.3.2. Visualization of Vesicles by Transition Electron Microscopy (TEM) and Cryo-Scanning Electron Microscopy (Cryo-SEM)

For transition electron microscopy (TEM) visualization, one day before the examination, the system was diluted 1:10 with suitable diluent and stained with 1% aqueous solution of phosphotungstic acid (PTA), dried at room temperature for 20 min, and viewed under the microscope (Philips TECHNAI CM 120 electron microscope, Eindhoven, The Netherlands) at 26.5–110 k-fold enlargement.

For cryo-scanning electron microscopy (cryo-SEM) visualization, specimen preparation was performed with a BAF-060 system (BalTec AG, Balzers, Liechtenstein). A small drop of the buspirone NDS was placed on an electron microscopy copper grid and sandwiched between two gold planchettes. The "sandwich" was plunged into liquid ethane at its freezing point, transferred into liquid nitrogen, and inserted into a sample fracture block that had been pre-cooled by liquid nitrogen. The block was split open to fracture the frozen sample drop. A Pt–C conductive thin film of 4 nm was deposited on the surfaces (at a 90° angle). The coated specimens were transferred under vacuum by a BalTec VCT100 shuttle that had been pre-cooled with liquid nitrogen into a Zeiss Ultra Plus High-Resolution Scanning Electron Microscope (HR-SEM) (Oberkochen, Germany), and maintained at −150 °C. The microscopic examination was performed under 3000-fold enlargement.

2.3.3. Vesicles Size Distribution by Dynamic Light Scattering (DLS)

Buspirone NDS was analyzed using a Malvern Zetasizer-nano, ZEN 3600, Malvern Instruments, Malvern, UK. The system was diluted 1:500 with suitable diluent one hour prior to measurement. Three batches of each system were tested. Each batch was analyzed by intensity, three times, at 25 °C. The duration and the set position of each measurement were fixed automatically by the apparatus.

2.3.4. Viscosity and pH of the System

The viscosity of the nanovesicular system was measured by Brookfield DV III Rheometer -LV (Brookfield engineering labs, Stoughton, MA, USA), spindle 18 and a small sample adaptor, at a rotation speed of 30 rpm.

The pH measurements were performed by a Fisher pH meter (Fisher Instruments, Pittsburgh, PA, USA). The system was diluted with double distilled water 1:5. All of the measurements were duplicated.

2.3.5. Stability Test for Buspirone NDS

Changes in drug chemical content, structure, and size distribution of the nanovesicles, viscosity, and pH of the system were measured and compared to zero time values following three months storage at room temperature (RT).

2.4. Pharmacodynamic Effect Evaluation in Animal Model

2.4.1. Animal Model

The protocol for the animal model and the experiments was conducted according to The National Institutes of Health regulations and approved by the Committee for Animal Care and Experimental Use of the Hebrew University of Jerusalem, as above in Section 2.2.

The effect of nasal administration of buspirone NDS on a hot flushes animal model was tested in bilateral ovariectomized rats (OVX). This is a model for estrogen deficiency-associated thermoregulatory dysfunction. The treatment effect was evaluated by monitoring the changes in tail skin temperature (TST) [2].

A total of 71 rats weighing 250–330 g underwent bilateral ovariectomies (OVX) ($n = 63$) or sham surgeries ($n = 8$) (which left their ovaries intact) at Harlan Biotech (Rehovot, Israel) followed by a recovery period of two weeks. No surgical or medical complications were observed.

Sixteen rats were used to test the animal model (including the eight sham and eight OVX), and 55 OVX rats were used for testing various treatments.

To test the reliability of the OVX animal model, the increase in the TST in OVX rats was assessed as compared with sham animals. The TST values for sham animals were considered the normal values [14].

2.4.2. Treatments and TST Measurements

For testing various treatments, 48 OVX animals were divided into six groups ($n = 8$/group) as follows: single administration of 3 mg/kg buspirone from NDS as compared to nasal aqueous solution (NAQ), oral aqueous solution (PO), and subcutaneous injection (SC). In addition, the effect of buspirone NDS was evaluated compared to the positive control, ethinylestradiol (EE), which was administrated subcutaneously to OVX rats at a dose of 0.3 mg/kg once daily for seven days. Untreated OVX rats served as control. A 3% w/w buspirone aqueous solution was used as the nasal or oral control system, while a 0.3% w/w buspirone solution in normal saline was used for SC administration. The 0.03% w/w ethinylestradiol SC solution was prepared in sesame oil. The administrated volumes were calculated to achieve a dose of 3 mg/kg buspirone and 0.3 mg/kg EE to each animal.

The experiments were carried out in two replicates; each replicate included four rats for each treatment group. The intra and interobserver variations were ≤4.6% and 3.9%, respectively. The drug dose was chosen following the evaluation of the dose- effect relationship (data is not shown).

TST was measured using Thermalert TH-5 (Physitemp Instruments Inc., Clifton, NJ, USA). A thermocouple skin sensor probe SST-1 (Physitemp Instruments Inc., Clifton, NJ, USA) was fixed on the dorsal surface of the tail approximately one cm away from the base, and the animals were retained in a flat-bottomed restraint during the 30–60 s sampling period. All of the measurements were performed from 10:00 to 15:00 and at 21.5 ± 0.1 °C.

On the day of the experiment, the rats were acclimatized in the experiment room for two hours. TST values were recorded before treatment (baseline) and 30 min, 60 min, 120 min, 180 min, and 240 min after treatment.

The following parameters were used to evaluate the effect of the various treatments: the average TST value (TSTave, °C) for each time point was the average of the readings recorded in the two experimental replicates for animals in the same treatment group [15]. The ΔTST value for each treatment at a certain time point was obtained by subtracting TSTave at baseline from the value at that time point. The duration of effect is the time period (min) in which TSTave is statistically different from the TST at baseline [16].

As a next step, we determined the onset of the action of buspirone NDS by measuring the TST values of OVX rats each minute following the treatment ($n = 7$).

2.5. Determination of Buspirone Levels in Rat Plasma and Brain

The concentration of buspirone in the plasma and brain tissue of normal animals at various time points was measured post-dose of 3 mg/kg drug nasal administration in NDS and oral administration (PO).

2.5.1. Drug Concentration in Plasma Measurement

Ten rats were randomly divided equally into two groups of five animals. Blood samples of 400–500 μL were collected from tail 5 min before treatment (zero-time point) and 5 min, 10 min, 20 min, 30 min, 60 min, 120 min, and 240 min after drug administration.

Briefly, blood samples were centrifuged at 3000 rpm for 10 min at room temperature, and plasma was transferred and stored at −20 °C until assayed. On the day of analysis, the samples were thawed, and buspirone was extracted from plasma by a modified protein precipitation method described by

Foroutan et al. [13]. One hundred microliters of plasma samples were extracted with 125 μL acetonitrile and diluted with 275 μL of water. Samples were centrifuged at 14,000 rpm for 5 min at room temperature. Supernatants were filtered and injected into LC-MS/MS (Thermo Scientific, San Jose, CA, USA).

2.5.2. Drug Concentration in Brain Tissue Measurement

Sixteen rats were randomly divided into four equal groups for testing two time points and two treatments. Animals were sacrificed 10 min or 30 min after administration. Brains were collected, immediately weighed, and kept at −70 °C until analysis. Brain tissues were purified by a modified liquid–liquid extraction method described by Lai et al. [17]. On the day of analysis, the brain tissues were thawed and homogenized with 2 mL of water/g brain tissue. The homogenates were alkalinized with 10% w/v NaOH solution. Buspirone was extracted with 5 mL a mixture (4:1) of hexane and ethyl acetate. Samples were then centrifuged at 4000 rpm for 45 min at 4 °C. Supernatants were collected and evaporated at room temperature. Dried residues were reconstituted with mobile phase, and centrifuged at 14,000 rpm for 10 min at room temperature. Final supernatants were filtered and injected into LC-MS/MS.

2.5.3. Buspirone LC-MS/MS Assay

Buspirone content in plasma and brain was quantified by a specific validated LC-MS/MS method according to the FDA regulation guidelines of bioanalytical validation. A Kinetex™ column (2.6 μm Minibore C18 50 × 2.1 mm, Phenomenex®, Torrance, CA, USA) was used. Flow rate and injection volume were 400 μL/min and 5 μL, respectively. At these defined conditions, the retention time of buspirone was 1.33 min. Buspirone plasma levels were expressed in ng/mL, and in ng/g in brain tissue. Standard calibration curves of buspirone hydrochloride were prepared with plasma and brain homogenates spiked with known amounts of drug (1–1000 ng/mL and 100–500 ng/g, respectively). For the standard calibration curve, each concentration was injected five times, and the experiment was duplicated. The inter-coefficients and intra-coefficients of variation were <2.2% and 4.0%, respectively. The sensitivity of the method was 1 ng/mL, and the recovery was 78% and 96.3% for plasma and brain, respectively.

The following parameters were used to evaluate the concentration profile in plasma: C_{max}, T_{max}, and AUC0-240 (from zero to 240 min). The AUC0−240 $_{[NDS]}$ and AUC0-240 $_{[PO]}$ represent the means of individual AUC0-240 from nasal and oral experimental groups, respectively. The area under the curve of plasma concentration was calculated using the linear trapezoidal rule. All of the pharmacokinetic parameters were calculated using a windows-based program for noncompartmental analysis of pharmacokinetic data, NCOMP; version 3.1 11-SEP-97 in (c) 1996-7 Fox Chase Cancer Center (Philadelphia, PA, USA).

The relative bioavailability (F %) was calculated according to the following equation:

$$F \% = [(AUC0 - 240 _{[NDS]} \times DOSE_{PO})]/[(AUC0 - 240 _{[PO]} \times DOSE _{NDS})] \times 100$$

2.6. Local Safety Assessment

In this experiment, we evaluated the effect of buspirone NDS on the nasal cavity in rats by a method previously described by Duchi et al. [7,8]. In brief, six rats were divided into three equal groups. Rats in the nasal administration groups received 15 μL of buspirone NDS or saline into both nostrils twice a day for seven days. Two rats were untreated and served as a negative control. At the end of the experiment, animals were sacrificed, and their nasal cavities were removed and fixed in 3.8% buffered formaldehyde, pH 7.4. Sections of the nasal cavity were cut serially at 7-μm thickness and stained with hematoxylin and eosin. The sections were examined by a professional histopathologist (Authority for Animal Facilities, Hebrew University of Jerusalem, Israel) by Zeiss Axioskop 2 plus (Oberkochen, Germany). Local toxicity was assessed by evaluating the histopathological alterations in different regions of the nasal cavity (cartilage and turbinate bone, lamina propria and submucosa, mucosal epithelium and lumen).

2.7. Statistical Analysis

Data is reported as mean $\pm$ SD and analyzed by one-way ANOVA with the Tukey–Kramer multiple comparisons post-test or by unpaired two-tailed t-test. $p < 0.05$ is considered significant in all cases.

3. Results

3.1. Buspirone NDS Characterization

The TE and cryo-SE micrographs presented in Figures 1 and 2 indicate the presence of nanovesicles in the tested samples.

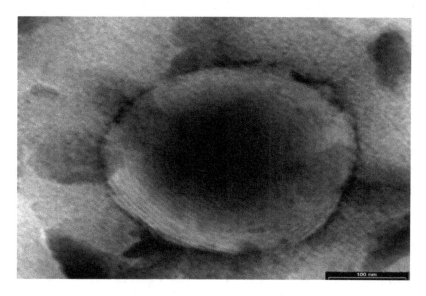

Figure 1. A multilamellar vesicle apparent in the transition electron (TE) micrograph of a buspirone nanovesicular delivery system (NDS) (110 k, Philips TEM CM 120 electron microscope).

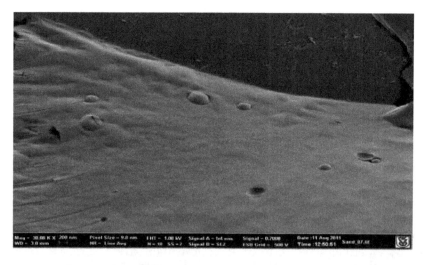

Figure 2. Cryo-scanning electron (cryo-SE) micrograph of a buspirone NDS (Zeiss Ultra Plus HR-SEM) showing multiple nanovesicles.

The micrograph in Figure 1 shows a spherical multilamellar nanovesicle.
The mean size distribution of the vesicles obtained by DLS measurements was 370.0 ± 68.8 nm. Other important system characteristics were viscosity 72.7 ± 8.1 cP and pH 5.8 ± 0.2.
Stability tests results for samples kept three months at room temperature are given in Table 1 and Figure 3.

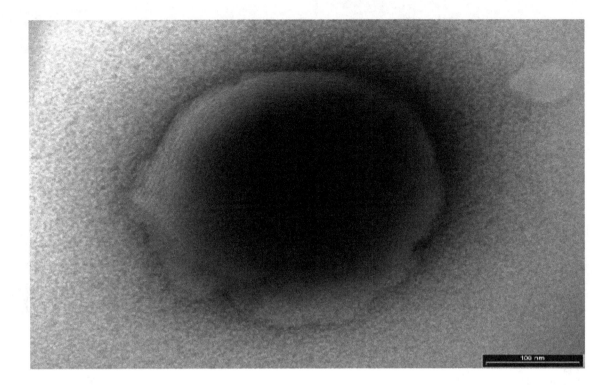

Figure 3. TE micrographs of buspirone NDS after three months of storage at room temperature (RT).

Table 1. Stability parameters for buspirone nasal nanovesicular delivery system (NDS) at zero time and after three months of storage at RT (mean ± SD).

Time	0 Time	Three Months	% of Initial after Three Months *
Drug Content, % w/w	3.13 ± 0.05	2.88 ± 0.02	92.0
Vesicles Mean Size Distribution, nm	395.1 ± 162.9	332.6 ± 111.1	84.0
Viscosity, cP	87.0 ± 3.1	91.0 ± 4.3	104.6
pH	5.73 ± 0.10	5.85 ± 0.05	102.1

* Calculated by the following equation: (value after three months/value at 0 time) × 100%.

As shown in Table 1, the percentage of change in drug content, viscosity, and pH after three months' storage at RT were less than 10% compared to the values at the initial time (zero time) storage. It is noteworthy that although the mean size distribution of vesicles decreased by 16%, the values remained in the initial nanosized range. No changes in the appearance of the vesicles were observed; the vesicles kept their spherical shape and multilamellar arrangement (Figure 3). These results suggest that the nanovesicular buspirone NDS preserved its characteristics and structure during the tested storage period.

3.2. Effect of Buspirone Nasal Administration on TST Values in Animal Model

The effect of buspirone NDS on TST values was tested in OVX animals.

The first step was to validate the OVX animal model by comparing the TST values in untreated OVX rats versus intact rats (sham-operated). The TSTave (°C) values in OVX rats at all of the tested time points were significantly higher than the values obtained in sham rats with an overall mean TST of 28.8 ± 0.3 °C vs. 26.1 ± 0.3 °C, respectively ($p < 0.001$) (Figure 4).

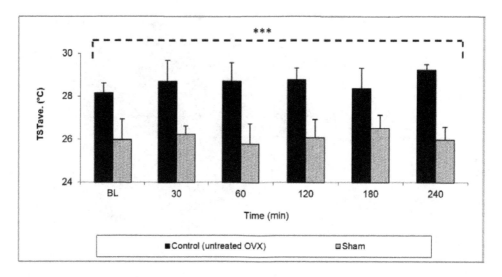

Figure 4. Tail skin temperature (TST) average values in untreated ovariectomized (OVX) Sprague–Dawley female rats and an untreated sham group. Data represent the mean ± SD, $n = 8$ for each group. *** $p < 0.001$ extremely significant by unpaired two-tailed t-test.

Buspirone was administrated at a dose of 3 m/kg as follows: in NDS, nasal aqueous solution, subcutaneous injection, and oral solution, and compared with results in untreated OVX rats. The TST baseline values were ≥28.5 °C in all of the OVX animal groups. The results in Figure 5 show that the nasal drug administration of buspirone NDS leads to a rapid and significant reduction in TST 30 min after treatment, achieving TSTave and ΔTST values of 26.26 ± 0.86 and −2.40 ± 0.48 °C, respectively. The treatment resulted in a statistically significant decrease in TST over the four hours of tested time as compared with PO, NAQ, or untreated OVX animals.

TST values reduction at 30 min was seen only in the treatment with buspirone NDS. At this time point, the TST values for all of the other controls were comparable to those of untreated OVX animals. At 60 min, low changes in TST were measured for the NAQ and PO groups. Further, the first significant reduction for the SC-treated group was at 60 min, indicating a relatively slow onset of action (Figure 5 and Table 2).

Table 2. Pharmacodynamic parameters of buspirone NDS administration to OVX rats as compared with controls ($n = 8$ for each group), mean ± SD.

System	Mean ΔTST, °C	Duration *, (min)	Max ΔTST, °C (Time, min)
NDS **	−2.61 ± 1.07	210	−3.88 ± 0.95 (120)
NAQ **	−0.46 ± 0.75	60	−1.16 ± 0.88 (60)
PO **	−0.39 ± 1.05	60	−0.58 ± 0.91 (120)
SC **	−1.86 ± 1.78	180	−3.71 ± 1.15 (180)
EE ***	−2.71 ± 0.47	240	−3.55 ± 0.20 (30)

TST, tail skin temperature; NDS, nasal nanovesicular delivery system; PO, oral administration; NAQ, nasal aqueous solution; SC, subcutaneous injection; EE, subcutaneous ethinylestradiol injection. * Duration of effect is the time at which the average TST is statistically different from the TST at baseline by one-way ANOVA, with the Tukey–Kramer multiple comparisons post-test. ** Buspirone administrated from systems at a single dose of 3 mg/kg. *** Subcutaneous ethinylestradiol administrated at a dose 0.3 mg/kg once daily for 7 days.

The calculated pharmacodynamic parameters of the above described experiments are presented in Table 2. The duration of a statistical significant effect on TST was 210 min for buspirone NDS administration and only 180 min and 60 min for SC and NAQ or PO, respectively. In addition, the absolute values of mean and maximum ΔTST were significantly higher in OVX rats treated with buspirone NDS than in the three control groups.

Further, it was interesting to compare the effect of one buspirone NDS treatment with one week of repeated subcutaneous EE.

The mean ΔTST values obtained were −2.61 ± 1.07 and −2.71 ± 0.47 for the nasal administration and the end of one week EE administration, respectively (Table 2). The TST values were near the baseline in the normal rat model.

Another important parameter is the onset of action of buspirone NDS. The evaluation was carried out by measuring the TST values of OVX rats each minute for the first 30 min following the treatment. The baseline TST value was 28.3 ± 0.5 °C; a slight increase was observed in the first five minutes following treatment, which could be a result of stress from anesthesia and administration procedures. At 10 min, a temperature reduction was measured followed by significant decrease at 15 min ($p < 0.05$) lasting to the end of experiment.

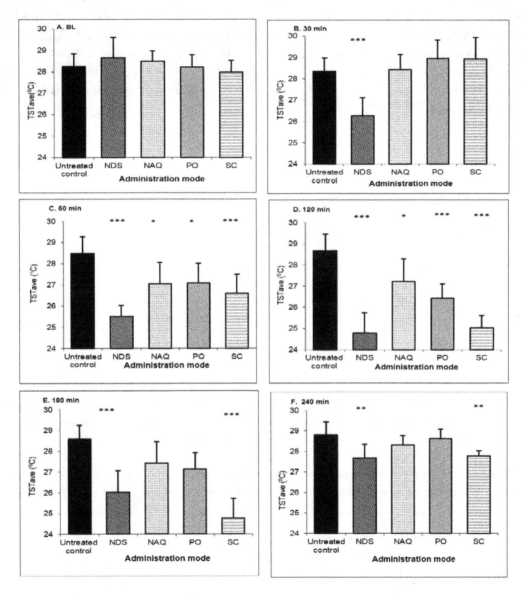

Figure 5. TST average values after buspirone NDS administration to OVX rats at dose 3 mg/kg compared to nasal aqueous solution (NAQ), oral administration (PO) and subcutaneous injection (SC) and in untreated control at: (**A**) baseline (BL); (**B**) 30 min; (**C**) 60 min; (**D**) 120 min; (**E**) 180 min; and (**F**) 240 min time points. Data represent the mean ± SD, $n = 8$ for each group. * $p < 0.05$, significant, ** $p < 0.01$ very significant, *** $p < 0.001$ extremely significant; compared to control (untreated OVX) by one-way ANOVA, with the Tukey–Kramer multiple comparisons post-test.

3.3. Buspirone Levels in Plasma and in Brain

Plasma and brain drug concentration as a function of time were measured following a single dose of 3 mg/kg buspirone nasal administration to normal rats from NDS and compared with a PO administration of a similar dose.

The results show that nasal drug administration produced a rapid increase in the drug plasma levels reaching concentrations of 764.2 ± 420.0 ng/mL and 478.2 ± 253.8 ng/mL at 5 min and 10 min post-administration, respectively. Then, the drug concentration decreased gradually 240 min after administration. Following oral administration, a relatively slow and mild increase in buspirone concentration was measured, 109.7 ± 74.9 ng/mL, 141.7 ± 95.3 ng/mL and 157.1 ± 102.9 ng/mL at 5 min, 10 min, and 20 min, respectively. A slow decrease occurred after 20 min, and the drug levels reached zero 240 min post-administration. The calculated parameters indicated that the drug nasal administration allowed for a four times higher C_{max} value than oral administration (764.2 ± 420.0 ng/mL and 181.5 ± 106.5 ng/mL, respectively) with a three times shorter T_{max} value (5.0 ± 0.0 min and 15.0 ± 7.1 min, respectively). The calculated $AUC0-240$ $_{[NDS]}$ and $AUC0-240$ $_{[PO]}$ values were 27515.3 ± 9104.4 and 12089.3 ± 8826.3, respectively, indicating a relative plasma bioavailability of 212.7% (Figure 6, Table 3).

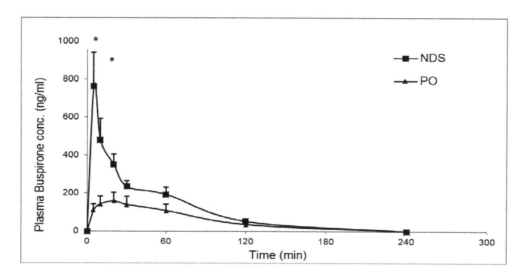

Figure 6. Plasma buspirone concentration-time profile after the administration of buspirone NDS to rat at a dose of 3 mg/kg compared with oral administration (PO). Data given as mean $\pm$ SD, $n = 5$ for each group. $*$ $p < 0.05$ significant by an unpaired two-tailed t-test.

Table 3. Pharmacokinetic parameters following the administration of 3 mg/kg buspirone in NDS and PO to rat at a similar dose ($n = 5$, for each group), mean $\pm$ SD.

Pharmacokinetic Parameter	Administration Mode	
	NDS	PO
T_{max} (min)	5.0 ± 0.0	15.0 ± 7.1
C_{max} (ng/mL)	764.2 ± 420.0	181.5 ± 106.5
$AUC0-240$ (ng $\times$ min/mL)	$25{,}715.3 \pm 9104.4$	$12{,}089.3 \pm 8826.3$

NDS: nasal nanovesicular delivery system; PO: oral administration. C_{max}: maximum plasma concentrations; T_{max}: time at which C_{max} is achieved; $AUC0-240$: area under the curve from zero time to 240 min.

Drug quantities measured in the brain tissue at 10 min and 30 min post-buspirone NDS administration were 688.4 ± 204.7 ng/g and 511.1 ± 149.4 ng/g, respectively. It is noteworthy that the drug concentrations that were detected in the brain tissue following PO administration were lower by five and two times (179.6 ± 58.8 ng/g and 258.9 ± 91.7 ng/g at 10 min and 30 min, respectively) (Figure 7).

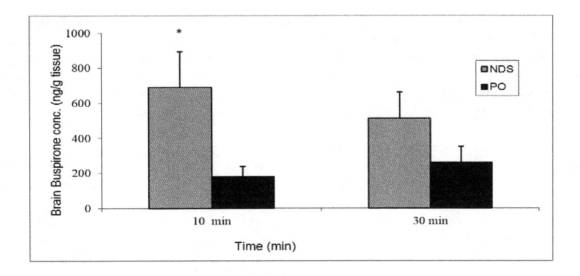

Figure 7. Brain buspirone concentrations after administration of buspirone NDS to rat at a dose of 3 mg/kg compared with oral administration (PO). Data represent the mean ± SD, $n = 5$ for each group. * $p < 0.05$ significant by unpaired two-tail t-test.

3.4. Local Safety

Histopathological analysis of the cavity and nasal tissue following sub-chronic buspirone NDS administration was assessed by comparing the nasal cavities treated with the new system or with saline and untreated rats.

No pathological findings were observed in the histopathological analysis of the nasal cavities excised from rats in the buspirone NDS and saline groups (images not shown). The results show intact mucosal epithelium, empty lumen, and no infiltration of inflammatory cells. Overall, there was no evidence of inflammation. Turbinate bone integrity was preserved. Epithelium was normal with no evidence of erosion or ulceration, and ciliated epithelium was intact. These findings are sustained by previous results obtained with tramadol NDS [7].

4. Discussion

Nasal administration is a nice alternative to improve the bioavailability of drugs that are poorly absorbed by the oral route. This mode of administration is generally associated with good patient compliance [4]. However, the nasal administration of some drugs may also result in low absorption due to their insufficient permeation across the nasal mucosa [18]. In previous publications, we proposed a new effective and safe nasal nanovesicular carrier for various drugs and treatments. The enhanced effect of drugs in pain and Multiple Sclerosis animal models was achieved following nasal administration using this delivery system [6–8].

In this work, we designed and characterized buspirone NDS, which is the nanovesicular carrier containing the drug. The effect of this system on hot flushes was evaluated in OVX rats. The OVX rat model used in the present study for pharmacodynamic evaluation is an acceptable model for estrogen deficiency-associated thermoregulatory dysfunction [2,14]. Subsequently, the elevation in TST is considered similar to menopausal hot flushes in women [19,20].

The ability of the new nasal nanovesicular system to enhance the systemic and brain delivery of buspirone was also investigated.

We found that the system is composed of spherical nanosized multilamellar vesicles, as evidenced by electron microscopy and DLS measurements. The pH of buspirone NDS was shown to be within the suitable range for nasal administration. Moreover, the system was stable for three months of storage at RT.

Treating OVX rats nasally with buspirone NDS lead to a significant reduction in TST. The effect was higher and over a longer time period than oral ornasal aqueous solutions, or subcutaneous injection.

The improved systemic and brain delivery of buspirone were proven by higher drug levels achieved in plasma and the brain (C_{max}), in addition to shorter T_{max} values following administration in the nanovesicular system compared with oral administration. The efficient delivery of buspirone to the brain via the nanovesicular NDS points toward the ability of the system to target the drug to the animal brain.

It is notable that other non-hormonal drugs including serotonin/norepinephrine reuptake inhibitors, gabapentinoids, and clonidine have been considered for the management of vasomotor symptoms (VMS) to overcome the side effects of HT [21]. These drugs are usually administered via the oral route.

The treatment we suggest here presents a new approach to be further investigated for hot flushes management in cases where women experience symptoms hourly, or suffer from night sweats and sleep disturbances. It is also suggested to be helpful in menopause women suffering from VMS associated with anxiety, owing to the approved anxiolytic effect of buspirone [22]. In addition, the nasal administration of buspirone could avoid drugs interaction in the gastrointestinal tract when the oral administration of other drugs is required.

5. Conclusions

Buspirone that was incorporated in the new nanovesicular carrier delivered nasally to the OXV animal model for hot flushes was more efficient than the administration of the same drug dose in nasal or oral aqueous solutions and subcutaneous injection. Buspirone levels in the brain and plasma of rats following nasal administration of the drug in the new carrier were superior to those measured in oral administration. Sub-chronic nasal administration of the buspirone nanosystem has shown no pathological changes in the mucosa for the tested period.

The feasibility data generated in this investigation point toward the possibility of considering buspirone NDS for further studies, and the development of a non-hormonal treatment of hot flushes.

6. Patents

Touitou, E.; Godin, B.; Duchi, S. Compositions for nasal delivery. 2014. US patent 8,911,751 B2.

Author Contributions: E.T. conceptualization, design, supervision, experimental design, writing, review editing, editing the final version. H.N. experimental, draft writing, contribution to the final version. S.D. experimental, draft preparation, assay validation, quantitative assay development.

Acknowledgments: We would like to thank Unipharm, Israel for kindly providing us buspirone hydrochloride.

References

1.   Krause, M.S.; Nakajima, S.T. Hormonal and nonhormonal treatment of vasomotor symptoms. *Obstet. Gynecol. Clin. N. Am.* **2015**, *42*, 163–179. [CrossRef] [PubMed]

2.   Shumilov, M.; Touitou, E. Buspirone transdermal administration for menopausal syndromes, in vitro and in animal model studies. *Int. J. Pharm.* **2010**, *387*, 26–33. [CrossRef] [PubMed]

3.   Mahmood, I.; Sahajwalla, C. Clinical pharmacokinetics and pharmacodynamics of buspirone, an anxiolytic drug. *Clin. Pharmacokinet.* **1999**, *36*, 277–287. [CrossRef] [PubMed]

4.   Touitou, E.; Illum, L. Nasal drug delivery. *Drug Deliv. Transl. Res.* **2013**, *3*, 1–3. [CrossRef] [PubMed]

5.   Lim, S.T.; Forbes, B.; Brown, M.B.; Martin, G.P. Physiological factors affecting nasal drug delivery. In *Enhancement in Drug Delivery*; Touitou, E., Barry, B.W., Eds.; CRC Press: Boca Raton, FL, USA, 2007; pp. 355–372. ISBN 0-8493-3203-6.

6.   Touitou, E.; Godin, B.; Duchi, S. Compositions for Nasal Delivery. U.S. Patent 8,911,751 B2, 16 December 2014.

7.   Duchi, S.; Touitou, E.; Pradella, L.; Marchini, F.; Ainbinder, D. Nasal tramadol delivery system: A new approach for improved pain therapy. *Eur. J. Pain Suppl.* **2011**, *5*, 449–452. [CrossRef]

8.   Duchi, S.; Ovadia, H.; Touitou, E. Nasal administration of drugs as a new non-invasive strategy for efficient treatment of multiple sclerosis. *J. Neuroimmunol.* **2013**, *258*, 32–40. [CrossRef] [PubMed]

9.   Khan, S.; Patil, K.; Yeole, P.; Gaikwad, R. Brain targeting studies on buspirone hydrochloride after intranasal administration of mucoadhesive formulation in rats. *J. Pharm. Pharmacol.* **2009**, *61*, 669–675. [CrossRef] [PubMed]

10. Khan, S.A.; Patil, K.S.; Yeole, P.G. Intranasal mucoadhesive buspirone formulation: In vitro characterization and nasal clearance studies. *Pharmazie* **2008**, *5*, 348–351.

11. Mittal, D.; Ali, A.; Md, S.; Baboota, S.; Sahni, J.K.; Ali, J. Insights into direct nose to brain delivery: Current status and future perspective. *Drug Deliv.* **2014**, *2*, 75–86. [CrossRef] [PubMed]

12. Mathure, D.; Madan, J.R.; Gujar, N.K.; Tupsamundre, A.; Ranpise, A.H.; Dua, K. Formulation and evaluation of niosomal in situ nasal gel of a serotonin receptor agonist, buspirone hydrochloride for the brain delivery via intranasal route. *Pharm. Nanotechnol.* **2018**, *1*, 69–78. [CrossRef] [PubMed]

13. Foroutan, S.M.; Zarghi, A.; Shafaati, A.R.; Khoddam, A. Simple high-performance liquid chromatographic determination of buspirone in human plasma. *Farmaco* **2004**, *59*, 739–742. [CrossRef] [PubMed]

14. Kobayashi, T.; Tamura, M.; Hayashi, M.; Katsuura, Y.; Tanabe, H.; Ohta, T.; Komoriya, K. Elevation of tail skin temperature in ovariectomized rats in relation to menopausal hot flushes. *Am. J. Physiol. Regul. Integr. Comp. Physiol.* **2000**, *278*, 863–869. [CrossRef] [PubMed]

15. Opas, E.E.; Rutledge, S.J.; Vogel, R.L.; Rodan, G.A.; Schmidt, A. Rat tail skin temperature regulation by estrogen, phytoestrogens and tamoxifen. *Maturitas* **2004**, *48*, 463–471. [CrossRef] [PubMed]

16. Sipe, K.; Leventhal, L.; Burroughs, K.; Cosmi, S.; Johnston, G.H.; Deecher, D.C. Serotonin 2A receptors modulate tail-skin temperature in two rodent models of estrogen deficiency-related thermoregulatory dysfunction. *Brain Res.* **2004**, *1028*, 191–202. [CrossRef] [PubMed]

17. Lai, C.T.; Tanay, V.A.; Rauw, G.A.; Bateson, A.N.; Martin, I.L.; Baker, G.B. Rapid, sensitive procedure to determine buspirone levels in rat brains using gas chromatography with nitrogen–phosphorus detection. *J. Chromatogr. B Biomed. Sci.* **1997**, *704*, 175–179. [CrossRef]

18. Arora, P.; Sharma, S.; Garg, S. Permeability issues in nasal drug delivery. *Drug Discov. Today* **2002**, *7*, 967–975. [CrossRef]

19. Holinka, C.F.; Brincat, M.; Coelingh Bennink, H.J. Preventive effect of oral estetrol in a menopausal hot flush model. *Climacteric* **2008**, *11* (Suppl. 1), 15–21. [CrossRef] [PubMed]

20. Bowe, J.; Li, X.F.; Kinsey-Jones, J.; Heyerick, A.; Brain, S.; Milligan, S.; O'Byrne, K. The hop phytoestrogen, 8-prenylnaringenin, reverses the ovariectomy-induced rise in skin temperature in an animal model of menopausal hot flushes. *J. Endocrinol.* **2006**, *191*, 399–405. [CrossRef] [PubMed]

21. Sicat, B.L.; Brokaw, D.K. Nonhormonal alternatives for the treatment of hot flashes. *Pharmacotherapy* **2004**, *24*, 79–93. [CrossRef] [PubMed]

22. Morrow, P.K.; Mattair, D.N.; Hortobagyi, G.N. Hot flashes: A review of pathophysiology and treatment modalities. *Oncologist* **2011**, *16*, 1658–1664. [CrossRef] [PubMed]

Dual pH/Redox-Responsive Mixed Polymeric Micelles for Anticancer Drug Delivery and Controlled Release

Yongle Luo [1,2], **Xujun Yin** [1], **Xi Yin** [1], **Anqi Chen** [1], **Lili Zhao** [1], **Gang Zhang** [1], **Wenbo Liao** [1], **Xiangxuan Huang** [1,*], **Juan Li** [3] **and Can Yang Zhang** [3,*]

[1]   School of Chemical Engineering and Energy Technology, Dongguan University of Technology, Dongguan 523808, China; luoyongle1988@gmail.com (Y.L.); yinxj96@gmail.com (X.Y.); yx3213331829@gmail.com (X.Y.); c18928489596@gmail.com (A.C.); 2017175@dgut.edu.cn (L.Z.); zhanggang@dgut.edu.cn (G.Z.); liaowenbo110@163.com (W.L.)

[2]   Safety Evaluation Department, Guangdong safety production technology center Co. Ltd., Guangzhou 510075, China

[3]   Advanced Research Institute for Multidisciplinary Science, Beijing Institute of Technology, Beijing 100081, China; jli@bit.edu.cn

*   Correspondence: huangxiangx@dgut.edu.cn (X.H.); canyang.zhang@wsu.edu (C.Y.Z.);

Abstract: Stimuli-responsive polymeric micelles (PMs) have shown great potential in drug delivery and controlled release in cancer chemotherapy. Herein, inspired by the features of the tumor microenvironment, we developed dual pH/redox-responsive mixed PMs which are self-assembled from two kinds of amphiphilic diblock copolymers (poly(ethylene glycol) methyl ether-b-poly(β-amino esters) (mPEG-b-PAE) and poly(ethylene glycol) methyl ether-grafted disulfide-poly(β-amino esters) (PAE-ss-mPEG)) for anticancer drug delivery and controlled release. The co-micellization of two copolymers is evaluated by measurement of critical micelle concentration (CMC) values at different ratios of the two copolymers. The pH/redox-responsiveness of PMs is thoroughly investigated by measurement of base dissociation constant (pK_b) value, particle size, and zeta-potential in different conditions. The PMs can encapsulate doxorubicin (DOX) efficiently, with high drug-loading efficacy. The DOX was released due to the swelling and disassembly of nanoparticles triggered by low pH and high glutathione (GSH) concentrations in tumor cells. The in vitro results demonstrated that drug release rate and cumulative release are obviously dependent on pH values and reducing agents. Furthermore, the cytotoxicity test showed that the mixed PMs have negligible toxicity, whereas the DOX-loaded mixed PMs exhibit high cytotoxicity for HepG2 cells. Therefore, the results demonstrate that the dual pH/redox-responsive PMs self-assembled from PAE-based diblock copolymers could be potential anticancer drug delivery carriers with pH/redox-triggered drug release, and the fabrication of stimuli-responsive mixed PMs could be an efficient strategy for preparation of intelligent drug delivery platform for disease therapy.

Keywords: mixed polymeric micelles; pH/redox-responsive; drug delivery; controlled release; anticancer

1. Introduction

With the rapid development of nanotechnology, a series of drug delivery systems (DDSs) such as liposomes [1], gels [2], polymeric micelles (PMs) [3,4], and nanoparticles (NPs) [5], etc., have been reported in cancer therapy [6]. However, major clinical barriers such as low accumulation at the tumor site, uncontrolled drug release, severe adverse effects, and high multidrug resistance still limit the efficacy of anticancer drugs and obstruct the step towards better cancer treatment [7–9]. To overcome these obstacles, efficient nanovehicles, which can efficiently deliver anticancer drug to tumor site with controlled drug release performance and enhanced therapeutic efficacy, urgently need to be developed. Among the aforementioned nanocarriers, PMs, which are self-assembled from amphiphilic copolymers, have shown great potential in anticancer drug-targeted delivery and controlled release due to superior advantages of technical ease, high drug-loading efficacy and biocompatibility, low cytotoxicity, and reduced side-effects [10–12].

The tumor metabolic profile is different from that of normal tissues, resulting in lots of features which are used as important hallmarks. For example, the pH value in the tumor microenvironment (TME) is generally lower than that in normal sites due to the elevated levels of lactic acid caused by poor oxygen perfusion [13,14]. Besides the weakly acidic conditions in the TME, the reductive characteristics of tumoral cytoplasm have attracted more and more attention in recent years [15–18]. As reported, the cellular glutathione (GSH) levels in solid tumors are much higher (~1000-times) than in normal cells [19,20]. Inspired by these specific features in the TME, a series of multi-functional stimuli-responsive PMs have been designed and prepared for drug targeted delivery and controlled release in cancer treatment [21–25]. For instance, Silva et al. reported a novel PM based on an amphiphilic derivative of chitosan-containing quaternary ammonium and myristoyl groups that might be a potential nanocarrier for curcumin in cancer therapy [26]. Zhang et al. designed and synthesized a novel pH-sensitive amphiphilic copolymer which could self-assemble into PMs together with a hydrophobic anticancer drug for targeted delivery and controlled release. The in vitro results demonstrated that the pH-responsive PMs may be a promising nanocarrier for encapsulated anticancer drug in cancer chemotherapy [14]. Lee's group developed redox/pH-responsive PMs self-assembled from amphiphilic copolymer poly(β-amino ester)-grafted disulfide methylene oxide poly(ethylene glycol) (PAE-g-DSMPEG), used as anticancer drug carriers in cancer chemotherapy [19]. Johnson and co-workers synthesized a series of bioreducible and pH-responsive zwitterionic/amphiphilic block copolymers bearing a degradable disulfide linker used as dual-stimuli-responsive drug delivery vehicle for a chemotherapeutic drug [27]. In addition, various stimuli-responsive PMs which can respond to other specific cues, such as dual pH/thermal-responsiveness [28,29] and dual photo/redox-responsiveness [30] in the TME, have also been thoroughly investigated and used as drug nanocarriers in cancer chemotherapy.

Herein, we design and prepare dual pH- and redox-responsive PMs which are self-assembled from two diblock copolymers: (1) pH-responsive copolymer poly(ethylene glycol) methyl ether-b-poly(β-amino esters) (mPEG-b-PAE); and (2) redox-responsive copolymer poly(ethylene glycol) methyl ether-grafted disulfide-poly(β-amino esters) (PAE-ss-mPEG). pH-sensitive segments form the polymeric micellar core, and the PEG shells are surrounded on the surface. Disulfide bonds are able to respond to reduction cues in the TME, such as GSH. Doxorubicin (DOX), which has been used extensively in various cancers as chemotherapy, is used as the model anticancer drug. As shown in Figure 1, two kinds of diblock copolymers are able to self-assemble into PMs, and DOX could be efficiently encapsulated into the core of mixed PMs (called DOX-PMs). The DOX-PMs are able to respond to the acid and GSH in the TME because of deprotonation/protonation (in acid conditions) of tertiary amine residues in the PAE segment and cleavage of disulfide bonds, respectively, resulting in rapid drug release from the PMs due to swelling and demicellization of the system. Furthermore, the other physicochemical characteristics of systems with different ratios of two kinds of diblock copolymers, including particle size, zeta-potential, loading efficacy, and cytotoxicity, are evaluated.

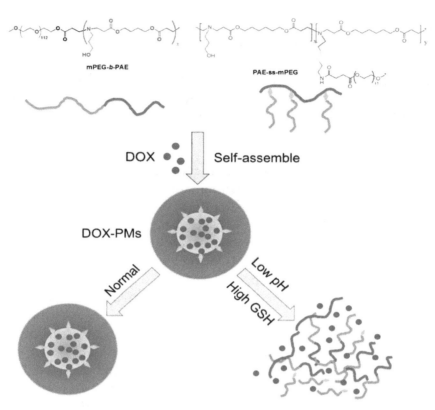

Figure 1. Co-micellization of pH/redox-responsive diblock copolymers for drug delivery and controlled release triggered by pH and glutathione (GSH). DOX: doxorubicin; PMs: polymeric micelles.

2. Materials and Methods

2.1. Material

Poly(ethylene glycol) methyl ether-grafted disulfide-poly(β-amino esters) (PAE3100-ss-mPEG2000) and poly(ethylene glycol) methyl ether-b-poly(β-amino esters) (mPEG5000-b-PAE4090) were synthesized as reported in our previous works [15,31]. Doxorubicin hydrochloride (DOX-HCl) was purchased from Wuhan Yuan Cheng Gong Chuang Co. Ltd. (Wuhan, China). Triethylamine (TEA, >99%), pyrene (99%), DL-dithiothreitol (DTT, which was used to replace GSH in this study), dichloromethane (DCM), dimethyl sulfoxide (DMSO), chloroform, and all other chemical reagents were used as received. Methylthiazoltetrazolium (MTT) was purchased from Sigma-Aldrich (St. Louis, MO, USA). Dulbecco's modified eagle media (DMEM) growth media, fetal bovine serum (FBS), trypsin, penicillin, and streptomycin were all purchased from Invitrogen (Carlsbad, NM, USA); HepG2 cell lines were obtained from the American Type Culture Collection (ATCC, Manassas, MA, USA) and all other reagents were used as received.

2.2. Preparation of Mixed PMs and DOX-PMs

The mixed PMs self-assembled from pH-sensitive and redox-responsive diblock copolymers were prepared using a dialysis method. In a typical experiment, the diblock copolymers (mPEG-b-PAE:PAE-ss-mPEG at mass ratios of 2:1, 1:1, or 1:2, here referred to as PMs-1, PMs-2, and PMs-3, respectively) were dissolved in 40 mL of DMSO with vigorous stirring for 2 h. The resulted copolymer solution was then transferred to a dialysis bag (Molecular weight cut-off MWCO 3500–4000) and dialyzed against 1 L deionized water at pH 7.4 for 48 h at room temperature. The deionized water was replaced every 2 h for the first 12 h and then every 6 h. After filtration using 0.45-μm filter and lyophilization, the mixed PMs were obtained in powder and stored at −20 °C for further experiments.

The DOX-loaded PMs (called DOX-PMs) were prepared similarly. In brief, 40 mg of mixed two diblock copolymers at different ratios and DOX (10 mg, 20 mg, or 40 mg) were dissolved in 40 mL

DMSO, and the solution was transferred to a dialysis bag. The dialysis process was carried out as aforementioned. After filtration and lyophilization as aforementioned, the DOX-PMs were obtained and stored at $-20\,°C$ for further experiments.

2.3. Characterization

The hydrodynamic diameter of PMs or DOX-PMs was measured by dynamic light scattering (DLS, Malvern Zetasizer Nano S, Malvern, UK). Briefly, the PMs were dissolved in phosphate buffer solution (PBS) at pH 8.0, 7.4, 6.5, 6.0, or 5.0 with or without DTT (10 mM) at a concentration of 1.0 mg/mL. As reported, a buffer solution with the addition of 10 mM DTT is commonly used to simulate the reductive microenvironment in tumor cells [32–35]. The samples were measured in a 1.0 mL quartz cuvette using a diode laser of 670 nm at room temperature. To evaluate the serum stability, the PMs were re-suspended into PBS with 20% FBS at a concentration of 1 mg/mL. After incubation at 37 °C for different time, the particle size of the sample was measured.

The morphology of PMs was determined by transmission electron microscopy (TEM, Hitachi H-7650, Hitachi-Science&Technology, Tokyo, Japan) with an acceleration voltage of 80 kV. The samples were prepared from PM solution at a concentration of 1 mg/mL onto copper grids coated with carbon. Briefly, the PM solution was re-suspended and dropped on the copper grid at atmospheric pressure and room temperature for 2 h. After drying, the sample was observed by TEM.

2.4. Drug Loading Efficacy

The drug loading content (LC) and entrapment efficiency (EE) were confirmed by a UV-vis spectrophotometer (UV-2450, Shimadzu, Japan) at 480 nm. In brief, 1 mg of DOX-PM powder was dissolved into 10 mL of dimethyl formamide (DMF) with vigorous stirring for 1 h. The DOX concentration of sample was measured and calculated according to the standard curve of pure DOX/DMF solution. The LC was defined as the weight ratio of encapsulated DOX to the DOX-PMs. The EE was defined as the weight ratio of encapsulated DOX to DOX in feed when preparation of DOX-PMs.

2.5. Critical Micelle Concentration (CMC) Measurement

The CMC values of the system (mixed diblock copolymers) were determined by the fluorescence probe technique using pyrene as a fluorescence probe. The two diblock copolymer mixtures at different ratios were first dissolved into acetone and then diluted by deionized water at a final concentration of 0.1 mg/mL. The acetone was removed using rotary evaporation with stirring for 4 h at room temperature. A series of copolymer solutions at concentrations from 0.0001 to 0.1 mg/mL were prepared. Pyrene/acetone solution (0.1 mL) was added to every vial and the acetone was allowed to evaporate to form a thin film at the bottom of the vial. The final concentration of pyrene was 6×10^{-7} M in water. The mixed solution was equilibrated at room temperature for 24 h in dark. And then, the fluorescence spectra of samples were obtained using a fluorescence spectrophotometer (F-4500, Hitachi-Science&Technology, Hitachi, Japan) with an emission wavelength of 373 nm.

2.6. Potentiometric Titration

To measure the base dissociation constant (pK_b) of system, potentiometric titrations were operated as reported. In brief, the mixed diblock copolymers were dissolved in deionized water, and the pH was adjusted to 3.0 with dilute hydrochloric acid. Then, NaOH solution (0.1 mol/L) was added dropwise in the mixed solution, and the real-time pH values were recorded by an automatic titration titrator (Hanon T-860, Jinan Hanon Instruments Co., Ltd., Jinan, China). The pK_b value of system was determined according to the plots of pH value against the volume of NaOH solution.

2.7. pH and Redox Responsiveness

To evaluate the pH- and redox-responsiveness of system, the PMs were firstly re-suspended in PBS at different pH values with or without DTT (10 mM). After incubation for 4 h at 37 °C, the hydrodynamic diameter of sample was measured by DLS as aforementioned.

2.8. In Vitro Release of DOX from PMs

The in vitro release of DOX from DOX-PMs was recorded using UV-vis spectrophotometer. To acquire sink conditions, in vitro drug release test was performed at low drug concentrations. In brief, 5 mg DOX-PMs were dissolved into 5 mL in PBS at pH 7.4 or 6.0 with or without the addition of DTT (10 mM), and the solution was transferred into a cellulose dialysis bag (MWCO 3500–4000). Then, the dialysis bag was placed in corresponding buffer (45 mL) in a beaker. The experiment was carried out at 37 °C with stirring at 110 rpm. At the desired time, 1 mL of solution was taken for measurement using UV-vis spectrophotometry, and 1 mL of fresh PBS was added. The cumulative drug release percent (E_r) was calculated according to our previous work [14]. Equation (1) is shown as follows:

$$E_r(\%) = \frac{V_e \sum_{1}^{n-1} C_i + V_0 C_n}{m_{DOX}} \times 100\% \tag{1}$$

where m_{DOX} is the amount of encapsulated drug in PMs, V_e is the volume of buffer in the dialysis bag, V_0 is the total volume of buffer in the beaker (50 mL), and C_i is the DOX concentration in the ith sample.

2.9. Cell Culture

The HepG2 cells were cultured in DMEM supplemented with 10% FBS, 100 units/mL penicillin, and 100 µg/mL streptomycin. The cells were incubated at 37 °C in a CO_2 (5%) incubator.

2.10. Cytotoxicity Test

The cytotoxicity of free DOX, blank PMs, and various DOX-PMs against HepG2 cells were evaluated by standard MTT assay [36–39]. In brief, HepG2 cells were seeded into a 96-well plate at an initial density of 1×104 cells/well in 200 µL DMEM medium and cultured in incubator for 24 h. The medium was removed, and 200 µL/well of free DOX, blank PMs, and DOX-PMs with different concentrations of DOX were added and cultured for 24 h. The wells without cells were used as blank, and the wells with cells but without treatment were used as control. After addition of 20 µL of MTT solution, the plate was shaken for 5 min at 150 rpm and then cultured for 4 h in incubator. After discarding the culture supernatants, 200 µL of DMSO were added to each well. The plate was gently agitated for 15 min, and the absorbance of sample was recorded by a microplate reader (Multiskan Spectrum, Thermo Scientific, Vantaa, Finland) at 490 nm. The cell viability (%) was defined as the absorbance ratio of difference between sample and blank and difference between control and blank.

2.11. Statistical Analysis

The experimental data were presented with an average values, expressed as the mean ± standard deviation (S.D.). Statistical analysis was conducted using two-sample Student's *t*-test of origin 8.5, and considered to be significant when $p < 0.05$.

3. Results and Discussions

3.1. Preparation and Chacracterization of PMs and DOX-Loaded PMs

Blank mixed PMs and DOX-loaded mixed PMs were prepared by the dialysis method. The particle size and morphology were measured and characterized by DLS (Figure 2A) and TEM (Figure 2B), respectively. As shown in Figure 2A, the particle sizes of mixed PMs-1, PMs-2, and PMs-3 were 160.7 nm, 138.6 nm, and 115.1 nm, respectively. The reason could be the much larger polymeric micellar core with increasing PAE segment in the system when the ratios of the linear diblock copolymer mPEG-b-PAE were enhanced. The particle size of DOX-PMs-2 (mixed copolymers:DOX = 2:1, mass ratio) was slightly higher (148.0 nm) than that of PMs-2 due to the loading of hydrophobic DOX molecules in the micellar core. In addition, the stability of three types of PMs in PBS containing 20% FBS at pH 7.4 was evaluated via the change of particle size, as shown in Figure S1 (Supporting Information). The results demonstrated that all of three mixed PMs showed high serum stability after incubation for 5 days. That indicated three mixed PMs possessed the potential to prolong the circulation time, thereby improving the accumulation of PMs in the site of tumor by enhanced permeability and retention (EPR) effect. Figure 2B presents the TEM images of DOX-PMs-2 after incubation in PBS at pH 7.4 for 2 h. The particle size was approximately 143.4 nm, and DOX-PMs-2 exhibited a uniformly spherical in shape with good dispersibility. The particle size measured by TEM was slightly lower compared with that determined by DLS, resulting from the shrinking of the polymeric micelles during drying process prior to TEM imaging. The TEM images of DOX-PMs-1 and DOX-PMs-3 are shown in Figure S2 (Supporting Information), and similar results were observed.

The particle size, polydispersity index (PDI), LC, and EE of the three types of DOX-PMs at different mass ratios of drug and carriers are shown in Table 1. As expected, the particle sizes of DOX-loaded PMs were increased compared with those of blank PMs. With increasing DOX in feed, the particle size was also enhanced due to more DOX molecules being encapsulated in the micellar core. When the mass ratio of drug and carriers was increased from 1:4 to 1:1, the LC was enhanced sharply and then tended to be gentle, while the EE was enhanced firstly and then reduced rapidly caused by the limitation of drug-loading capability of mixed PMs. Besides, at the same mass ratio of drug and carriers, the mixed PMs-1 had the highest drug loading efficacy, attributed to the much bigger micellar core. Therefore, DOX-PMs at the drug:carrier mass ratio of 1:2 for the three types of mixed PMs were selected for further study.

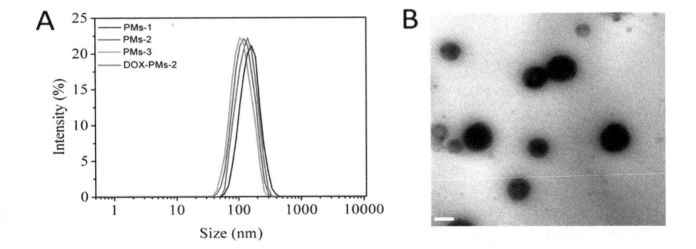

Figure 2. (**A**) Hydrodynamic diameter of different mixed PM and DOX-loaded PMs-2 measured by dynamic light scattering (DLS). (**B**) TEM image of DOX-PMs-2 after incubation in PBS at pH 7.4 for 2 h. Scale bar, 100 nm.

Table 1. Particle size, polydispersity index (PDI), loading content (LC), and entrapment (EE) of DOX-PMs at different mass ratios of drug and carriers.

PMs (40 mg)	DOX (mg)	Size (nm) [a]	PDI [a]	LC (%) [b]	EE (%) [b]
	10	165	0.25	13.60	61.18
PMs-1	20	171	0.22	27.71	73.45
	40	178	0.35	28.67	53.76
	10	143	0.21	14.21	60.43
PMs-2	20	148	0.23	26.85	77.64
	40	155	0.33	29.11	55.70
	10	121	0.23	12.77	59.08
PMs-3	20	125	0.31	23.90	71.54
	40	130	0.33	25.69	52.77

[a] measured by DLS, [b] measured by UV-vis.

3.2. CMC Measurement

The CMC value is related to the thermodynamic stability of polymeric micelles and affects the initial release of the drug when introduced into the bloodstream by intravenous administration. The low CMC value indicated the system could self-assemble easily into polymeric micelles. The CMC values of three types of mixed systems were measured by fluorescence spectroscopy using pyrene as the probe, as shown in Figure 3. The CMC values of mixed PMs-1, PMs-2, and PMs-3 were determined as 3.1 mg/L, 4.2 mg/L, and 6.4 mg/L, respectively, which were values much lower than those of PMs self-assembled from single amphiphilic copolymer [40], indicating the much higher stability. Furthermore, the result showed that the stability of mixed PMs-1 is slightly superior to PMs-2 and PMs-3. The reason could be that a lower CMC value was resulted from the more hydrophobic PAE segment in mixed diblock copolymer. In summary, the three types of mixed copolymers were able to self-assemble into mixed polymeric micelles with low CMC values, indicating that these PMs could be potential efficient hydrophobic drug carriers with high stability.

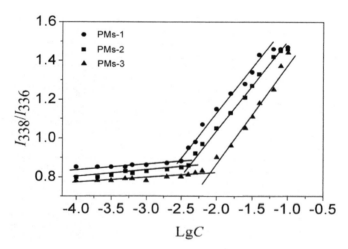

Figure 3. Plot of intensity ratios (I_{338}/I_{336}) as a function of logarithm of the mixed copolymers at various concentrations (mg/mL).

3.3. pH Sensitivity of Three Types of PMs

The pK_b value of mixed PMs was defined as the pH value at 50% neutralization of protonated amine groups according to the reference [41]. Here, the pK_b values of the three types of system were measured by acid–base titration, and the corresponding titration curves are shown in Figure 4. As expected, the pH value increased sharply with the addition of NaOH solution, then reached a plateau, and then increased rapidly again. The reason could be that the tertiary amine residues in the

PAE segment were protonated in acidic environment and were transferred to deprotonation in basic environment. As shown in Figure 4, the pK_b values of PMs-1, PMs-2, and PMs-3 were measured as 6.45, 6.57, and 6.72, respectively, owing to different amount of pH-sensitive PAE segment in the system. PMs-1 showed the lowest pK_b value due to the ratio of diblock copolymer mPEG-b-PAE in the mixed system. With the increase of diblock copolymer PAE-ss-mPEG, the pK_b value of sysem increased from 6.45 to 6.72. The results suggested that pK_b values of three types of mixed PMs were in the range of weakly acidic range, indicating the suitable and potential pH-responsiveness of mixed PMs used as anticancer drug carriers.

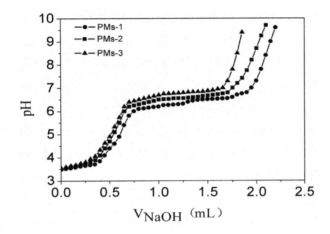

Figure 4. The potentiometric titration of the mixed copolymer solution with the mass ratios of mPEG-b-PAE and PAE-ss-mPEG at 2:1, 1:1, and 1:2. PAE-ss-mPEG: poly(ethylene glycol) methyl ether-grafted disulfide-poly(β-amino esters); mPEG-b-PAE: poly(ethylene glycol) methyl ether-b-poly(β-amino esters).

3.4. pH- and Redox-Responsiveness

Next, the pH- and redox-responsiveness of mixed PMs were evaluated through measurement of size and zeta-potential change of system at different pH conditions, as shown in Figure 5. Figure 5A shows the particle size of three mixed PMs depended on the pH value. When the pH of the mixed diblock copolymer solution was higher than 7.0, the particle sizes of the three mixed PMs increased slightly with the pH increase. The reason could be the few tertiary amine residues in the PAE segment with protonation, resulting in slight swelling of PMs. When the pH value decreased to the range of 7.0–5.5, the particle sizes of three mixed PMs increased sharply. The reason may be that the tertiary amine residues in PAE segment were fully protonated in acidic conditions, leading to the transition from hydrophobic PAE to a hydrophilic one that transformed the PMs from dense to swollen structures, so that the particle size was increased. The PMs-1 with the most tertiary amine residues were the biggest and exhibited the most dramatic size change compared with the other two mixed PMs. As expected, the PMs-3 with the lowest segment ratio of PAE had the smallest particle size and change, consistent with the results in Figure 2. Thus, the more pH-sensitive and hydrophobic PAE content, the greater the micelle particle size and the greater the size change when pH decreased from base to acid. The reason could be that the tertiary amine residues in the PAE segment were transferred from deprotonated to protonated, resulting in a hydrophilic PAE segment in the system and swollen nanoparticles. When the pH value decreased below pH 6.0 sequentially, the particle sizes of three types of mixed PMs were reduced slightly because of disassembly of few polymeric micelles. Figure 5B shows the zeta-potential of PMs at different pH conditions. The zeta-potential of three mixed PMs increased significantly with pH value decrease as a result of the tertiary amine residues in the PAE segment being transferred from deprotonation to protonation. The zeta-potential was positive, indicating the high cellular uptake due to the charge interactions, as reported in references [42,43]. When the pH was higher than 7.0, the zeta-potential was decreased with the pH increase due to the uncharged PEG shield on the surface of the polymeric micelles. In summary, three types of mixed PMs showed effective pH sensitivity. The redox-responsiveness of PMs was next investigated, as shown in Figure 5C. After incubation in PBS with DTT (10 mM) for 2 h, particle sizes of three types of mixed PMs were obviously increased, attributed to the cleavage of disulfide bonds which resulted in detachment of hydrophilic PEG segment that might lead to the aggregation of nanoparticles. Furthermore, the left hydrophobic PAE segment was entrapped into the micellar core, which led to the increase of particle size. PMs-3 with the most diblock copolymer brush PAE-ss-mPEG, including disulfide bonds, showed much greater size changes compared to the other mixed PMs. In conclusion, the prepared three mixed PMs showed pH- and redox-responsiveness.

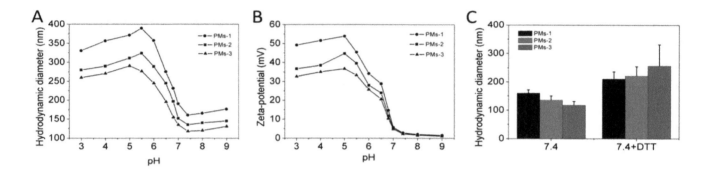

Figure 5. Particle size (**A**) and zeta-potential (**B**) of the mixed PM dependence on pH value in PBS. (**C**) Particle size of the mixed PMs in PBS with or without DTT (10 mM) after incubation for 2 h.

3.5. pH- and Redox-Triggered DOX Rlease In Vitro

After effective accumulation of drug-loaded system at the targeted site, the controlled drug release from carries triggered by specific microenvironmental cues are of great importance. Next, the in vitro DOX release from mixed PMs in different conditions (pH 7.4, pH 6.0, pH 7.4 with DTT and pH 6.0 with DTT) was investigated, as shown in Figure 6. It could be observed that the release rates of DOX from PMs were markedly influenced by pH values and DTT. At pH 7.4, the mixed PMs were tight and compact; the release rates of DOX were very slow for the three DOX-PMs. The cumulative release of DOX was less than 30% after 48 h for DOX-PMs-1, DOX-PMs-2, and DOX-PMs-3, indicating that the DOX molecules could be well protected in the micellar core and with reduced burst release. When the pH decreased to 6.0, the DOX release rate was obviously accelerated, and the cumulative release of DOX was approximately 70%, 67%, and 60% after 48 h for DOX-PMs-1 (Figure 6A), DOX-PMs-2 (Figure 6B), and DOX-PMs-3 (Figure 6C), respectively, due to the swelling of polymeric micelles caused by deprotonation/protonation (in acid conditions) of tertiary amine residues in PAE segment. The cumulative release of DOX for DOX-PMs-3 was the highest, attributed to the greater PAE segment in the system compared to the others. At pH 7.4 with DTT, the drug release rates and cumulative release were also significantly improved, resulting from the cleavage of disulfide bonds and the detachment of the PEG segment which led to the increase in porosity. Moreover, the cumulative release of DOX at 48 h for DOX-PMs-3 (75%, Figure 6C) was higher compared to DOX-PMs-1 (63%, Figure 6A) and DOX-PMs-2 (65%, Figure 6B), due to the higher mass ratio of diblock copolymer PAE-ss-mPEG in the system. At pH 6.0 with DTT, the DOX release rates of three DOX-loaded PMs were obviously enhanced, and the cumulative release of DOX was almost 100% for three DOX-PMs, caused by the acid and DTT in the solution. In summary, the DOX was of controlled release from the mixed PMs triggered by the pH and DTT, indicating the DOX might have controlled release in the tumor microenvironment by responding to the acid and reducing agent glutathione (GSH).

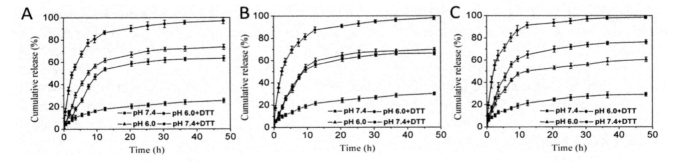

Figure 6. In vitro drug release profiles of DOX-loaded PMs-1 (**A**), DOX-loaded PMs-2 (**B**), or DOX-loaded PMs-3 (**C**) in PBS at pH 7.4, pH 6.0, pH 7.4 with 10 mM DTT, and pH 6.0 with 10 mM DTT ($n = 3$, mean $\pm$ SD).

3.6. Cytotoxicity Assay

Next, the cytotoxic effects of the blank PMs, free DOX, and DOX-PMs for HepG2 cells were evaluated using MTT assay, as shown in Figure 7. Since their cytotoxic effect increased slightly with the increasing PM concentration after incubation of 24 h, the cell viability for treatment of PMs-1, PMs-2, and PMs-3 was higher than 95% even at the highest concentration of PMs (400 mg/L) (Figure 7A). The result demonstrated that all of three types of mixed PMs had negligible cytotoxicity for HepG2 cells. Figure 7B shows the cytotoxicity of free DOX and three DOX-PMs against HepG2 cells for 24 h. The half maximal inhibitory concentration (IC50) values of free DOX, DOX-PMs-1, DOX-PMs-2, and DOX-PMs-3 were measured as 1.85 mg/L, 1.50 mg/L, 0.91 mg/L, and 0.75 mg/L, respectively. The cytotoxicity of DOX-PMs for HepG2 cells was higher than that of free DOX, possibly resulting from the enhanced cellular uptake and reduced active efflux of DOX molecules. Compared with the other DOX-PMs, the DOX-PMs-3 showed the highest cytotoxicity against HepG2 cells due to the rapid drug release rate and high cumulative release at 24 h, as shown in Figure 6. Conclusively, the three mixed PMs had very low cytotoxicity and the DOX-PMs could efficiently inhibit the suppressed HepG2 cell growth.

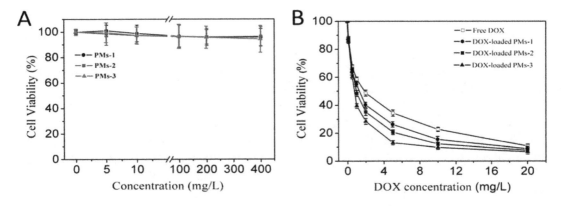

Figure 7. In vitro cytotoxicity of blank three PMs (**A**) and DOX-loaded PMs (**B**) at different concentrations in HepG2 cells after incubation for 24 h.

4. Conclusions

Three types of PMs were self-assembled from mixture of two kinds of diblock copolymers. The particle sizes of three PMs were in the range of 100–200 nm with a spherical shape. The three types of PMs showed low CMC values, indicating the self-assembly and high stability of system in aqueous solution. DOX, one of the most effective drugs against a wide range of cancers, was efficiently encapsulated into the micellar core via the hydrophobic interaction. The pH- and redox-responsiveness of mixed PMs were thoroughly investigated by recording the particle size and zeta-potential at different conditions. In vitro drug release profiles and cytotoxicity assay demonstrated that the DOX was released from mixed PMs triggered by acidic pH and high concentration of DTT, and the released DOX molecules were able to inhibit the HepG2 cell growth. Furthermore, the structure–activity relationship of mixed PMs based on different mass ratios of two diblock copolymers were preliminarily studied. These results suggested that the dual pH- and redox-responsive polymeric micelles might be promising as a potential efficient drug delivery carrier for cancer chemotherapy, and mixed polymeric micelles self-assembled from two or more kinds of stimuli-responsive copolymers could be an effective method to prepare multi-functional drug delivery vehicles.

Author Contributions: Conceptualization, X.H. and C.Y.Z.; methodology, Y.L.; software, X.Y. (Xi Yin) and J.L.; validation, X.Y. (Xujun Yin), Y.L., and A.C.; formal analysis, L.Z.; investigation, G.Z.; resources, W.L.; data curation, Y.L.; writing—original draft preparation, Y.L., X.H., and C.Y.Z.; writing—review and editing, Y.L., X.H., J.L., and C.Y.Z.; visualization, Y.L., X.H., and C.Y.Z.; supervision, X.H. and C.Y.Z.; project administration, X.H. and C.Y.Z.; funding acquisition, X.H.

References

1. Allen, T.M.; Cullis, P.R. Liposomal Drug Delivery Systems: From Concept to Clinical Applications. *Adv. Drug Deliv. Rev.* **2013**, *65*, 36–48. [CrossRef]
2. Zha, L.; Banik, B.; Alexis, F. Stimulus Responsive Nanogels for Drug Delivery. *Soft Matter* **2011**, *7*, 5908–5916. [CrossRef]
3. Kwon, G.S.; Okano, T. Polymeric Micelles as New Drug Carriers. *Adv. Drug Deliv. Rev.* **1996**, *21*, 107–116. [CrossRef]
4. Amjad, M.W.; Kesharwani, P.; Mohd Amin, M.C.I.; Iyer, A.K. Recent Advances in the Design, Development, and Targeting Mechanisms of Polymeric Micelles for Delivery of siRNA in Cancer Therapy. *Prog. Polym. Sci.* **2017**, *64*, 154–181. [CrossRef]
5. Cho, K.; Wang, X.; Nie, S.; Chen, Z.; Shin, D.M. Therapeutic Nanoparticles for Drug Delivery in Cancer. *Clin. Cancer Res.* **2008**, *14*, 1310–1316. [CrossRef] [PubMed]
6. Wolinsky, J.B.; Colson, Y.L.; Grinstaff, M.W. Local Drug Delivery Strategies for Cancer Treatment: Gels, Nanoparticles, Polymeric films, Rods, and Wafers. *J. Control. Release* **2012**, *159*, 14–26. [CrossRef]
7. Jones, C.H.; Chen, C.-K.; Ravikrishnan, A.; Rane, S.; Pfeifer, B.A. Overcoming Nonviral Gene Delivery Barriers: Perspective and Future. *Mol. Pharm.* **2013**, *10*, 4082–4098. [CrossRef]
8. von Roemeling, C.; Jiang, W.; Chan, C.K.; Weissman, I.L.; Kim, B.Y. Breaking Down the Barriers to Precision Cancer Nanomedicine. *Trends Biotechnol.* **2017**, *35*, 159–171. [CrossRef]
9. Wicki, A.; Witzigmann, D.; Balasubramanian, V.; Huwyler, J. Nanomedicine in Cancer Therapy: Challenges, Opportunities, and Clinical Applications. *J. Control. Release* **2015**, *200*, 138–157. [CrossRef] [PubMed]
10. Biswas, S.; Kumari, P.; Lakhani, P.M.; Ghosh, B. Recent Advances in Polymeric Micelles for Anti-Cancer Drug Delivery. *Eur. J. Pharm. Sci.* **2016**, *83*, 184–202. [CrossRef] [PubMed]
11. Nishiyama, N.; Matsumura, Y.; Kataoka, K. Development of Polymeric Micelles for Targeting Intractable Cancers. *Cancer Sci.* **2016**, *107*, 867–874. [CrossRef]
12. Gothwal, A.; Khan, I.; Gupta, U. Polymeric Micelles: Recent Advancements in the Delivery of Anticancer Drugs. *Pharm. Res.* **2016**, *33*, 18–39. [CrossRef]
13. Kurisawa, M.; Yui, N. Gelatin/Dextran Intelligent Hydrogels for Drug Delivery: Dual-Stimuli-Responsive Degradation in Relation to Miscibility in Interpenetrating Polymer Networks. *Macromol. Chem. Phys.* **1998**, *199*, 1547–1554. [CrossRef]
14. Zhang, C.Y.; Yang, Y.Q.; Huang, T.X.; Zhao, B.; Guo, X.D.; Wang, J.F.; Zhang, L. Self-Assembled pH-Responsive MPEG-b-(PLA-co-PAE) Block Copolymer Micelles for Anticancer Drug Delivery. *Biomaterials* **2012**, *33*, 6273–6283. [CrossRef]

15. Li, J.; Ma, Y.J.; Wang, Y.; Chen, B.Z.; Guo, X.D.; Zhang, C.Y. Dual Redox/pH-Responsive Hybrid Polymer-Lipid Composites: Synthesis, Preparation, Characterization and Application in Drug Delivery with Enhanced Therapeutic Efficacy. *Chem. Eng. J.* **2018**, *341*, 450–461. [CrossRef]

16. Curcio, M.; Blanco-Fernandez, B.; Diaz-Gomez, L.; Concheiro, A.; Alvarez-Lorenzo, C. Hydrophobically Modified Keratin Vesicles for GSH-Responsive Intracellular Drug Release. *Bioconjug. Chem.* **2015**, *26*, 1900–1907. [CrossRef]

17. Li, Q.; Chen, M.; Chen, D.; Wu, L. One-Pot Synthesis of Diphenylalanine-Based Hybrid Nanospheres for Controllable pH-and GSH-Responsive Delivery of Drugs. *Chem. Mater.* **2016**, *28*, 6584–6590. [CrossRef]

18. Ling, X.; Tu, J.; Wang, J.; Shajii, A.; Kong, N.; Feng, C.; Zhang, Y.; Yu, M.; Xie, T.; Bharwani, Z.; et al. Glutathione-Responsive Prodrug Nanoparticles for Effective Drug Delivery and Cancer Therapy. *ACS Nano* **2019**, *13*, 357–370. [CrossRef]

19. Bui, Q.N.; Li, Y.; Jang, M.-S.; Huynh, D.P.; Lee, J.H.; Lee, D.S. Redox- and pH-Sensitive Polymeric Micelles Based on Poly(β-amino ester)-Grafted Disulfide Methylene Oxide Poly(ethylene glycol) for Anticancer Drug Delivery. *Macromolecules* **2015**, *48*, 4046–4054. [CrossRef]

20. Russo, A.; DeGraff, W.; Friedman, N.; Mitchell, J.B. Selective Modulation of Glutathione Levels in Human Normal Versus Tumor Cells and Subsequent Differential Rsponse to Chemotherapy Drugs. *Cancer Res.* **1986**, *46*, 2845–2848.

21. Chen, J.; Qiu, X.; Ouyang, J.; Kong, J.; Zhong, W.; Xing, M.M.Q. pH and Reduction Dual-Sensitive Copolymeric Micelles for Intracellular Doxorubicin Delivery. *Biomacromolecules* **2011**, *12*, 3601–3611. [CrossRef]

22. Yang, H.Y.; Jang, M.-S.; Gao, G.H.; Lee, J.H.; Lee, D.S. Construction of Redox/pH Dual Stimuli-Responsive PEGylated Polymeric Micelles for Intracellular Doxorubicin Delivery in Liver Cancer. *Polym. Chem.* **2016**, *7*, 1813–1825. [CrossRef]

23. Huang, X.; Liao, W.; Zhang, G.; Kang, S.; Zhang, C.Y. pH-Sensitive Micelles Self-Assembled from Polymer Brush (PAE-g-cholesterol)-b-PEG-b-(PAE-g-cholesterol) for Anticancer Drug Delivery and Controlled Release. *Int. J. Nanomed.* **2017**, *12*, 2215–2226. [CrossRef]

24. Zhang, C.Y.; Chen, Q.; Wu, W.S.; Guo, X.D.; Cai, C.Z.; Zhang, L.J. Synthesis and Evaluation of Cholesterol-grafted PEGylated Peptides with pH-Triggered Property as Novel Drug Carriers for Cancer Chemotherapy. *Colloids Surf. B* **2016**, *142*, 55–64. [CrossRef]

25. Alsuraifi, A.; Curtis, A.; Lamprou, A.D.; Hoskins, C. Stimuli Responsive Polymeric Systems for Cancer Therapy. *Pharmaceutics* **2018**, *10*, 136. [CrossRef]

26. Silva, S.D.; dos Santos, D.M.; Almeida, A.; Marchiori, L.; Campana-Filho, P.S.; Ribeiro, J.S.; Sarmento, B. N-(2-Hydroxy)-propyl-3-trimethylammonium, O-Mysristoyl Chitosan Enhances the Solubility and Intestinal Permeability of Anticancer Curcumin. *Pharmaceutics* **2018**, *10*, 245. [CrossRef]

27. Johnson, R.P.; Uthaman, S.; Augustine, R.; Zhang, Y.; Jin, H.; Choi, C.I.; Park, I.K.; Kim, I. Glutathione and Endosomal pH-Responsive Hybrid Vesicles Fabricated by Zwitterionic Polymer Block poly(l-aspartic acid) as a Smart Anticancer Delivery Platform. *React. Funct. Polym.* **2017**, *119*, 47–56. [CrossRef]

28. Soppimath, K.S.; Tan, D.W.; Yang, Y.Y. pH-Triggered Thermally Responsive Polymer Core–Shell Nanoparticles for Drug Delivery. *Adv. Mater.* **2005**, *17*, 318–323. [CrossRef]

29. Soppimath, K.S.; Liu, L.H.; Seow, W.Y.; Liu, S.Q.; Powell, R.; Chan, P.; Yang, Y.Y. Multifunctional Core/Shell Nanoparticles Self-Assembled from pH-Induced Thermosensitive Polymers for Targeted Intracellular Anticancer Drug Selivery. *Adv. Funct. Mater.* **2007**, *17*, 355–362. [CrossRef]

30. Shao, Y.; Shi, C.; Xu, G.; Guo, D.; Luo, J. Photo and Redox Dual Responsive Reversibly Cross-Linked Nanocarrier for Efficient Tumor-Targeted Drug Delivery. *ACS Appl. Mater. Interface* **2014**, *6*, 10381–10392. [CrossRef]

31. Huang, X.; Liao, W.; Xie, Z.; Chen, D.; Zhang, C.Y. A pH-Responsive Prodrug Delivery System Self-Assembled from Acid-Labile Doxorubicin-Conjugated Amphiphilic pH-Sensitive Block Copolymers. *Mater. Sci. Eng. C* **2018**, *90*, 27–37. [CrossRef]

32. Yin, M.; Bao, Y.; Gao, X.; Wu, Y.; Sun, Y.; Zhao, X.; Xu, H.; Zhang, Z.; Tan, S. Redox/pH Dual-Sensitive Hybrid Micelles for Targeting Delivery and Overcoming Multidrug Resistance of Cancer. *J. Mater. Chem. B* **2017**, *5*, 2964–2978. [CrossRef]

33. Bao, Y.; Guo, Y.; Zhuang, X.; Li, D.; Cheng, B.; Tan, S.; Zhang, Z. D-α-tocopherol Polyethylene Glycol Succinate-Based Redox-Sensitive Paclitaxel Prodrug for Overcoming Multidrug Resistance in Cancer Cells. *Mol. Pharm.* **2014**, *11*, 3196–3209. [CrossRef]

34. Teranishi, R.; Matsuki, R.; Yuba, E.; Harada, A.; Kono, K. Doxorubicin Delivery Using pH and Redox Dual-Responsive Hollow Nanocapsules with a Cationic Electrostatic Barrier. *Pharmaceutics* **2017**, *9*, 4. [CrossRef]

35. Pan, Y.-J.; Chen, Y.-Y.; Wang, D.-R.; Wei, C.; Guo, J.; Lu, D.-R.; Chu, C.-C.; Wang, C.-C. Redox/pH Dual Stimuli-Responsive Biodegradable Nanohydrogels with Varying Responses to Dithiothreitol and Glutathione for Controlled Drug Release. *Biomaterials* **2012**, *33*, 6570–6579. [CrossRef]

36. Laaksonen, T.; Santos, H.; Vihola, H.; Salonen, J.; Riikonen, J.; Heikkila, T.; Peltonen, L.; Kumar, N.; Murzin, D.Y.; Lehto, V.-P.; et al. Failure of MTT as a Toxicity Testing Agent for Mesoporous Silicon Microparticles. *Chem. Res. Toxicol.* **2007**, *20*, 1913–1918. [CrossRef]

37. Zhang, C.Y.; Wu, W.S.; Yao, N.; Zhao, B.; Zhang, L.J. pH-Sensitive Amphiphilic Copolymer Brush Chol-g-P(HEMA-co-DEAEMA)-b-PPEGMA: Synthesis and Self-Assembled Micelles for Controlled Anti-Cancer Drug Release. *RSC Adv.* **2014**, *4*, 40232–40240. [CrossRef]

38. Ma, W.; Guo, Q.; Li, Y.; Wang, X.; Wang, J.; Tu, P. Co-assembly of Doxorubicin and Curcumin Targeted Micelles for Synergistic Delivery and Improving Anti-Tumor Efficacy. *Eur. J. Pharm. Biopharm.* **2017**, *112*, 209–223. [CrossRef]

39. Thambi, T.; Son, S.; Lee, D.S.; Park, J.H. Poly(ethylene glycol)-b-poly(lysine) Copolymer Bearing Nitroaromatics for Hypoxia-Sensitive Drug Delivery. *Acta Biomater.* **2016**, *29*, 261–270. [CrossRef]

40. Zhang, C.Y.; Xiong, D.; Sun, Y.; Zhao, B.; Lin, W.J.; Zhang, L.J. Self-Assembled Micelles Based on pH-Sensitive PAE-g-MPEG-cholesterol Block Copolymer for Anticancer Drug Delivery. *Int. J. Nanomed.* **2014**, *9*, 4923–4933. [CrossRef]

41. Shen, Y.; Tang, H.; Zhan, Y.; Van Kirk, E.A.; Murdoch, W.J. Degradable Poly(β-amino ester) Nanoparticles for Cancer Cytoplasmic Drug Delivery. *Nanomed. Nanotechnol. Biol. Med.* **2009**, *5*, 192–201. [CrossRef]

42. Hui, Y.; Wibowo, D.; Liu, Y.; Ran, R.; Wang, H.F.; Seth, A.; Middelberg, A.P.J.; Zhao, C.X. Understanding the Effects of Nanocapsular Mechanical Property on Passive and Active Tumor Targeting. *ACS Nano* **2018**, *12*, 2846–2857. [CrossRef]

43. Ran, R.; Wang, H.; Liu, Y.; Hui, Y.; Sun, Q.; Seth, A.; Wibowo, D.; Chen, D.; Zhao, C.X. Microfluidic Self-Assembly of A Combinatorial Library of Single- and Dual-Ligand Liposomes for in vitro and in vivo Tumor Targeting. *Eur. J. Pharm. Biopharm.* **2018**, *130*, 1–10. [CrossRef]

Photo-Magnetic Irradiation-Mediated Multimodal Therapy of Neuroblastoma Cells Using a Cluster of Multifunctional Nanostructures

Rohini Atluri [1,2], **Rahul Atmaramani** [1,3], **Gamage Tharaka** [4], **Thomas McCallister** [1], **Jian Peng** [4], **David Diercks** [5], **Somesree GhoshMitra** [1] **and Santaneel Ghosh** [1,4,*]

[1]   Nano-Bio Engineering Laboratory, Southeast Missouri State University, Cape Girardeau, MO 63701, USA; atluri.rohini@gmail.com (R.A.); rratmaramani1s@semo.edu (R.A.); tgmccallister@gmail.com (T.M.); somesree@gmail.com (S.G.)

[2]   Mechanical and Energy Engineering Department, University of North Texas, Denton, TX 76207, USA

[3]   Department of Bioengineering, The University of Texas at Dallas, Richardson, TX 75080, USA

[4]   Department of Physics and Engineering Physics, Southeast Missouri State University, Cape Girardeau, MO 63701, USA; tharakarcbb13@gmail.com (G.T.); jpeng@semo.edu (J.P.)

[5]   Department of Metallurgical and Materials Engineering, Colorado School of Mines, Golden, CO 80401, USA; ddiercks@mines.edu

*   Correspondence: sghosh@semo.edu;

Abstract: The use of high intensity chemo-radiotherapies has demonstrated only modest improvement in the treatment of high-risk neuroblastomas. Moreover, undesirable drug specific and radiation therapy-incurred side effects enhance the risk of developing into a second cancer at a later stage. In this study, a safer and alternative multimodal therapeutic strategy involving simultaneous optical and oscillating (AC, Alternating Current) magnetic field stimulation of a multifunctional nanocarrier system has successfully been implemented to guide neuroblastoma cell destruction. This novel technique permitted the use of low-intensity photo-magnetic irradiation and reduced the required nanoparticle dose level. The combination of released cisplatin from the nanodrug reservoirs and photo-magnetic coupled hyperthermia mediated cytotoxicity led to the complete ablation of the B35 neuroblastoma cells in culture. Our study suggests that smart nanostructure-based photo-magnetic hybrid irradiation is a viable approach to remotely guide neuroblastoma cell destruction, which may be adopted in clinical management post modification to treat aggressive cancers.

Keywords: photo-magnetic actuation; cisplatin; nanoparticle; MYCN; multimodal therapy

1. Introduction

Neuroblastoma is a childhood cancer that is diagnosed at a median age of 17 months [1], with an incidence rate of 10.2 per million children under 15 years of age [2]. There are about seven hundred new cases each year in the United States, and in two out of three cases, the disease usually spreads to the lymph nodes or other parts of the body at the time of diagnosis. This is an embryonal tumor of the autonomic nervous systems [3], and it is the most common extra cranial tumor of childhood with long term survival rates of only about 15% [4]. Theoretically, tumors can appear anywhere along the sympathetic nervous system, but in reality, a majority of the tumors are detected in the adrenal medulla [5]. Other sites for tumors include the upper chest, neck, and paraspinal spaces. Often, metastasis can be seen in regional lymph nodes and in the bone marrow, and during an advanced stage of the disease, it can infiltrate a local organ such as with a celiac axis tumor [6,7]. Overexpression and dominance of cell survival pathways are mainly responsible for the malignant transformation and metastasis of neural crest derived cells [8]. There are several factors that define specific cases of neuroblastoma, but high risk ones include stage, age, MYCN oncogene amplification, chromosome 11q status, metastasis, histologic category, and deoxyribonucleic acid (DNA) ploidy [5].

Due to biological heterogeneity of neuroblast tumors, different therapeutic strategies are pursued. While reduced intensity therapeutic approaches, such as surgery alone or in combination with moderate intensity chemotherapy, are the usual line of treatment for less aggressive tumors, high intensity chemo-radiotherapies are usually favored for tumors with more aggressive features [5]. For high risk neuroblastoma, the current treatment is divided into three phases: (1) induction of remission, (2) consolidation of remission, and (3) maintenance. The most commonly used induction regimen includes cycles of cisplatin and etoposide as well as alternate use of vincristine, doxorubicin, and cyclophosphamide [9]. Additionally, two types of radiation therapies are used: (1) external beam radiation therapy, and (2) Metaiodobenzylguanidine (MIBG) radiotherapy [10]. Myeloablative chemotherapy with autologous hematopoietic stem-cell rescue [4,11] and isotretinoin with anti-GD2 immunotherapy [12] is also considered for high-risk neuroblastoma treatment.

Although the use of high-intensity chemo-radiotherapies have demonstrated only modest improvement in the treatment of high-risk neuroblastoma, undesirable side effects include mouth sores, nausea, hair loss, and most importantly, increased chance of infection [10]. In addition to these, there may be several drug-specific side effects, for example, cisplatin and carboplatin can affect kidneys [13], doxorubicin is a cardiotoxic agent [14], and cyclophosphamide can damage bladder as well as ovaries and testicles [15], which may affect future fertility. Short-term side effects of radiation therapy are nausea, diarrhea, burns, and fatigue [10], while long-term side effects may lead to damage in DNA, which has a risk of developing into a second cancer many years after completion of radiotherapy. Unfortunately, despite implementing all advanced treatment modalities, 50–60% patients in high-risk groups have a relapse, and there is no known curative treatment available to date [5]. Use of anti-GD2 monoclonal antibodies to prevent relapse is a good example of an immunotherapeutic approach to lessen the side effects of chemo [16], as well as radiotherapies. A future trend is to develop antibody-based treatment guidelines as well as synergistic combination therapies.

From the above discussion, it is evident that innovative approaches possessing a novel therapeutic potential need to be implemented in order to overcome the existing challenges to treat high-risk neuroblastoma. An innovative technique that holds promise in the area of cancer diagnosis and therapeutics to perform precise drug delivery, multimodal therapy, and detection of circulating or residual cancer cells, all of which can play crucial roles in the treatment of high-risk neuroblastoma, is the development of novel nanostructures coupled with smart actuation strategies [17–24]. Nanostructured materials and smart surfaces carry excellent treatment potential for the development of novel clinical solutions because they can be designed to target/detect specific cancer cells and be remotely tuned to release measured doses of therapeutic agents, which in turn may improve treatment efficacy, decrease therapy time, and decrease the quantities of the therapeutic agent necessary for effective treatment by 10–50-fold [25]. In order to meet these goals cumulatively, "combinatorial therapeutics" approaches consisting of various nanostructures and advanced instrumentation are becoming one of the most exciting forefront fields, but it has been in its infancy until now. Oscillating magnetic field induced hyperthermia [26–28] or photothermal destruction of cancer cells [29] are among the most promising approaches among these; however, both fall short of addressing several concerns, including the use of high intensity magnetic or optical irradiation coupled with a lower yield at a clinically viable dose level. As discussed earlier, the rapid emergence of treatment resistance is a formidable challenge that needs a multimodal treatment approach, and unfortunately, the aforementioned approaches do not address this concern. Recently reported [30] "multimodal chemo-radiotherapy of glioblastoma" demonstrated encouraging outcomes, which has the potential of addressing this challenge; however, the technique needs further investigation before successful implementation, especially where the use of potent γ–rays is involved.

Therefore, we set ourselves the goal of enhancing the treatment efficacy by combining a group of smart nanostructures, each of which are capable of performing a specific task with a novel strategy that has been unexplored thus far, namely simultaneous photo-magnetic actuation. In this study, three different types of nanostructures have been used to accomplish the objectives: (1) core-shell magnetic nanospheres (CSMNSs), (2) Polyvinylpyrrollidone (PVP)-capped gold nanoparticles (AuNPs), and (3) cisplatin loaded thermo-responsive nanoparticles (CPNPs). The first two protagonists (i.e., the CSMNS and the AuNPs) induce a coupled hyperthermia and oxidative stress under the hybrid photo-magnetic irradiation, whereas the CPNPs cause sustained release of the imbibed cisplatin during the treatment. These augmented the cisplatin and photo-magnetic hyperthermia mediated cytotoxicity inducing mechanisms, and intensified the oxidative stress induced damage, all at a relatively lower irradiation and nanoparticle exposure level, which led to complete ablation of the B35 neuroblastoma cells in culture. Additionally, by using this technique, exposures to the high energy γ-rays have been avoided. Our study suggests that smart nanostructure-based photo-magnetic hybrid irradiation is a viable approach to remotely guide neuroblastoma cell destruction, which may be adopted as an efficient technique in clinical management post modification. Although we have explored this technique for neuroblastoma cell destruction in this study, it can be further modified and extended to treat other aggressive cancers.

2. Materials and Methods

2.1. Photo-Magnetic Actuator Design

A unique photo-magnetic actuator was designed to perform simultaneous optical and AC magnetic field stimulation of cultured mammalian cells or dispersed nanocarrier systems (Figure 1a,b). The incubator (Figure 1b) consisted of a sample chamber for placing TPP tissue culture tubes, AC/DC magnetic field generating coil, a cage for the placement of light-emitting diodes (LEDs) for low-level optical irradiation, and a high-performance glass window at the front wall of the incubator for transmitting the laser irradiation during moderate/high level optical stimulation. Inside the sample chamber, the B35 neuroblastoma cells were cultured or the nanocarriers were colloidally dispersed, as needed. The circuit utilized a capacitor bank in series with the inductor coil and a 0.5 Ω resistor. A magnetic field in the range of 10–150 Oe and 60–150 kHz could be produced as needed by changing the capacitor and/or the coil inductance. A temperature controlling unit was attached to stabilize the incubator temperature in the range of 36–37 °C during the experiments, and the top and the bottom panels of the incubator were designed to be removable to allow easy swapping of the samples. The incubator was attached to the base of the class 3B laser (520 nm, 300 mW), and a laser stop was placed to the rear of the incubator to inhibit reflection. Further, black absorbent tape material was used to confine the laser exposure to only necessary areas. A fiber optic thermometer was used to measure precise temperature change during heating of the nanocarriers.

2.2. Nanocarrier Design

Magnetite (Fe_3O_4) core-polymeric shell nanospheres (CSMNS) were synthesized as reported in our previous work [31]. In brief, a double-layered shell consisting of a thermo-activated polymer network of poly(ethylene glycol) ethyl ether methacrylate-co-poly(ethylene glycol) methyl ether methacrylate (PEGEEMA-co-PEGMEMA) was synthesized first using a precipitation polymerization method. One batch of these designed spheres was used to induct the magnetic nanocrystals inside the outer shell, while the other batch was freeze dried and later loaded with the anticancer drug cisplatin (Sigma Aldrich, Bellefonte, PA, USA), as described below. Polyvinylpyrrollidone (PVP)-capped gold nanoparticles (0.05 mg/mL, 5 nm diameter) were obtained from nano Composix. All nanocarrier morphology was assessed by performing scanning and transmission electron microscopy (SEM and TEM: FEI NOVA 230 NANOSEM, Tustin, CA, USA, accelerating voltage 5–20 kV; Philips EM 420 TEM, Port Elizabeth, South Africa-120 kV electron beam) [31].

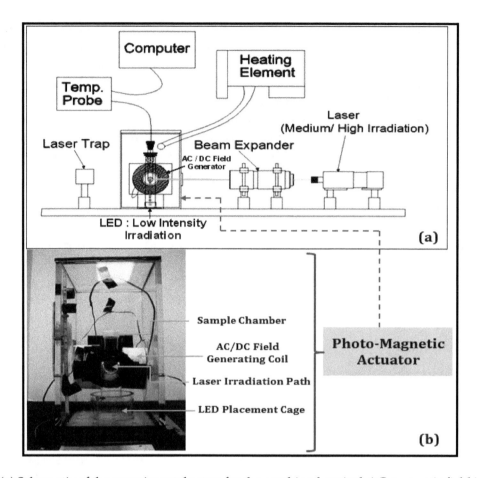

Figure 1. (a) Schematic of the experimental setup for the combined optical-AC magnetic field irradiation of nanocarriers and B35 neuroblastoma cells (electronics not shown). (b) Various components of the incubator with a TPP tissue culture tube mounted inside.

2.3. Loading the Drugs in Polymeric Nanocarriers and Characterization of Release Profile

An aqueous solution of cisplatin (2 mg/mL) was added to the previously prepared freeze-dried (non-magnetic) nanospheres. The solution was stirred for 24 h at room temperature and the cisplatin-loaded nanoparticles (CPNPs) were collected by centrifugation. A specialized diffusion chamber (PermeGear Static Franz cell,) with two compartments was used for the in vitro release kinetics measurement. The two compartments communicate through an opening 2 cm in diameter. A semipermeable membrane (mol. wt. cut-off 13,000 Da) was used to cover the opening. The CPNP solution was placed in the donor compartment and the receiver compartment was filled with the deionized (DI) water. To determine the concentration of the released cisplatin (at room temperature and at 37 °C) in the receiving compartment, samples were withdrawn at definite time intervals (20, 40, 60, 80, and 100 h) and the absorbance was measured using UV-visible spectroscopy at a wavelength of 301 nm.

2.4. Light Scattering and Magnetic Measurements

Dynamic light scattering (DLS) measurements were performed to examine the volumetric transition behavior using a Malvern NanoZS system equipped with a helium-neon laser (632.8 nm) as the light source. The hydrodynamic radius distribution of the nanospheres in water was measured at a scattering angle of 60°. A magnetic property [M(H)] of the nanospheres was measured using a Lakeshore model 7300 (Westerville, Ohio, USA) Vibrating Sample Magnetometer (VSM), at ambient temperature and at 38 °C.

2.5. Cell Culture and Treatment

B 35 rat neuroblastoma cells (ATCC, Manassas, VA, USA) were routinely cultured at 37 °C in 5% CO_2 and 85% relative humidity by using Dulbecco's modified Eagle's medium (DMEM, Invitrogen, Carlsbad, CA, USA) derived complete media that contains 90% DMEM, and 10% fetal bovine serum (FBS). For the experiments, about 10,000 cells/cm^2 were seeded in TPP tissue culture tube flasks (10 cm^2 growth surface area) containing 2 mL of DMEM complete media and were allowed to grow for 48 h or more until a 70% confluence was observed. All the experiments were performed in triplicates.

For the treatment with nanoparticles, after 48 h of cell growth and attachment, the cells were washed with serum-free DMEM and were exposed to the NPs (various concentrations of MNPs (Magnetic Nano-Particle) and/or AuNPs), which were colloidally suspended in the culture media. During the nanoparticle exposure, cultures were placed into serum-free DMEM to prevent particle aggregation. After 4 h of exposure, the cells were washed with serum-free DMEM and were cultured back into 2 mL complete DMEM media until the beginning of the next exposure cycle. The treatment was repeated thrice for every 24 h. At the end of the final exposure, live cell imaging was performed to assess the cell proliferation.

For the AC magnetic field exposure, optical irradiation, and hybrid optical-AC magnetic field exposure, the cells were cultured and exposed to the NPs as mentioned earlier. Immediately after the addition of NPs (MNPs and/or AuNPs), the cells were exposed to AC magnetic field exposure/optical irradiation/hybrid optical-AC magnetic field exposure (magnetic field intensity 60 Oe, frequency 120 kHz, laser power 300 mW) for 15 min. Following irradiation, the cells were placed in the incubator for 3 h and 45 min as part of the treatment. After 4 h of NP exposure and irradiation, the cells were washed with serum-free DMEM and were cultured back into 2 mL complete DMEM media until the beginning of the next exposure cycle. The treatment was repeated thrice for every 24 h. At the end of the final exposure, live cell imaging was performed to assess cell proliferation.

For the treatment with cisplatin-loaded thermo-responsive nanoparticles (CPNPs), after 48 h of cell growth and attachment, the cells were washed with serum-free DMEM and were exposed to the CPNPs (200 µg/mL), which were colloidally suspended in the culture media for 4 h. After 4 h of exposure, the cells were washed with serum-free DMEM and were cultured back into 2 mL complete DMEM media until the beginning of the next exposure cycle. The treatment was repeated thrice for every 24 h. At the end of the final exposure, live cell imaging was performed to assess cell proliferation.

For hybrid optical-AC magnetic field exposure in the presence of CPNPs and NPs, the cells were treated (with CPNPs and NPs) as mentioned earlier. After the addition of the nanocarriers, the cells were exposed to hybrid optical-AC magnetic field exposure (magnetic field intensity 60 Oe, frequency 120 kHz, laser power 300 mW) for 15 min. Following irradiation, the cells were placed in the incubator for 3 h and 45 min as part of the treatment. After 4 h of nanocarrier exposure and irradiation, the cells were washed with serum-free DMEM and were cultured back into 2 mL complete DMEM media until the beginning of the next exposure cycle. The treatment was repeated thrice for every 24 h. At the end of the final exposure, live cell imaging was performed to assess cell proliferation.

Nuclear morphology was assessed using confocal images captured through a 64× objective from cells (cultured on the coverglasses, which were inserted into the TPP tissue culture tube flasks and fixed) labeled with 4',6-diamidino-2-phenylindole (DAPI, Ex = 405 nm, Em = 450/35 nm), following various treatments.

2.6. Flow Cytometry Analysis: Annexin V Apoptosis Assay

Upon treatment under various conditions, the cells were washed with serum-free DMEM, trypsinized, centrifuged, and suspended in 500 µL 1× binding buffer. Cells were further incubated with FITC (Fluorescein isothiocyanate) Annexin V apoptosis detection reagent for 20 min at room temperature in darkness (100 µL of cell suspension was mixed with 5 µL of FITC Annexin V and 5 µL of PI), followed by flow cytometry analysis.

3. Results

A simultaneous optical and AC magnetic field assisted therapeutic strategy was unexplored thus far, despite having a huge potential of generating synergetic effects, which may be especially beneficial for the destruction of aggressive cancer cells. This innovative setup (Figure 1a,b) enabled high-risk neuroblastoma cell exposure to varying combinations of optical and magnetic field excitation in the presence of specifically designed nanocarriers, thereby augmenting the positive outcomes of separate actuation strategies and the nanocarrier functionalities. The maximum field strength generated by the coils ($\approx$150 Oe) is approximately 200 times weaker than that produced by a magnetic resonance imaging (MRI) machine ($\approx 3 \times 10^4$ Oe), which are known to be safe for use by people with medical implants such as pacemakers [32]. It may be noted that a Helmholtz coil-based design can be adopted for conducting experimentation with animal models and to obtain deeper penetration, a near infrared (NIR) laser can be used [22]. However, for low-level photo-magnetic therapy requiring LED irradiation in vivo, further modification is needed in the instrumentation.

No recognizable physicochemical interactions or clustering (and thereby precipitation) were observed among these three types of nanocarriers when they were (simultaneously) dispersed for 48 h in: (i) aqueous solution (DI H_2O), and in (ii) phosphate buffered saline (PBS). This indicates that the encapsulation (shell) formed by the polymerized, stable, and higher mechanical strength-possessing PEG-derivative biopolymer chains protected the embedded magnetic nanoparticles from being exposed to the proteins, salts, and other potential reactive agents present in the colloidal suspensions. Similarly, the polyvinylpyrollidone surface-tethered gold-nanoparticles were protected from potential (damaging) interactions with the media constituents, and therefore, did not facilitate agglomeration. The synthesized magnetic nanocarriers (CSMNSs) exhibited good colloidal stability, strong magnetic properties, and no precipitation after several days. From the SEM imaging, slightly oval shaped particles (arising from the surface roughness of the carbon film during sample preparation), were observed (Figure 2a). The mean diameter of the nanocarriers was found to be 268 ± 24 nm. Particle encapsulation was assessed using TEM imaging at 120 kV. The resulting TEM micrographs (Figure 2b) revealed that the magnetic nanocrystals were located near each other, which is very typical for magnetic nanoparticle-based systems, as observed earlier by several researchers [26,33,34]. Due to their size and structure, the nanomagnets were expected to exhibit super-paramagnetic behavior at a moderate field and frequency (0–150 Oe, 0–1000 kHz) range [31,35], which was assessed at 311 K, or above the volumetric transition temperature (Figure 2c). No to minimal hysteresis response was observed, unlike the ferromagnetic nanoparticle-based systems [28,34], even after the volumetric shrinkage of the spheres, which indicated super-paramagnetic behavior and the absence of nanocrystal agglomeration at elevated temperatures. Under the measured field intensity of 60 Oe, created by a permanent magnet at the adjacent wall of the flask, the CSMNSs moved in the direction of the field and formed a film on the flask wall close to the magnet (Figure 2d). Almost all particles were completely separated from the solution, even with the application of a moderately intense field, which demonstrated their controllability under a magnetic field. It may be noted that the CSMNS response to an external magnetic field was much stronger than that of the individual magnetic nanodots due to a much higher magnetization value per carrier. Slight agitation brought the nanospheres back into the solution once the magnetic field was removed. This behavior further indicated that it will be possible to trap and maintain these nanocarriers in the targeted tissue regions without being washed away by the blood flow during in vivo applications. TEM imaging of the AuNPs demonstrated the particle distribution (Figure 2e) in the culture media and the high absorption in the range of 520 ± 15 nm (Figure 2f) facilitated coupled hyperthermia under hybrid optical-AC magnetic field exposure, as assessed later. The CPNPs consisted of two polymer shells with varying degrees of hydrophilicity, as described in the previous section (nanocarrier design), the inner one having a diameter of 162 ± 24 nm (not shown here). Multi-shell nanocarriers were designed to expand the volumetric transition range [31], which in turn facilitated the release of the imbibed therapeutic agents. Morphology of the CPNPs was assessed by performing SEM imaging (Figure 2g) and the mean diameter of the double shell nanocarriers was found to be 341 ± 32 nm. The temperature-dependent volumetric transition behavior of these cisplatin loaded nanocarriers is shown in Figure 2h, which demonstrates a broader (31–38 °C) volumetric transition range, and consequently, sustained release of the imbibed cisplatin (Figure 2i).

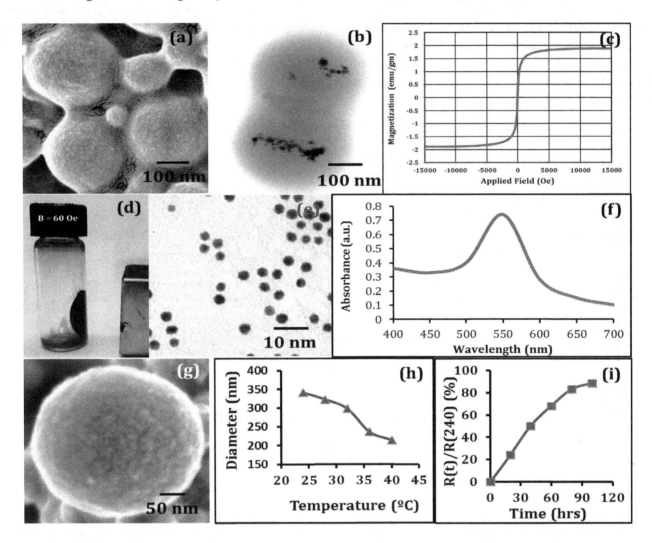

Figure 2. Morphology of designed CSMNSs: (**a**) SEM analysis demonstrating the polymer shell, and (**b**) TEM analysis demonstrating the distribution of the encapsulated MNPs. (**c**) Applied field vs magnetization plot for CSMNSs at 311 K, demonstrating super-paramagnetic behavior, even at the collapsed state of the polymeric shell. (**d**) Response of the CSMNSs to an applied DC magnetic field of 60 Oe by a permanent magnet at the adjacent wall of the flask. Characterization of the AuNPs: (**e**) TEM analysis demonstrating the particle distribution in cell culture media, ruling out the possibility of agglomeration, and (**f**) UV-visible spectrum of the dispersed AuNPs in the culture media. (**g**) SEM imaging of the CPNP demonstrating nanocarrier morphology. (**h**) Temperature dependence of hydrodynamic diameter of the CPNPs. (**i**) Drug release profile from the CPNPs. R(t) represents the mass released at any time t, and R(240) represents total mass released over 240 h (10 days).

The remote heating response of the nanocarriers was observed under AC magnetic fields (Figure 3a,b), optical irradiation (Figure 3c), and under hybrid optical-AC magnetic field exposure (Figure 3d). Upon field application, the nanocarrier-suspended culture media temperature increased in a concentration-dependent manner and reached a near steady state after approximately 20–30 min of irradiation. For AC magnetic field modulation, MNP concentration was varied between 200–400 μg/mL, and the temperature change was observed to be in the range of 1.5–3.5 K at 40 Oe, and between 3–5 K at 60 Oe field intensities, respectively. The optical irradiation-induced temperature change was found to be in the range of 3.7 and 8 K, respectively, when the concentration of the AuNPs were changed from 2 to 4 µg/mL in the culture media. A significantly stronger heating response was observed under the hybrid optical-AC magnetic field, in the range of 8–10.5 K, even with a mixture consisting of only 2 µg/mL AuNPs and 400 µg/mL MNPs. During all measurements, observed joule heating was found to be minimal, in the range of 0.5–1.25 K. Observing the heating response under coupled optical-AC magnetic field and considering clinically viable dose levels of the nanocarriers, 400 µg/mL MNPs and 2 µg/mL AuNPs were chosen as the mixture composition for executing acute hyperthermia towards the development of a multi modal therapy for the destruction of the neuroblastoma cells.

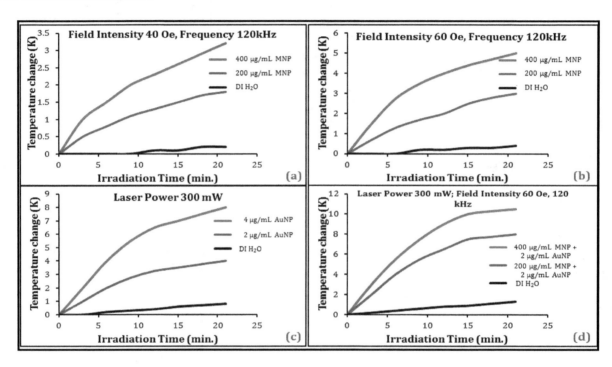

Figure 3. Remote heating response under AC magnetic field exposure as a function of CSMNS concentration at (**a**) 40 Oe, and (**b**) at 60 Oe. Frequency of the magnetic field was kept at 120 kHz. Heating response (**c**) under optical irradiation as a function of AuNP concentration, and (**d**) under hybrid optical-AC magnetic field irradiation using CSMNSs and AuNPs together in the media at various concentrations.

B35 neuroblastoma cell proliferation was observed post hyperthermia treatments and compared with the control (Figure 4a), and with only nanoparticle exposure (Figure 4b) conditions. The dose level of the CSMNSs and AuNPs used in this study were found to have a very low cytotoxicity, as observed in Figure 4b and quantified later (Figure 4i). Hybrid optical and AC magnetic field irradiation did not inhibit cell proliferation in the absence of the nanocarriers, as observed in Figure 4c, although a slight reduction in cell proliferation was observed in the presence of the nanocarriers under separate (i.e., magnetic or optical) actuations (Figure 4d,e). Under combined photo-magnetic actuation in the presence of the nanocarriers, severe inhibition in proliferation with cytoplasmic blebbing and irregularities in shape were observed (Figure 4f), which even surpassed the culture condition with the CPNP exposure in the media (Figure 4g). Finally, complete ablation of the B35 neuroblastoma cells in culture was observed under photo-magnetic combined actuation in the presence of the magnetic, gold, and the cisplatin loaded nanocarriers (Figure 4h). One-way analysis of variance (ANOVA) depicted statistically significant differences (p-value < 0.01) in the cell density values between the control and hybrid photo-magnetic actuation in the presence of nanocarriers with and without the presence of the cisplatin loading, as well as between control and 200 µg/mL CPNP treatments (Figure 4i).

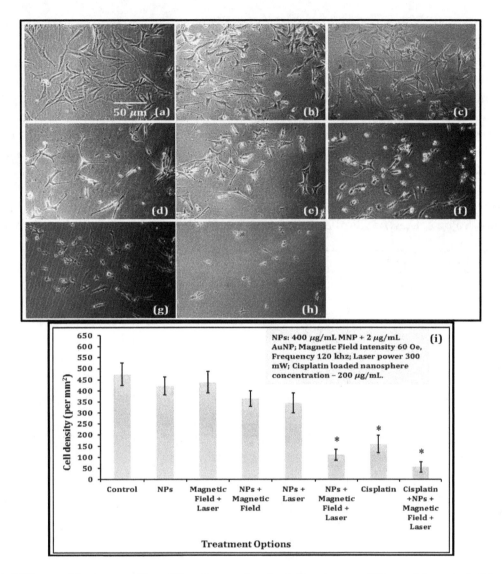

Figure 4. B35 neuroblastoma cell proliferation under the following conditions: (**a**) control; (**b**) presence of NPs (400 μg/mL MNP + 2 μg/mL AuNP) in the culture media; (**c**) combined optical-AC magnetic field irradiation in the absence of NPs; (**d**) presence of NPs under AC magnetic field irradiation; (**e**) presence of NPs under optical irradiation; (**f**) combined optical-AC magnetic field irradiation in the presence of NPs; (**g**) presence of 200 μg/mL CPNPs; and (**h**) combined optical-AC magnetic field irradiation in the presence of NPs and CPNPS. The AC magnetic field intensity was 60 Oe, frequency was 120 kHz, and laser power was 300 mW (at 520 nm). Scale bar is 50 μm in (**a**), and is also applicable for (**b–h**). (**i**) Bar chart displaying quantification of average cell densities (cell number/mm^2), indicative of cell proliferation for B35 neuroblastoma cells under all treatment options. Data are means ± SEM from four separate experiments and * indicates statistically significant differences, compared to cells cultured as the control, at $p < 0.01$ (ANOVA and LSD post-hoc).

In apoptotic cells, the membrane phospholipid phosphatidylserine (PS) is translocated from the inner to the outer leaflet of the plasma membrane, thereby exposing PS to the external cellular environment. Annexin V is a 35–36 kDa Ca^{2+} dependent phospholipid-binding protein (conjugated to FITC) that has a high affinity for PS, and binds to cells with exposed PS. Staining with FITC Annexin V is typically used in conjunction with a vital dye, such as propidium iodide (PI) or 7-amino-actinomycin (7-AAD), to identify early apoptotic cells. Cells that are considered viable are FITC Annexin V and PI negative; cells that are in early apoptosis are FITC Annexin V positive and PI negative; and cells that are in late apoptosis or already dead are both FITC Annexin V and PI positive. Results demonstrated more than 95% viable cells for the control (Figure 5a), post nanoparticle exposure (Figure 5b), and hybrid photo-magnetic irradiation in the absence of the nanocarriers (Figure 5c), thereby revealing the innate biocompatibility of the nanocarriers, as well as the irradiation exposure. Slight elevation of apoptosis (15–20% in the suspended cells) was observed in the presence of the nanocarriers under separate (i.e., magnetic or optical) actuations (Figure 5d,e). However, 98% early/late apoptotic cells were observed under combined photo-magnetic actuation in the presence of the nanocarriers (Figure 5f), which was found to be significantly greater than that of the 200 μg/mL CPNP exposure (65% apoptotic/necrotic cells, Figure 5g), demonstrating the extent of induced cytotoxicity by this hybrid actuation-nanocarrier combination. Figure 5h demonstrates a severe degree of induced apoptosis (99% apoptotic or necrotic cells) under photo-magnetic combined actuation in the presence of the magnetic, gold, and the cisplatin loaded nanocarriers. It should be noted that the apoptosis trend was found to be somewhat similar to the previously observed cell proliferation results.

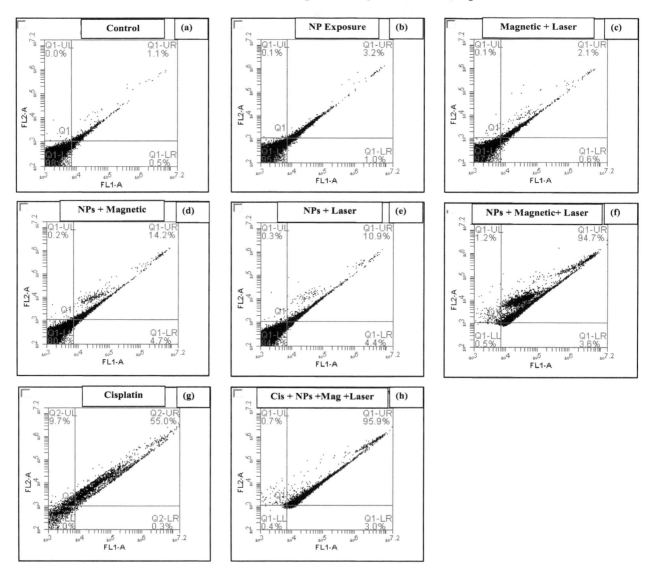

Figure 5. Apoptosis detection by the Annexin V assay. In four windows of each plot, the lower left indicates normal cells, the lower right indicates early apoptotic cells, the upper right indicates middle phase apoptotic cells, and the upper left indicates late phase apoptotic cells or necrotic cells. Irradiation/exposure parameters where applied: AC magnetic field intensity was 60 Oe, frequency was 120 kHz, and laser power was 300 mW (at 520 nm); NPs: (400 μg/mL MNP + 2 μg/mL AuNP); CPNPs 200 μg/mL.

Nuclear changes, such as condensation of the nucleus and/or DNA fragmentation, are the typical characteristics of later stages of the apoptotic program. Induction of apoptosis was further investigated by observing DAPI stained cell nuclei for the conditions that severely inhibited B35 neuroblastoma cell proliferation (Figure 6a–d). While in the control (Figure 6a), the cells had round and homogeneous nuclei, exposure to CPNPs (200 μg/mL) launched the apoptotic machinery of the cell, as observed from the deformed and condensed nuclei and apoptotic bodies (Figure 6b). Under combined photo-magnetic actuation in the presence of the gold and magnetic nanocarriers, severe chromatin condensation and nuclear fragmentation was evident (Figure 6c), indicating the potency of photo-magnetic hyperthermia-mediated cytotoxicity at a relatively lower irradiation and nanoparticle exposure level. Even a higher degree of damage was observed under photo-magnetic combined actuation in the presence of the CSMNSs, AuNPs, and CPNPs (Figure 6d), thereby demonstrating the effectiveness of the multimodal therapeutic strategy. Quantification of pyknotic nuclei, which is indicative of cell death [36], is displayed in Figure 6e, depicting statistically significant differences (p-value < 0.01) between the control and 200 μg/mL CPNP treatment, as well as between the control and hybrid photo-magnetic actuation in the presence of nanocarriers with and without the presence of the cisplatin loading.

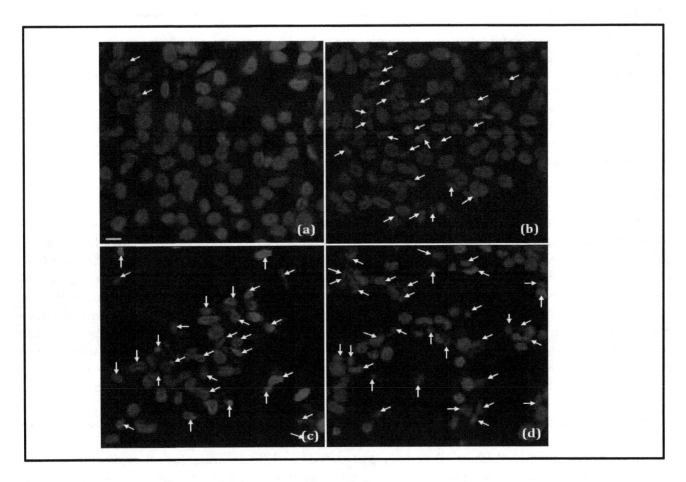

Figure 6. *Cont.*

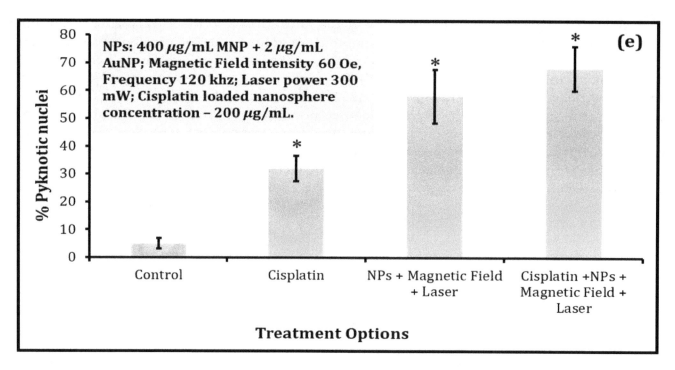

Figure 6. Nuclear condensation and fragmentation (white arrows) under the following conditions: (**a**) control, (**b**) presence of 200 µg/mL CPNPs, (**c**) combined optical-AC magnetic field irradiation in the presence of NPs (400 µg/mL MNP + 2 µg/mL AuNP), and (**d**) combined optical-AC magnetic field irradiation in the presence of NPs and CPNPS. AC Magnetic field intensity was 60 Oe, frequency was 120 kHz, and laser power was 300 mW (at 520 nm). Scale bar is 10 µm in (**a**), and is also applicable for (**b–d**). (**e**) Bar chart displaying quantification of pyknotic nuclei, indicative of cell death. Data are means ± SEM from four separate experiments and * indicates statistically significant differences, compared to cells cultured as the control, at $p < 0.01$ (ANOVA and LSD post-hoc).

4. Discussion

Combined photo-magnetic stimulation has successfully been implemented on the cluster of complementing nanocarriers to develop a multimodal therapy to guide the neuroblastoma cell destruction (Figure 7). This novel strategy permitted the use of a less intense AC magnetic field in combination with optical irradiation during the treatment, thus removing the safety concerns associated with the AC magnetic field-assisted therapies. Although a green laser (300 mW) has been used in this study as the light source for the optical irradiation as a proof of concept, it can be replaced by a near infrared (NIR) laser to obtain deeper penetration, since the gold nanoparticles can be tuned to possess high NIR absorption [22]. The penetration depth of the optical irradiation can be further enhanced by the use of free-space or even a fiber-optic Bessel beam [37], thus eliminating the use of high-intensity radiotherapy, which has the potential to incur severe DNA damage and has a risk of developing into a second cancer at a later stage. Moreover, the treatment efficacy has been achieved at a reduced nanoparticle dose level [28,38]. In our recent reports [21,24], various strategies for targeting and delivery of therapeutic agents for the central nervous system (CNS)-related conditions have been identified: (i) endocytosis based, and (ii) laminin (or other disease specific surface proteins) binding peptide based. The later strategy is gaining huge traction for specific targeting at present, and coupled with the impressive development of the target-specific synthetic oligonucleotides/aptamer design [39], provides a viable option for delivery of these nanocarriers, since all these vectors can be surface-functionalized with appropriate functional groups (such as –COOH, –NH$_2$, or –SH) for the conjugation of biomolecules. Another recent work by Jeong et al. [40] demonstrated the feasibility of administering these types of nanocarriers intravenously to treat spinal cord injury in mice. Prior observations indicate that these aforementioned strategies will increase the concentration of the nanocarriers at the target tissue. Site-specific injection is also another route that needs to be explored with these types of nanocarriers depending on the location and accessibility of the tumor. In our previous studies [24,31,41], the nanocarriers were found to be highly non-reactive, stable in physiological solutions, and were minimally toxic at even a higher dose level than the dose administered here. Reduced dose level can potentially render them as ideal candidates for photo-magnetic combination therapy.

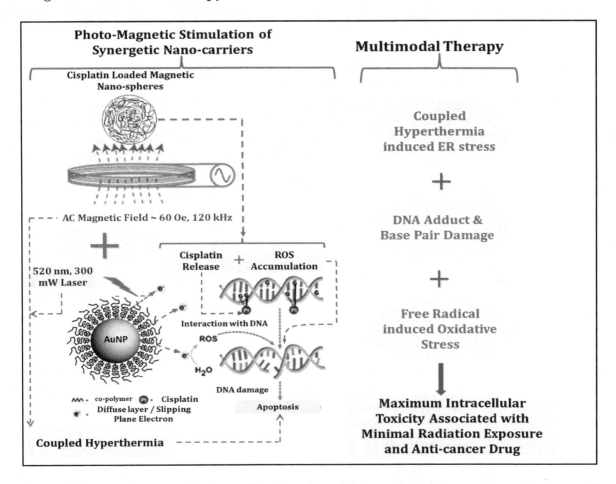

Figure 7. Photo-magnetic irradiation mediated multimodal therapeutic strategy of neuroblastoma cells using clusters of nanostructures: coupled hyperthermia, DNA damage, and reactive oxygen species (ROS) -induced apoptosis of B35 neuroblastoma cells in culture. Note that in this experiment, cisplatin has been loaded in a separate non-magnetic nanocarrier.

For tumorigenesis and malignant transformation, responsible molecular mechanisms are: (1) overexpression of cell survival pathways, and (2) downregulation of apoptosis [8]. The molecular factors of cell survival pathways include protein kinases (protein kinase B (AKT/PKB); anaplastic lymphoma kinase (ALK); phosphatidylinositide 3-kinases (PI3K); and focal adhesion kinase (FAK)), transcription factors (NF-κB, MYCN, and p53), and growth factors (insulin-like growth factor (IGF); epidermal growth factor (EGF); platelet-derived growth factor (PDGF); and vascular endothelial growth factor (VEGF)). Manipulation of the cell survival pathways may reduce the malignant potential of the tumor, which in turn may provide reduction of required dosages and the dose-related side effects of the conventional therapies in clinical practice. Moreover, since the presence of residual cancer cells in the hematopoietic compartment is the plausible explanation for tumor relapse [5], highly sensitive methods to detect and isolate rare circulating tumor cells may lead to improved treatment efficacy. The cluster of nanostructures used in this study carries the potential to act as effective modulators of these pathways and selectively target the tumor cells due to their controllability under hybrid photo-magnetic field and temperature-sensitive behavior. A temperature-dependent hydrophilic–hydrophobic transition behavior renders them suitable for drug delivery applications as well, in which triggered release is necessary.

Kinases are enzymes to phosphorylate, thus they act as on-off switches for activating other factors in cell signaling pathways. One well known kinase is AKT kinase, which regulates important cellular functions like cell growth, proliferation, survival, and angiogenesis [8,42]. In human tissue samples, it was observed that the AKT phosphorylation was more prevalent in primary neuroblastoma than in benign ganglioma or in normal adrenal tissue [8]. Downregulation of AKT to increase apoptosis is one of the many ways to address the neuroblastoma tumor growth, and two main strategies are being pursued: (1) long-term exposure of SH-SY5Y cells to interferon β, which decreased activation of the P13K-AKT pathway [43,44], thereby increasing the apoptosis, and (2) Rapamycin-induced mTOR (a downstream effector of AKT) inhibition [45], which is related to decreased tumor growth, angiogenesis, and increased apoptosis. Similarly, inhibition of FAK by siRNA [46] or small molecule inhibitors, such as NVP-TAE 226 [47] and Y15 [48] results in decreased cell survival, increased apoptosis, and G2 cell cycle arrest. NVP-TAE 226 (mol. wt. 468.94) and Y15 (mol. wt. 284.01) are ideal candidates to be loaded into these designed nanocarriers due to their low molecular weight and adequate water solubility, which will be extremely beneficial for controlled release into the tumor cells under photo-magnetic stimulation. Among transcription factors, NF-κB has important roles in neuroblastoma chemo-resistance as doxorubicin and VP16 have both been shown to trigger NF-κB activation in neuroblastoma cells, inhibiting apoptosis [49]; nevertheless, siMYCN (siRNA against MYCN) has been found to increase caspase-3 mediated apoptosis [50]. Selective inhibition of MYCN can be achieved using an anti-gene peptide nucleic acid (PNA) [51], which can either be covalently attached to the nanocarrier surface, or can be loaded inside for on-demand release when the target site is reached. Targeted therapy to modulate the growth factors is another direction for the treatment of high risk neuroblastoma [52]. Imatinib, a tyrosine kinase inhibitor of PDGFR (PDGF receptor) has been shown to inhibit the growth of a number of human neuroblastoma cell lines in vitro and xenograft in vivo [53]. We recently demonstrated a nanocarrier mediated neurite growth factor (NGF) delivery to neuronal model cells for promoting neurite outgrowth [28,41]. A similar strategy can be adopted for the delivery of a selected growth factor mediated cell survival pathway modulators to the targeted cancer cells.

For high-risk neuroblastoma treatment, identification and targeting of the rare circulating tumor cells or removal of the nucleic acids from such cells is extremely important to prevent the tumor relapse. We have recently designed Förster resonance energy transfer (FRET)-based multifunctional nanocarriers [41], which are capable of performing organelle specific binding for detection of damaged cells and can provide on-demand release of a specific drug or a combination of drugs. Combined with the photo-magnetic actuation, these nanocarriers have the potential to perform detection at the single cell level, which may lead to a greater understanding of how to handle residual tumor cells. Further, since most of these aforementioned tasks can be performed with various types of magnetically controllable nanocarriers, it will be possible to prevent the diffusion out of the targeted area using a concentrated DC magnetic field during in vivo localization. Use of a Halbach cylinder [54] can extend the penetration depth of the applied magnetic field during clinical applications.

5. Conclusions

In conclusion, an optical and AC magnetic field-assisted therapeutic strategy for high risk neuroblastoma treatment was developed. Multifunctional nanostructures CSMNSs, AuNPs, and CPNPs at a reduced dose level were used to create coupled hyperthermia and induce sustained release of the imbibed cisplatin, which caused complete ablation of the B35 neuroblastoma cells. This enabled replacement of high energy γ–ray and high-intensity AC magnetic field exposure. The developed technique can potentially further combine the modulation of cell survival pathways and the detection of rare circulating tumor cells, thereby leading to a greater understanding and comprehensive solution to overcome the existing challenges to treat high-risk neuroblastoma. The results of this study suggest that photo-magnetic irradiation based multimodal therapy is a viable approach to remotely guide neuroblastoma cell destruction and the technique may be extended to treat other aggressive cancers.

Author Contributions: S.G. (Santaneel Ghosh) and S.G. (Somesree GhoshMitra) designed the experiments. T.M. synthesized and characterized the nanostructures, and R.A. (Rohini Atluri) and R.A. (Rahul Atmaramani) performed PC12 cell related experiments. D.D. performed the electron microscopy and the analysis. G.T. performed the photo-magnetic actuation of the nanocarriers and temperature regulation measurements. S.G. (Santaneel Ghosh) and J.P. supervised the design of the photo-magnetic actuator. S.G. (Santaneel Ghosh) directed the project and supervised this work. All authors have read and approved the final manuscript.

Acknowledgments: This work was supported by grants from the Research Corporation—Single Investigator Cottrell College Science Award (SG); Grants and Research Funding Committee, Southeast Missouri State University (SG). The authors declare no conflict of interests.

References

1. London, W.B.; Castleberry, R.P.; Matthay, K.K.; Look, A.T.; Seeger, R.C.; Shimada, H.; Thorner, P.; Brodeur, G.; Maris, J.M.; Reynolds, C.P.; et al. Evidence for an age cutoff greater than 365 days for neuroblastoma risk group stratification in the Children's Oncology Group. *J. Clin. Oncol.* **2005**, *23*, 6459–6465. [CrossRef] [PubMed]

2. Ries, L.A.; Smith, M.A.; Gurney, J.G.; Linet, M.; Tamra, T.; Young, J.L.; Bunin, G. *Cancer Incidence and Survival among Children and Adolescents: United States SEER Program 1975–1995*; NIH: Bethesda, MD, USA, 1999.

3. Hoehner, J.C.; Wester, T.; Pahlman, S.; Olsen, L. Localization of neurotrophins and their high-affinity receptors during human enteric nervous system development. *Gastroenterology* **1996**, *110*, 756–767. [CrossRef] [PubMed]

4. Matthay, K.K.; Villablanca, J.G.; Seeger, R.C.; Stram, D.O.; Harris, R.E.; Ramsay, N.K.; Swift, P.; Shimada, H.; Black, C.T.; Brodeur, G.M.; et al. Treatment of high-risk neuroblastoma with intensive chemotherapy, radiotherapy, autologous bone marrow transplantation, and 13-cis-retinoic acid. *N. Engl. J. Med.* **1999**, *341*, 1165–1173. [CrossRef] [PubMed]

5. Maris, J.M. Recent advances in neuroblastoma. *N. Engl. J. Med.* **2010**, *362*, 2202–2211. [CrossRef] [PubMed]

6. Rees, H.; Markley, M.A.; Kiely, E.M.; Pierro, A.; Pritchard, J. Diarrhea after resection of advanced abdominal neuroblastoma: A common management problem. *Surgery* **1998**, *123*, 568–572. [CrossRef] [PubMed]

7. Bousvaros, A.; Kirks, D.R.; Grossman, H. Imaging of neuroblastoma: An overview. *Pediatr. Radiol.* **1986**, *16*, 89–106. [CrossRef] [PubMed]

8. Megison, M.L.; Gillory, L.A.; Beierle, E.A. Cell survival signaling in neuroblastoma. *Anticancer Agents Med. Chem.* **2013**, *13*, 563–575. [CrossRef] [PubMed]

9. Kushner, B.H.; LaQuaglia, M.P.; Bonilla, M.A.; Lindsley, K.; Rosenfield, N.; Yeh, S.; Eddy, J.; Gerald, W.L.; Heller, G.; Cheung, N.K. Highly effective induction therapy for stage 4 neuroblastoma in children over 1 year of age. *J. Clin. Oncol.* **1994**, *12*, 2607–2613. [CrossRef] [PubMed]

10. American Cancer Society, Inc. Neuroblastoma. Available online: www.cancer.org/cancer/neuroblastoma (accessed on 25 August 2018).

11. Berthold, F.; Boos, J.; Burdach, S.; Erttmann, R.; Henze, G.; Hermann, J.; Klingebiel, T.; Kremens, B.; Schilling, F.H.; Schrappe, M.; et al. Myeloablative megatherapy with autologous stem-cell rescue versus oral maintenance chemotherapy as consolidation treatment in patients with high-risk neuroblastoma: A randomised controlled trial. *Lancet Oncol.* **2005**, *6*, 649–658. [CrossRef]

12. Yu, A.L.; Gilman, A.L.; Ozkaynak, M.F.; London, W.B.; Kreissman, S.G.; Chen, H.X.; Smith, M.; Anderson, B.; Villablanca, J.G.; Matthay, K.K.; et al. Anti-GD2 antibody with GM-CSF, interleukin-2, and isotretinoin for neuroblastoma. *N. Engl. J. Med.* **2010**, *363*, 1324–1334. [CrossRef] [PubMed]

13. Arany, I.; Safirstein, R.L. Cisplatin nephrotoxicity. *Semin. Nephrol.* **2003**, *23*, 460–464. [CrossRef]

14. Buzdar, A.U.; Marcus, C.; Blumenschein, G.R.; Smith, T.L. Early and delayed clinical cardiotoxicity of doxorubicin. *Cancer* **1985**, *55*, 2761–2765. [CrossRef]

15. Travis, L.B.; Curtis, R.E.; Glimelius, B.; Holowaty, E.J.; Van Leeuwen, F.E.; Lynch, C.F.; Hagenbeek, A.; Stovall, M.; Banks, P.M.; Adami, J.; et al. Bladder and kidney cancer following cyclophosphamide therapy for non-Hodgkin's lymphoma. *J. Natl. Cancer Inst.* **1995**, *87*, 524–530. [CrossRef] [PubMed]

16. Barker, E.; Mueller, B.M.; Handgretinger, R.; Herter, M.; Yu, A.L.; Reisfeld, R.A. Effect of a chimeric anti-ganglioside GD2 antibody on cell-mediated lysis of human neuroblastoma cells. *Cancer Res.* **1991**, *51*, 144–149. [PubMed]

17. Islam, M.; Atmaramani, R.; Mukherjee, S.; Ghosh, S.; Iqbal, S.M. Enhanced proliferation of PC12 neural cells on untreated, nanotextured glass coverslips. *Nanotechnology* **2016**, *27*, 415501. [CrossRef] [PubMed]

18. Yuan, G.; Yuan, Y.; Xu, K.; Luo, Q. Biocompatible PEGylated Fe_3O_4 nanoparticles as photothermal agents for near-infrared light modulated cancer therapy. *Int. J. Mol. Sci.* **2014**, *15*, 18776–18788. [CrossRef] [PubMed]

19. You, C.C.; Miranda, O.R.; Gider, B.; Ghosh, P.S.; Kim, I.B.; Erdogan, B.; Krovi, S.A.; Bunz, U.H.; Rotello, V.M. Detection and identification of proteins using nanoparticle–fluorescent polymer "chemical nose" sensors. *Nat. Nanotechnol.* **2007**, *2*, 318–323. [CrossRef] [PubMed]

20. Mendes, R.; Pedrosa, P.; Lima, J.C.; Fernandes, A.R.; Baptista, P.V. Photothermal enhancement of chemotherapy in breast cancer by visible irradiation of Gold nanoparticles. *Sci. Rep.* **2017**, *7*, 11491–11498. [CrossRef] [PubMed]

21. GhoshMitra, S.; Ghosh, S. A novel nano-structure for central nervous system drug delivery:Sustained release of Therapeutic agents from Core-Multi-Shell nano-carriers. *JSM Nanotechnol. Nanomed.* **2016**, *4*, 1040.

22. Gu, L.; Koymen, A.R.; Mohanty, S.K. Crystalline magnetic carbon nanoparticle assisted photothermal delivery into cells using CW near-infrared laser beam. *Sci. Rep.* **2014**, *4*, 5106. [CrossRef] [PubMed]

23. Chowdhury, S.M.; Surhland, C.; Sanchez, Z.; Chaudhary, P.; Kumar, M.S.; Lee, S.; Peña, L.A.; Waring, M.; Sitharaman, B.; Naidu, M. Graphene nanoribbons as a drug delivery agent for lucanthone mediated therapy of glioblastoma multiforme. Nanomedicine Nanotechnology. *Biol. Med.* **2015**, *11*, 109–118.

24. GhoshMitra, S.; Diercks, D.R.; Mills, N.C.; Hynds, D.L.; Ghosh, S. Role of engineered nanocarriers for axon regeneration and guidance: Current status and future trends. *Adv. Drug Deliv. Rev.* **2012**, *64*, 110–125. [CrossRef] [PubMed]

25. Ellis-Behnke, R. Nano Neurology and the Four P's of Central Nervous System Regeneration: Preserve, Permit, Promote, Plasticity. *Med. Clin. N. Am.* **2007**, *91*, 937–962. [CrossRef] [PubMed]

26. Kumar, C.S.S.R.; Mohammad, F. Magnetic Nanomaterials for Hyperthermia-based Therapy and Controlled Drug Delivery. *Adv. Drug Deliv. Rev.* **2011**, *63*, 789–808. [CrossRef] [PubMed]

27. Orel, V.; Shevchenko, A.; Romanov, A.; Tselepi, M.; Mitrelias, T.; Barnes, C.H.; Burlaka, A.; Lukin, S.; Shchepotin, I. Magnetic properties and antitumor effect of nanocomplexes of iron oxide and doxorubicin. Nanomedicine Nanotechnology. *Biol. Med.* **2015**, *11*, 47–55.

28. Ghosh, S.; GhoshMitra, S.; Cai, T.; Diercks, D.R.; Mills, N.C.; Hynds, D.A.L. Alternating Magnetic Field Controlled, Multifunctional Nano-Reservoirs: Intracellular Uptake and Improved Biocompatibility. *Nanoscale Res. Lett.* **2010**, *5*, 195–204. [CrossRef] [PubMed]

29. Huang, X.; El-Sayed, I.H.; Qian, W.; El-Sayed, M.A. Cancer cell imaging and photothermal therapy in the near-infrared region by using gold nanorods. *J. Am. Chem. Soc.* **2006**, *128*, 2115–2120. [CrossRef] [PubMed]

30. Setua, S.; Ouberai, M.; Piccirillo, S.G.; Watts, C.; Welland, M. Cisplatin-tethered gold nanospheres for multimodal chemo-radiotherapy of glioblastoma. *Nanoscale* **2014**, *6*, 10865–10873. [CrossRef] [PubMed]

31. McCallister, T.; Gidney, E.; Adams, D.; Diercks, D.R.; Ghosh, S. Engineered, thermoresponsive, magnetic nanocarriers of oligo (ethylene glycol)-methacrylate-based biopolymers. *Appl. Phys. Express* **2014**, *7*, 117003. [CrossRef]

32. 3B Sci. Inc. 2015. Available online: https://www.a3bs.com/ (accessed on 25 August 2018).

33. Rubio-Retama, J.; Zafeiropoulos, N.E.; Serafinelli, C.; Rojas-Reyna, R.; Voit, B.; Cabarcos, E.L.; Stamm, M. Synthesis and Characterization of Thermosensitive PNIPAM Microgels Covered with Superparamagnetic γ-Fe_2O_3 Nanoparticles. *Langmuir* **2007**, *23*, 10280–10285. [CrossRef] [PubMed]

34. Ghosh, S.; Yang, C.; Cai, T.; Hu, Z.; Neogi, A. Oscillating magnetic field-actuated microvalves for micro-and nanofluidics. *J. Phys. D* **2009**, *42*, 135501. [CrossRef]

35. Fortin, J.P.; Wilhelm, C.; Servais, J.; Ménager, C.; Bacri, J.C.; Gazeau, F. Size-sorted anionic iron oxide nanomagnets as colloidal mediators for magnetic hyperthermia. *J. Am. Chem. Soc.* **2007**, *129*, 2628–2635. [CrossRef] [PubMed]

36. Adams, C.F.; Rai, A.; Sneddon, G.; Yiu, H.H.P.; Polyak, B.; Chari, D.M. Increasing magnetite contents of polymeric magnetic particles dramatically improves labeling of neural stem cell transplant populations. Nanomedicine Nanotechnology. *Biol. Med.* **2015**, *11*, 19–29.

37. Mohanty, S.K.; Mohanty, K.S.; Berns, M.W. Manipulation of mammalian cells using a single-fiber optical microbeam. *J. Biomed. Opt.* **2008**, *13*, 54047–54049. [CrossRef] [PubMed]

38. Alkilany, A.M.; Murphy, C.J. Toxicity and cellular uptake of gold nanoparticles: What we have learned so far? *J. Nanoparticle Res.* **2010**, *12*, 2313–2333. [CrossRef] [PubMed]

39. Wagner, K.; Kautz, A.; Roder, M.; Schwalbe, M.; Pachmann, K.; Clement, J.H.; Schnabelrauch, M. Synthesis of oligonucleotide-functionalized magnetic nanoparticles and study on their in vitro cell uptake. *Appl. Organometal. Chem.* **2004**, *18*, 514–519. [CrossRef]

40. Jeong, S.J.; Cooper, J.G.; Ifergan, I.; McGuire, T.L.; Xu, D.; Hunter, Z.; Sharma, S.; McCarthy, D.; Miller, S.D.; Kessler, J.A. Intravenous immune-modifying nanoparticles as a therapy for spinal cord injury in mice. *Neurobiol. Dis.* **2017**, *108*, 73–82. [CrossRef] [PubMed]

41. GhoshMitra, S.; Diercks, D.R.; Mills, N.C.; Hynds, D.A.L.; Ghosh, S. Excellent biocompatibility of semiconductor quantum dots encased in multifunctional poly (*N*-isopropylacrylamide) nanoreservoirs and nuclear specific labeling of growing neurons. *Appl. Phys. Lett.* **2011**, *98*, 103702. [CrossRef]

42. Song, G.; Ouyang, G.; Bao, S. The activation of Akt/PKB signaling pathway and cell survival. *J. Cell. Mol. Med.* **2005**, *9*, 59. [CrossRef] [PubMed]

43. Hennessy, B.T.; Smith, D.L.; Ram, P.T.; Lu, Y.; Mills, G.B. Exploiting the PI3K/AKT pathway for cancer drug discovery. *Nat. Rev. Drug Discov.* **2005**, *4*, 988–1004. [CrossRef] [PubMed]

44. Wang, L.; Yang, H.-J.; Xia, Y.-Y.; Feng, Z.-W. Insulin-like growth factor 1 protects human neuroblastoma cells SH-EP1 against MPP -induced apoptosis by AKT/GSK-3β/JNK signaling. *Apoptosis* **2010**, *15*, 1470–1479. [CrossRef] [PubMed]

45. Johnsen, J.I.; Segerström, L.; Orrego, A.; Elfman, L.; Henriksson, M.; Kågedal, B.; Eksborg, S.; Sveinbjörnsson, B.; Kogner, P. Inhibitors of mammalian target of rapamycin downregulate MYCN protein expression and inhibit neuroblastoma growth in vitro and in vivo. *Oncogene* **2008**, *27*, 2910–2922. [CrossRef] [PubMed]

46. Beierle, E.A.; Trujillo, A.; Nagaram, A.; Kurenova, E.V.; Finch, R.; Ma, X.; Vella, J.; Cance, W.G.; Golubovskaya, V.M. N-MYC regulates focal adhesion kinase expression in human neuroblastoma. *J. Biol. Chem.* **2007**, *282*, 12503–12516. [CrossRef] [PubMed]

47. Beierle, E.A.; Trujillo, A.; Nagaram, A.; Golubovskaya, V.M.; Cance, W.G.; Kurenova, E.V. TAE226 inhibits human neuroblastoma cell survival. *Cancer Investig.* **2008**, *26*, 145–151. [CrossRef] [PubMed]

48. Beierle, E.A.; Ma, X.; Stewart, J.; Nyberg, C.; Trujillo, A.; Cance, W.G.; Golubovskaya, V.M. Inhibition of focal adhesion kinase decreases tumor growth in human neuroblastoma. *Cell Cycle* **2010**, *9*, 1005–1015. [CrossRef] [PubMed]

49. Ammann, J.U.; Haag, C.; Kasperczyk, H.; Debatin, K.; Fulda, S. Sensitization of neuroblastoma cells for TRAIL-induced apoptosis by NF-κB inhibition. *Int. J. Cancer* **2009**, *124*, 1301–1311. [CrossRef] [PubMed]

50. Kang, J.-H.; Rychahou, P.G.; Ishola, T.A.; Qiao, J.; Evers, B.M.; Chung, D.H. MYCN silencing induces differentiation and apoptosis in human neuroblastoma cells. *Biochem. Biophys. Res. Commun.* **2006**, *351*, 192–197. [CrossRef] [PubMed]

51. Tonelli, R.; Purgato, S.; Camerin, C.; Fronza, R.; Bologna, F.; Alboresi, S.; Franzoni, M.; Corradini, R.; Sforza, S.; Faccini, A.; et al. Anti-gene peptide nucleic acid specifically inhibits MYCN expression in human neuroblastoma cells leading to cell growth inhibition and apoptosis. *Mol. Cancer Ther.* **2005**, *4*, 779–786. [CrossRef] [PubMed]

52. Byrne, A.M.; Bouchier-Hayes, D.J.; Harmey, J.H. Angiogenic and cell survival functions of vascular endothelial growth factor (VEGF). *J. Cell. Mol. Med.* **2005**, *9*, 777. [CrossRef] [PubMed]

53. Beppu, K.; Jaboine, J.; Merchant, M.S.; Mackall, C.L.; Thiele, C.J. Effect of imatinib mesylate on neuroblastoma tumorigenesis and vascular endothelial growth factor expression. *J. Natl. Cancer Inst.* **2004**, *96*, 46–55. [CrossRef] [PubMed]

54. Riegler, J.; Lau, K.D.; Garcia-Prieto, A.; Price, A.N.; Richards, T.; Pankhurst, Q.A.; Lythgoe, M.F. Magnetic cell delivery for peripheral arterial disease: A theoretical framework. *Med. Phys.* **2011**, *38*, 3932–3943. [CrossRef] [PubMed]

Development of Parvifloron D-Loaded Smart Nanoparticles to Target Pancreatic Cancer

Ana Santos-Rebelo [1,2], Catarina Garcia [1,2], Carla Eleutério [3], Ana Bastos [3,4] (ID),
Sílvia Castro Coelho [5], Manuel A. N. Coelho [5] (ID), Jesús Molpeceres [2], Ana S. Viana [6],
Lia Ascensão [7] (ID), João F. Pinto [3,4], Maria M. Gaspar [3,4] (ID), Patrícia Rijo [1,4] (ID) and
Catarina P. Reis [3,4,8,*] (ID)

[1] Centro de Investigação em Biociências e Tecnologias da Saúde (CBIOS),
    Universidade Lusófona de Humanidades e Tecnologias, Campo Grande 376, 1749-024 Lisboa, Portugal;
    ana.rebelo1490@gmail.com (A.S.-R.); catarina.g.garcia@gmail.com (C.G.); p1609@ulusofona.pt (P.R.)
[2] Department of Biomedical Sciences, Faculty of Pharmacy, University of Alcalá,
    Ctra. A2 km33,600 Campus Universitario, 28871 Alcalá de Henares, Spain; jesus.molpeceres@uah.es
[3] Faculdade de Farmácia, Universidade de Lisboa (FFUL), Av. Prof. Gama Pinto, 1649-003 Lisboa, Portugal;
    carlavania@ff.ul.pt (C.E.); anacarrerabastos@gmail.com (A.B.); jfpinto@ff.ulisboa.pt (J.F.P.);
    mgaspar@ff.ulisboa.pt (M.M.G.)
[4] iMed.ULisboa-Faculdade de Farmácia, Universidade de Lisboa, Av. Prof. Gama Pinto,
    1649-003 Lisboa, Portugal
[5] Laboratory for Process Engineering, Environment (LEPABE), Department of Chemical Engineering,
    Faculty of Engineering, University of Porto, 4200-135 Porto, Portugal; silviac@fe.up.pt (S.C.C.);
    mcoelho@fe.up.pt (M.A.N.C.)
[6] Centro de Química e Bioquímica (CQB), Centro de Química Estrutural (CQE), Faculdade de Ciências,
    Universidade de Lisboa, Campo Grande 1749-016 Lisboa, Portugal; apsemedo@fc.ul.pt
[7] Centre for Environmental and Marine Studies (CESAM), Faculdade de Ciências, Universidade de Lisboa,
    Campo Grande 1749-016 Lisboa, Portugal; lmpsousa@fc.ul.pt
[8] Institute of Biophysics and Biomedical Engineering (IBEB), Faculdade de Ciências, Universidade de Lisboa,
    1749-016 Lisboa, Portugal
*   Correspondence: catarinareis@ff.ulisboa.pt;

Abstract: Pancreatic cancer is the eighth leading cause of cancer death worldwide. For this reason, the development of more effective therapies is a major concern for the scientific community. Accordingly, plants belonging to *Plectranthus* genus and their isolated compounds, such as Parvifloron D, were found to have cytotoxic and antiproliferative activities. However, Parvifloron D is a very low water-soluble compound. Thus, nanotechnology can be a promising delivery system to enhance drug solubility and targeted delivery. The extraction of Parvifloron D from *P. ecklonii* was optimized through an acetone ultrasound-assisted method and isolated by Flash-Dry Column Chromatography. Then, its antiproliferative effect was selectivity evaluated against different cell lines (IC_{50} of 0.15 ± 0.05 μM, 11.9 ± 0.7 μM, 21.6 ± 0.5, 34.3 ± 4.1 μM, 35.1 ± 2.2 μM and 32.1 ± 4.3 μM for BxPC3, PANC-1, Ins1-E, MCF-7, HaCat and Caco-2, respectively). To obtain an optimized stable Parvifloron D pharmaceutical dosage form, albumin nanoparticles were produced through a desolvation method (yield of encapsulation of 91.2%) and characterized in terms of size (165 nm; PI 0.11), zeta potential (-7.88 mV) and morphology. In conclusion, Parvifloron D can be efficiently obtained from *P. ecklonii* and it has shown selective cytotoxicity to pancreatic cell lines. Parvifloron D nanoencapsulation can be considered as a possible efficient alternative approach in the treatment of pancreatic cancer.

Keywords: *Plectranthus ecklonii*; Parvifloron D; cytotoxicity; pancreatic cancer; nanoparticles

1. Introduction

Pancreatic cancer is one of the most deadly oncologic disease and it is estimated that it will be the second most common cause of death due to cancer in the United States (USA) in 2030 [1].

This type of cancer is difficult to diagnose early, and currently, the treatment options available are very limited, being surgical resection the only potentially curative treatment. Nevertheless, surgery may be not possible in 80—90% of the cases, and long-term survival after surgical resection is very low [2–4].

Chemotherapy has demonstrated a positive impact on overall survival when prescribed after surgery with curative intent, and may reduce the risk of recurrence [5]. Gemcitabine and erlotinib are some examples of approved drugs in use and nab-paclitaxel has been approved in the USA and in Europe for metastasis [6]. However, chemotherapy with classical therapeutic agents has many side effects, such as nausea and vomiting, loss of appetite, hair loss, ulcers nozzles and higher chance of infection, as it promotes a shortage of white blood cells. In order to improve the long-term survival and improve the quality of life of patients with pancreatic cancer, it is imperative to find new therapeutic agents.

The use of medicinal plants and their constituents has proved their potential as clinical alternatives to synthetized drugs, leading to the discovery of new bioactive compounds [7]. These compounds have generated a strong interest in pharmacological research, towards the development of new anticancer agents. In fact, more than 50% of the compounds with different mechanisms of action used in chemotherapy are extracted from plant materials [4,6].

Many *Plectranthus* species are used as plants with medicinal interest against a variety of diseases, such as cancer. Abietane diterpenoids have been reported as the main constituents of some species in this *genus* and are responsible for its potential therapeutic value [8]. These naturally occurring compounds display a vast array of biological activities including cytotoxic and antiproliferative activities against human tumor cells [8,9]. Diterpenoids containing an abietane skeleton have proven to be strongly cytotoxic against human leukemia cells [10].

Burmistrova et al. confirmed that Parvifloron D (Figure 1) has strong cytotoxic properties against several human tumor cell lines [8]. Parvifloron D was isolated from *P. ecklonii* and thus, this plant can be associated as a good source of this abietane diterpenoid. In addition, it was also found that Parvifloron D anti-proliferative effect is generally associated with an increase in the intracellular level of Reactive Oxygen Species (ROS) that seems to play a crucial role in the apoptotic process of cells [11].

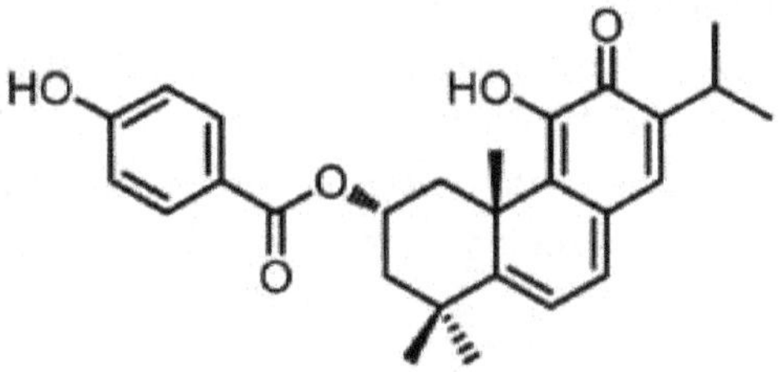

Figure 1. Molecular structure form Parvifloron D.

Nanotechnology has the potentiality of controlling and manipulating matter at the nanoscale by designing and engineering new systems [4]. Advances in nanoscience and nanotechnology can transform what has been done until today since new strategies will enhance and upgrade solutions to the formulation problems raised [12]. Besides improving solubility and stability of active compounds, nanoparticles may extend a formulation's action and successfully combine active substances with different degrees of hydrophilicity [12–14]. Its targeting abilities to deliver drugs directly to the affected organs and tissues are another advantage of these systems that can be used in medicine [12,15].

Nanocarriers can improve the efficiency of drugs by changing their body distribution, decreasing acute toxicity, increasing their dissolution rate and in vivo stability concerning the risk of earlier metabolism and degradation [12,14,16,17].

The present study focuses on the optimization of the extraction and isolation of Parvifloron D, given its cytotoxic potential. Therefore, new approaches to target pancreatic cancer cells will be performed to improve its selectivity. Moreover, the development of a novel diterpene-encapsulated nanosystem will be done in order to optimize the Parvifloron D stability.

2. Materials and Methods

2.1. Materials

Plant material *P. ecklonii* Benth was given by the Faculty of Pharmacy of the University of Lisbon and it was collected from seeds provided by the herbarium of the National Botanical Garden of Kirstenbosch, South Africa. Voucher specimens (S/No. LISC) have been deposited in the herbarium of the Tropical Research Institute in Lisbon [8]. Acetone, hexane and ethyl acetate were supplied by VWR Chemicals (VWR international S.A.S., Briare, France); Silica was obtained from Merck (grade 60, 230–400 mesh, Merck KGaA, Darmstadt, Germany); Bovine serum albumin was purchased to Sigma-Aldrich (Steinheim, Germany). Culture media and antibiotics were obtained from Invitrogen (Life Technologies Corporation, Carlsbad, CA, USA). All cell lines were obtained from the American Type Culture Collection (LGC Standards S.L.U. Barcelona, Spain). Reagents for cell proliferation assays were purchased from Promega (Madison, WI, USA). All reagents used for the nanoparticles preparation were of analytical grade and purified water obtained by a Millipore system (Millipore, Burlington, MA, USA).

2.2. Extraction and Isolation

2.2.1. Extraction

The whole plant-dried powdered *P. ecklonii* (197.55 g) was used to perform the Parvifloron D exhaustive extraction followed by thin-layer chromatography (TLC) (hexane: ethyl acetate, 7:3 (v/v)). The ultrasound-assisted extraction was performed using the acetone (10 × 600 mL) as the extraction solvent. The extract was obtained (28.54 g) by filtration and evaporation of acetone under vacuum (<40 °C) [9].

2.2.2. Isolation

Repeated Flash-Dry Column Chromatography of *P. ecklonii* extract (25 g), over silica gel (Merck 9385, 75 g), using n-hexane: ethyl acetate mixtures of increasing polarity, allowed the isolation of pure Parvifloron D (0.882 g) [18]. The chemical structure of Parvifloron D was elucidated comparing the ^{1}H-NMR spectroscopic data (Table S1: NMR data of PvD, (CDCl3, [1]H 400 MHz, [13]C 100 MHz; δ in ppm, J in Hz) and Table S2: Significant assignments observed on Heteronuclear Multiple Bond Correlation (HMBC) experiment for Parvifloron D) which was almost identical to those in the literature [9,19].

2.3. Parvifloron D Quantification by HPLC-DAD Analysis

The High-Performance Liquid Chromatography (HPLC) quantification of Parvifloron D from *P. ecklonii* extract was carried out as previously described [20]. It was used as a Liquid Chromatograph Agilent Technologies 1200 Infinity Series Liquid Chromatography (LC) System equipped with diode array detector (DAD), using a ChemStation Software (Agilent Technologies, Waldbronn, Germany) and a LiChrospher, 100 RP-18 (5 mm) column from Merck (Darmstadt, Germany). Parvifloron D was determined and quantified by injecting 20 µL of the sample at 1 mg/mL, using a gradient composed of Solution A (methanol), Solution B (acetonitrile) and Solution D (0.3% trichloroacetic acid in water) as follows: 0 min, 15% A, 5% B and 80% D; 20 min, 80% A, 10% B and 10% D; 25 min, 80% A, 10% B and 10% D. The flow rate was set at 1 mL/min. The authentic sample of Parvifloron D was run under the same conditions in methanol, and the detection was carried out between 200 and 600 nm with a diode array detector (DAD). All analyses were performed in triplicate.

2.4. Cell Culture and Cytotoxicity Assays

In order to evaluate Parvifloron D selectivity and antiproliferative effects against human tumor cells, different cell lines were tested: three pancreatic (BxPC3, PANC-1 and Ins1-E) and three non-pancreatic (MCF-7, HaCat and Caco-2) cell lines.

All cell lines tested, BxPC3 (human pancreas adenocarcinoma), PANC-1 (human pancreas adenocarcinoma), Ins1-E (rat pancreas insulinoma), MCF-7 (human breast cancer), HaCat (human keratinocyte) and Caco-2 (colon adenocarcinoma), are typically adherent cell cultures. Evaluations were made in different conditions regarding the different types of cells. Thus, BxPC3 cells were maintained in Roswell Park Memorial Institute (RPMI)-1640 medium with 10% heat-inactivated FBS; Ins1-E cells were maintained in RPMI medium supplemented with 10% fetal bovine serum, 100 IU/mL of penicillin, 100 µg/mL streptomycin and β-mercaptoethanol (50 µM) 1:1000; MCF-7, PANC-1 and HaCat cells were maintained in Dulbecco's Modified Eagle's medium (DMEM) with high-glucose (4500 mg/L), supplemented with 10% fetal bovine serum and 100 IU/mL of penicillin and 100 µg/mL streptomycin; and Caco-2 cells were maintained in RPMI medium supplemented with 10% fetal bovine serum and 100 IU/mL of penicillin and 100 µg/mL streptomycin all at 37 °C in a humidified atmosphere of 5% CO_2 incubator.

The effects of Parvifloron D on cell growth were evaluated by different assays, namely, for BxPC3 cells, the sulforhodamine B (SRB) assay (colorimetric) was used [21] and for Ins1-E, MCF-7, PANC-1, HaCat and Caco-2 cells the MTT test was used [10]. Briefly, cells were seeded in 96-well plates (using a cell concentration of 800 cells per well for BxPC3, 1×10^4 cell/mL per well for Ins1-E, MCF-7, PANC-1, HaCat and Caco-2) under normal conditions (5% CO_2 humidified atmosphere at 37 °C) and allowed to adhere for 24 h. The cells were then incubated with Parvifloron D at different concentrations: between 0.5 and 25.0 µM for BxPC3 and to Ins1-E, MCF-7, PANC-1, HaCat and Caco-2 between 10.0 and 60.0 µM. Following this incubation period, and once the cells were analyzed through different assays, they were processed under different conditions. BxPC3 cells were fixed with 10% trichloroacetic acid for 1 h on ice, and washed and stained with 50 µL 0.4% SRB dye for 30 min. The cells were then washed repeatedly with 1% acetic acid to remove unbound dye. After, the cells were dried, and the protein-bound stain was solubilized with 10 mM Tris solution.

The SRB absorbance was measured at 560 nm using the microplate reader Model 680 (Bio-Rad, Hercules, CA, USA). The concentration that inhibits cell survival in 50% (IC_{50}) was determined using the SRB assay. The absorbance of the wells containing the drug and the absorbance of the wells containing untreated cells, following a 24 h incubation period, were subsequently compared with that of the wells containing the cells that had been fixed at time zero (when Parvifloron D was added). Similarly, Ins1-E, MCF-7, PANC-1, HaCat and Caco-2 cells medium was removed, and the wells were washed with Phosphate-Buffered Saline (PBS). Then, 50 µL of a 10% MTT solution was added to the cells and the plates were incubated for 4 h. After the incubation time, 100 µL of DMSO were added to each well to solubilize the formazan crystals formed during the incubation period.

The absorbance of all samples was again measured at 570 nm using the microplate reader and IC_{50} was determined.

The cytotoxic effect was evaluated by determining the percentage of viable/death cells for each Parvifloron D studied concentration. Based on these values, the IC_{50} (Parvifloron D concentration that induces a 50% inhibition of cell growth) was calculated, according to an equation proposed by Hills and co-workers [22]. For IC_{50} determination, two concentrations, X_1 and X_2, and the respective cell densities, Y_1 and Y_2, that correspond to higher or lesser than half cell density in negative control (Y_0), were established, according to the following equation:

$$\text{Log } IC_{50} = \text{Log } X_1 + \{[(Y_1 - (Y_0)/2)]/(Y_1 - Y_2)\} \times (\text{Log } X_2 - \text{Log } X_1) \tag{1}$$

where, $Y_0/2$ is the half-cell density of the negative control; Y_1 is the cell density above $Y_0/2$; X_1 is the concentration corresponding to Y_1; Y_2 is the cell density below $Y_0/2$; X_2 is the concentration corresponding to Y_2; The IC_{50} was determined by linear interpolation between X_1 and X_2.

2.5. Parvifloron D Solubility Assays

Parvifloron D solubility in PBS (pH 7.4, European Pharmacopoeia 7.0) was determined at two different temperatures, 25 °C and 37 °C, by measuring the amount of compound dissolved in a saturated solution (~30 µg/mL) after 24 h, with constant stirring (200 rpm). Three independent measurements at each condition were conducted ($n = 3$) [23].

2.6. Parvifloron D Encapsulation into a Biocompatible and Hydrophilic Nanomaterial

In previous studies, Parvifloron D has showed low water-solubility, probably due to its long carbon chains and the presence of aromatic rings, giving Parvifloron D lipophilic characteristics [24,25], along with an apparent lack of selectivity to cancer cells [23]. Therefore, the encapsulation of Parvifloron D into a biocompatible and hydrophilic nanomaterial as a drug delivery system had the main objective of the achievement of optimized bioavailability and stability of the drug and thus, optimal drug loading and release properties, a long shelf life and higher therapeutic efficacy, with lower side effects [26].

Albumin was chosen as the encapsulating material to Parvifloron D due to its biocompatibility and affinity to the liver. The technology used to produce nanoparticles was the desolvation method, suitable to a wide range of polymers, especially heat-sensitives ones such as albumin, being the main advantage that it does not require an increase in temperature [27,28]. Briefly, bovine serum albumin was dissolved in purified distilled water with the pH adjusted to 8.2 with NaOH 0.1 M. Subsequently, Parvifloron D was dissolved in acetone and added to the albumin solution, which was added dropwise into a solution of absolute ethanol under magnetic stirring (500 rpm). After stirring, an opalescent suspension was spontaneously formed at room temperature. After this desolvation process, glucose in water (1.8%, v/v) was added to cross-link the desolvated albumin nanoparticles. The cross-linking process was performed under stirring of the colloidal suspension over a time period of 30 min. Measurement of pH was conducted with a pH electrode meter (827 pH lab Metrohm) calibrated daily with buffer solutions pH 4.00 ± 0.02 and 7.00 ± 0.02 (25 °C).

2.7. Determination of the Parvifloron D Encapsulation Efficiency by HPLC Analysis

Parvifloron D encapsulation efficiency ($EE\%$) was determined using a reverse-phase HPLC chromatographic method (stationary phase—LiChrospher RP 18 (5 µm), Lichrocart 250–4.6) for the drug quantification at a detection wavelength of 254 nm. Briefly, a HPLC (Hitachi system LaCrom Elite, Column oven, Diode Array Detector (UV-Vis) (Hitachi High Technologies America, San Jose, CA, USA)) was used with a mobile phase comprising methanol and trichloroacetic acid 0.1% (80:20, v/v) (flow rate of 1.0 mL/min). Column conditions were maintained at 30 °C, with an injection volume of 20 µL and a run-time of 15 min. Measurements were carried out in duplicate and according to the described formula:

$$EE\ (\%) = (\text{Amount of encapsulated drug/Initial drug amount}) \times 100\% \qquad (2)$$

2.8. In Vitro Release Studies

After determining Parvifloron D solubility, to maintain sink conditions during the in vitro release studies, empty nanoparticles and Parvifloron D-loaded nanoparticles were freeze-dried (24 h at −50 ± 2 °C, Freezone 2.5 L Benchtop Freeze Dry System, Labconco, MO, USA) and weighted according to the drug solubility. As an approximation to the blood pH, each sample of weighted nanoparticles was placed in a glass recipient, containing 250 mL of PBS (pH 7.4, European Pharmacopoeia 7.0), under constant stirring (200 rpm), in order to simulate the in vivo conditions [23]. At appropriate time intervals, aliquots of the release medium were collected from three different points of the dissolution medium, in order to obtain a homogenous collection of the sample. Nanoparticles were isolated from the supernatant by centrifugation (20,000 rpm for 15 min). The Parvifloron D amount collected from the in vitro release medium, at each time point, was determined by HPLC (see Section 2.7). The assay was conducted for 72 h, to assure that all Parvifloron D was released. ($n = 3$, mean $\pm$ SD).

2.9. Physical and Morphological Characterization of the Nanoparticles: Dynamic Light Scattering (DLS), Scanning Electron Microscopy (SEM) and Atomic Force Microscopy (AFM)

Freshly prepared empty nanoparticles and Parvifloron D-loaded nanoparticles were studied in terms of their structure, surface morphology, shape and size by DLS, SEM and AFM.

Physical characterization of the nanoparticles was carried out by evaluation of mean particle size, polydispersity index (PI) and zeta potential by DLS and electrophoretic mobility (Coulter nano-sizer Delsa Nano™ (Beckman Coulter, Brea, CA, USA)) of the nanoparticles' concentrated suspension ($n = 3$).

For SEM, the aqueous suspensions containing empty and loaded nanoparticles were fixed with 2.5% glutaraldehyde in 0.1 M sodium phosphate buffer at pH 7.2 (European Pharmacopoeia 7.0) during 1 h. After centrifugation, the pellets were washed three times in the fixative buffer. Then, aliquots (10 μL) of the two samples suspensions were scattered over a round glass coverslip previously coated with poly-L-lysine and left to dry in a desiccator. Subsequently, the material was coated with a thin layer of gold and observed on a JEOL 5200LV scanning electron microscope (JEOL Ltd., Tokyo, Japan) at an accelerating voltage of 20 kV. Images were recorded digitally.

AFM images were acquired on an atomic force microscope, Multimode 8 coupled to Nanoscope V Controller, from Bruker, UK, by using peak force tapping and ScanAssist mode. In order to offer a clean and flat surface for AFM analysis, an aliquot of each sample (~30 μL) was mounted on a freshly cleaved mica sheet and left to dry before being analyzed. The images were obtained in ambient conditions, at a sweep rate close to 1 Hz, using scanasyst-air 0.4 N/m tips, from Bruker.

2.10. Physicochemical Characterization of Nanoparticles Interaction Analysis by Fourier Transform Infrared (FT-IR)

To study the possible interactions between Parvifloron D and bovine serum albumin polymer of the developed nanoparticles, FT-IR spectroscopy was conducted on freeze-dried nanoparticles samples and on each isolated compound, using potassium bromide (KBr). The FT-IR spectra was recorded by using a Nicolet FT-IR Spectrometer (Thermo Electron Corporation, Beverly, MA, USA) from 4000 to 400 cm^{-1}, at a scanning speed of cm^{-1} for 256 scans by placing the KBr pellet on the attenuated total reflection objective. The final data is reported as a data average of 256 scans. The pellet was prepared in a ratio of 1:10 (w/w) of KBr to sample (nanoparticles or other component) and left to dry in a desiccator for 24 h before the analysis. The following samples were compared: empty nanoparticles (i.e., without Parvifloron D), Parvifloron D-loaded nanoparticles, physical mixture of Parvifloron D and bovine serum albumin (1:1, w/w), the polymer (bovine serum albumin), the cross-linking agent (glucose) and the drug (Parvifloron D).

2.11. Differential Scanning Calorimetry

In an attempt to check the purity of the drug and to confirm possible physicochemical interactions between nanoparticles and their raw components, thermal transformations and phase transitions of the nanoparticles were studied by calorimetry (Diferential Scanning Calorimetry, Q200, TA Instruments, New Castle, DE, USA) under a nitrogen gas flow of 50 mL/min (AirLiquide, Algés, Portugal). Samples (1–5 mg) were analyzed in hermetic aluminum pans at a heating rate of 10 °C /min from 40 to 400 °C. The endothermic and exothermic events were analyzed using TA-Universal Analysis software (Universal Analysis 2000 version 4.7A, TA Instruments, New Castle, DE, USA).

3. Results and Discussion

3.1. Extraction and Isolation

The diterpenoid Parvifloron D was isolated from a *P. ecklonii* extract in a total amount of 166.1 µg/mg, quantified by HPLC. This extraction yield of Parvifloron D with acetone was optimized when compared with Burmistrova et al. extraction (136.75 µg/mg) [8]. Here, the ultrasound-assisted extraction showed a higher extraction yield when compared with the previous described maceration method. The optimized isolation of Parvifloron D (882 mg, 0.45% on the dry plant) showed to be a successful isolation process which presented a higher yield of Parvifloron D in comparison with M Simões et al. results (0.27% on the dry plant) [9].

The isolated compound peak was verified by HPLC, as Figure 2 shows.

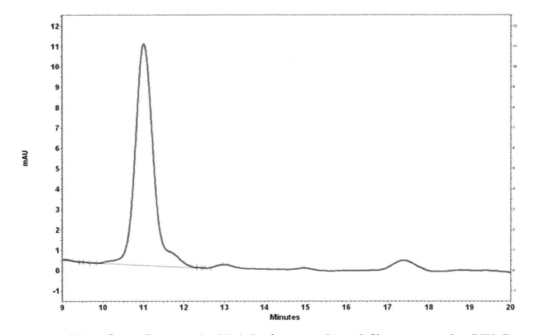

Figure 2. Isolated Parvifloron D spectra by High-Performance Liquid Chromatography (HPLC) analysis.

3.2. Parvifloron D Quantification by HPLC-DAD

The phytochemical analysis of *P. ecklonii* extract was performed by HPLC-DAD as represented in Figure 3. The presence of Parvifloron D was revealed (Retention Time (RT) = 27.63 min) as the principal constituent was obtained and its absorption spectra was performed, as previously described [29].

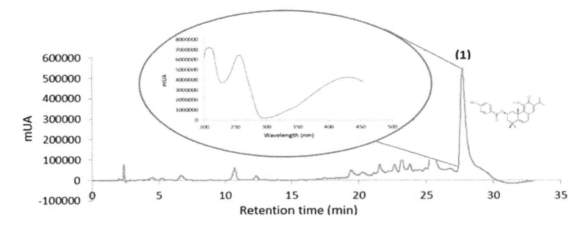

Figure 3. HPLC profile of *P. ecklonii* extract (254 nm): (1) Parvifloron D peak and absorption spectra.

3.3. Cell culture and Cytotoxicity Assays

To study the cytotoxicity of free Parvifloron D, SRB and MTT assays were conducted. The results have shown that free Parvifloron D was more cytotoxic to pancreatic cell lines (BxPC3, PANC-1 and Ins1-E) than to non-pancreatic cell lines (MCF-7, Caco-2 and HaCat), displaying more selectivity to our target tumor cells than to others. Parvifloron D presented the lowest value of IC_{50} of 0.15 ± 0.05 μM for BxPC3 (human pancreatic tumor cells), and a high value of 32.1 ± 4.3 μM for Caco-2 cells (colon adenocarcinoma) according Table 1. Even in tumor cells, Parvifloron D had a higher selectivity to human tumor pancreatic cells. Cell viability in different time points, 24 h and 48 h, for Ins1-E, MCF7 and Caco-2 cells were measured and the results were added to supplementary material (Table S3—IC_{50} (μM) values in different time points, 24 h and 48 h, of different cell lines–cytotoxicity assays).

Table 1. IC_{50} ($\pm$ Standard deviation (SD)) values of different cell lines—cytotoxicity assays.

Cell line	IC_{50} (μM) $\pm$ SD
MCF-7 (breast cancer)	35.1 ± 2.2
HaCat (human keratinocyte)	34.3 ± 4.1
Caco-2 (Colon adenocarcinoma)	32.1 ± 4.3
INS-1E (rat pancreatic insulinoma)	21.6 ± 0.5
BxPC3 (human pancreatic adenocarcinoma)	0.15 ± 0.1
PANC-1 (human pancreatic adenocarcinoma)	11.9 ± 0.7

Considering some previously published results such as X. Yu et al. (IC_{50} = 0.2 μM to gemcitabine in BxPC3 cell line) [30], A. Singh et al. (IC_{50} = 123.9 μM to gemcitabine in PANC-1 cell line) [31], A. Acuna et al. (IC_{50} = 46.5 μM to PH-427 in BxPC3 cell line) [32], S. Mukai et al. (IC_{50} = 19.5 μM and 20.4 μM to gefitinib in BxPC3 and PANC-1 cell lines, respectively) [33], L. Wang et al. (IC_{50} = 39.86 μM and 83.76 μM to Pemetrexed in BxPC3 and PANC-1 cell lines, respectively) [34] or even A. Wright et al. (IC_{50} = 70.9 μM and 22.8 μM to Aphrocallistin in BxPC3 and PANC-1 cell lines, respectively) [35], we can suggest that Parvifloron D has a higher cytotoxic potential (IC_{50} = 0.15 ± 0.05) to these pancreatic tumor cells.

Despite these results and concerning the Parvifloron D mechanism of action, our group work is studding Parvifloron D-induced cell death and they have observed that Parvifloron D induces an increase in Sub-G1 and a reduction of G2/M populations in MDA-MB-231 (human breast tumor cells), as Burmistrova et al. already described in leukemia HL-60 and U-937 cells [8]. These results lead us to believe that Parvifloron D-induced cell death can be through this mechanism independently of the cell line tested. Although, this data is still in progress, and thus it has not been published yet. Nevertheless, our group has tested the internalization of polymeric nanoparticles with Parvifloron D, observing that it had occurred by endocytosis within 2 h [23]. Moreover, according to the literature, seven membrane-associated albumin-binding proteins have been discovered, namely: albondin/glycoprotein60 (gp60), glycoprotein18 (gp18), glycoprotein30 (gp30), the neonatal Fcreceptor (FcRn), heterogeneous nuclear ribonucleoproteins (hnRNPs), calreticulin, cubilin, and megalin [36]. This leads us to believe that our nanoparticles may internalize via endocytosis [37]. This assumption must be confirmed with future experiments of nanoparticles co-localization and nanoparticles cellular quantification.

3.4. Nanoparticles Encapsulation Efficiency by HPLC Analysis

In order to determine Parvifloron D encapsulation efficiency, a calibration curve was made using previously isolated Parvifloron D as a calibration standard. Parvifloron D standards ranging from 3 to 75 µg/mL were evaluated and a calibration curve (y = 7589.9x − 12798) was obtained with R^2 = 0.999. Limit of Detection (LOD) and Limit of Quantification (LOQ) were calculated to be 2.6 µg/mL and 7.9 µg/mL, respectively.

Encapsulation efficiency (%) was determined by measuring the non-encapsulated drug. Non-encapsulated drug was measured (8.79 µg/mL) (i.e., indirect quantification) and the value obtained was subtracted from the amount of drug initially added, being the encapsulation efficiency value for Parvifloron D 91.2 ± 5.51% (mean value ± SD, n = 3).

3.5. Parvifloron D Solubility Assays and In Vitro Release Studies

HPLC studies were carried out to determine the solubility of Parvifloron D in PBS (pH 7.4) before performing in vitro release studies of Parvifloron D after entrapment into the albumin nanoparticles.

After 24h incubation in PBS pH 7.4, at two different temperatures, 25 °C and 37 °C, Parvifloron D solubility was 3.7 ± 0.8 µg/mL and 4.9 ± 0.3 µg/mL, respectively (n = 3).

Concerning the in vitro release studies, all entrapped Parvifloron D was released from albumin nanoparticles in 72 h in PBS at pH 7.4. As illustrated in Figure 4, after 24 h, approximately 40% of Parvifloron D was released from the nanoparticles and no burst release was observed. Besides, Parvifloron D degradation was evaluated as the in vitro release studies went by. The release profile was continually sustained over the assay and all of the drug was been released in less than 72 h.

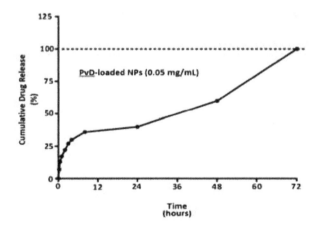

Figure 4. In vitro drug release of Parvifloron D-loaded nanoparticles at 0.05 mg/mL, for 72 h, in phosphate buffered saline (PBS) pH 7.4 solution. Results are expressed as mean of measurements of three independent nanoparticles lots ± Standard Deviation (SD) (n = 3).

3.6. Physical and Morphological Characterization of the Nanoparticles: DLS, AFM, SEM

In terms of mean size value, Parvifloron D-loaded nanoparticles were smaller than empty nanoparticles (165 nm (PI 0.11) and 250 nm (PI 0.37), respectively). This fact is probably due to electrostatic interactions, which may reduce and compact the particle structure. It should also be noted that there was a color change of nanoparticles from white to orange, when Parvifloron D was entrapped inside the particles. The pH value was around 8.5 in both formulations. Zeta potential was negative in both cases (−19.65 and −7.88 mV to empty nanoparticles and Parvifloron D-loaded nanoparticles, respectively) and the difference might be attributed to the presence of Parvifloron D, suggesting some interaction between the albumin and the drug, which can be related to the intrinsic charge of Parvifloron D (pKa values of 8.9, 9.9, calculated values by ChemDraw Professional).

AFM analysis has confirmed particles size. Figure 5 shows that the particle size of the prepared nanoparticles was approximately 210 nm and 190 nm for empty and Parvifloron D-loaded nanoparticles, respectively, as measured by DLS. AFM can offer a significant contribution to understand surface and interface properties, thus allowing for the optimization of biomaterials performance, processes, and physical and chemical properties even at the nanoscale [38]. In addition, we can notice that particles, especially the empty nanoparticles, were monodispersed. Figure 6 shows the 3D images highlighting the shape and morphology of the prepared nanoparticles.

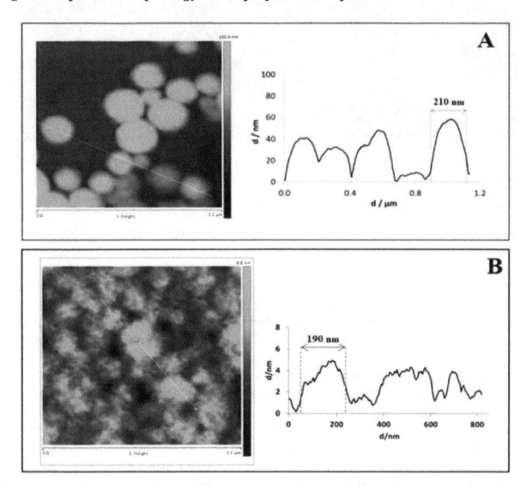

Figure 5. Atomic Force Microscopy (AFM) sectorial analysis of: (**A**) Albumin empty nanoparticles and (**B**) Parvifloron D-loaded nanoparticles. Particle sizes of 210 nm and 190 nm are also represented, for A and B, respectively.

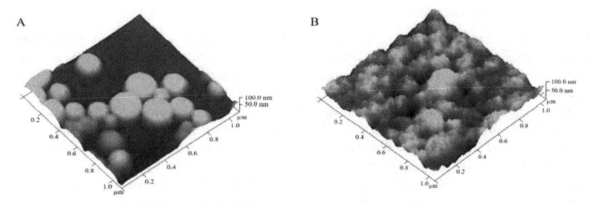

Figure 6. Atomic Force Microscopy (AFM) analysis 3D images of: (**A**) Albumin empty nanoparticles and (**B**) Parvifloron D-loaded nanoparticles.

In the current study, SEM observations showed that nanoparticles in both formulations had a uniform distribution and exhibited a spherical shape with a smooth surface. It is also clearly seen that the particles size is different, the empty nanoparticles being slightly larger than the Parvifloron D-loaded nanoparticles (Figure 7). Here, SEM provides information on surface topography, size, and size distribution of nanoparticles [39].

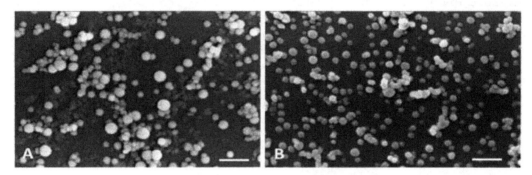

Figure 7. Scanning Electron Microscopy (SEM) micrographs of: (**A**) Albumin empty nanoparticles (scale bar: 1 μm) and (**B**) Parvifloron D-loaded nanoparticles (scale bar: 1 μm).

3.7. Physicochemical Characterization of Nanoparticles Interaction Analysis by FT-IR

FT-IR spectra main peaks and the corresponding functional groups were identified for all tested samples. For physical mixtures and nanoparticles, the peaks were identified based on the functional groups of the raw components (wavenumbers: 4000–400 cm^{-1}), as it is shown in Table 2. This analysis has demonstrated to be a useful method to interpret intra- and inter-material interactions in raw materials and their combination to obtain nanoparticles.

After the analysis of the spectra, it was confirmed the bovine serum albumin structure by the presence of specific bands for amides (I and II). Also, Parvifloron D analysis showed its specific bands, confirming its structure previously done by NMR (supplementary material). When albumin empty nanoparticles were analyzed, the same specific bands were identified in the raw bovine serum albumin spectra, although the N–H amide II band has shifted, suggesting some structure modification of bovine serum albumin chains when aggregated to provide nanoparticles. In addition, a new band at 3000 cm^{-1} appears in empty nanoparticles, probably due to the cross-linking with glucose. As for the interactions between drug and nanoparticles, it was possible to differentiate the spectra of albumin nanoparticles loaded with Parvifloron D and the physical mixture of bovine serum albumin and free Parvifloron D (at 1:1, *w/w*). This fact can indicate that the drug was successfully entrapped inside the nanoparticles, and observing the distinct peaks in the nanostructures analysis, some kind of drug–albumin interaction during nanoparticles formation might have occurred.

3.8. Differential Scanning Calorimetry

Differential scanning calorimetry was used to characterize the different properties of the developed nanosystems, such as Parvifloron D polymorphism, interactions between drug and nanoparticles and the effect on their thermal events, compared to raw materials. Figure 8 shows an exothermic peak near to 170 °C, indicating a crystallization and an endothermic peak close to 300 °C, which can represent a crystal melting, suggesting that Parvifloron D is a polymorphic drug. Anyway, to better understand the thermal behavior of Parvifloron D, more crystallographic studies have to be conducted in the future. Bovine serum albumin endothermic peaks were observed around 215 °C while exothermic peaks appeared around 310 °C. Analyzing albumin at nanoparticles form, its spectra changed, showing a lower melting point, once the endothermic peak appeared near to 190 °C, suggesting some structure modification of albumin chains to organize nanoparticles arrangement. For albumin nanoparticles loaded with Parvifloron D, the spectra show two endothermic peaks which probably represents both bovine serum albumin and Parvifloron D melting points, but due to some rearrangement between these raw materials into nanoparticles, these endothermic events had occurred at lower temperatures (136 °C and 219 °C).

Table 2. FT-IR analysis of spectra of all tested samples (cm^{-1}).

Functional Groups Compound	O–H Carboxylic Acid (Stretching)	C–H Alkane (Stretching)	C=O Carbonyl (Stretching)	C=O Amide I (Stretching)	N–H Amide II (Bending)	C=C Aromatic (Stretching)	C–H Alkane (Bending)	C–O Alcohol (Stretching)	=C–H Alkene (Bending)
BSA [1]	—	—	—	1654	1590	—	—	—	—
PvD [2]	—	2871	1693	—	—	1510	—	—	850
Glucose	3350	—	—	—	—	—	1456	1032	—
Physical mixture BSA + PvD	—	2871	1690	1658	1590	1515	—	—	—
Empty BSA-NPs [3]	3000	—	—	1654	1540	—	—	—	—
BSA-NPs loaded With PvD	3000	2873	—	1654	1540	1540	—	—	910

[1] BSA: Bovine serum albumin; [2] PvD: Parvifloron D; [3] NPs: nanoparticles.

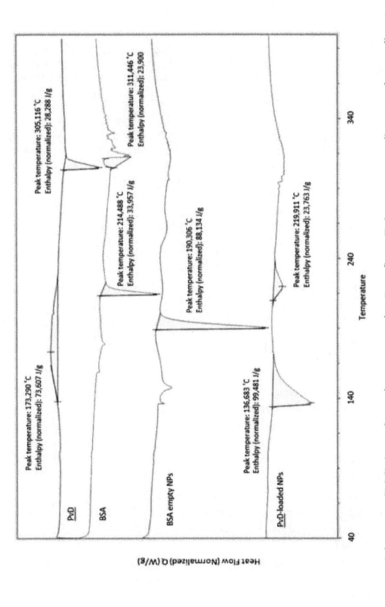

Figure 8. Differential Scanning Calorimetry (DSC) thermal transformations in free Parvifloron D, bovine serum albumin polymer, albumin empty nanoparticles and Parvifloron D-loaded nanoparticles, respectively. The major peak temperatures (°C) and the difference in Gibbs energy (J/g), for each sample, are also represented.

4. Conclusions

Parvifloron D has been efficiently extracted and isolated from *P. ecklonii*. Cell cultures have shown that Parvifloron D may have more selectivity to human pancreatic tumor cells than healthy cells or breast cancer cells. Parvifloron D-loaded small and spherical nanoparticles (water soluble particles) have been formulated with high encapsulation efficiency. Those nanoparticles led to a controlled release of the drug encapsulation over 72 h. Parvifloron D nanoparticles were stable, and therefore, they can be considered a suitable and promising carrier to deliver the drug to the tumor site, improving the treatment of pancreatic cancer.

Author Contributions: Conceptualization: A.S.-R. and C.P.R.; methodology and formal analysis: A.S.-R., C.G., C.E., A.B., S.C.C., M.A.N.C., J.M., A.S.V., L.A., J.F.P., M.M.G., P.R. and C.P.R.; investigation: A.S.-R.; writing—original draft preparation, A.S.-R.; writing, review and editing: C.P.R., J.M., J.F.P., A.S.V., M.M.G. and L.A.; supervision, C.P.R., P.R. and J.M.; project administration: A.S.-R. and C.P.R.; funding acquisition: ULHT/CBIOS and UAH.

Acknowledgments: The authors would like to thank to P. Fonte for kindly donating the Ins1-E cell line used in this paper, and to A. S. Fernandes and N. Saraiva (CBIOS/ULHT) for sharing their unpublished results, allowing us to better discuss the mechanism of action of Parvifloron D. The authors would also like to thank to M. Minas da Piedade and C. Bernardes for their help in FT-IR analysis.

References

1.   Rahib, L.; Smith, B.D.; Aizenberg, R.; Rosenzweig, A.B.; Fleshman, J.M.; Matrisian, L.M. Projecting cancer incidence and deaths to 2030: The unexpected burden of thyroid, liver, and pancreas cancers in the united states. *Cancer Res.* **2014**, *74*, 2913–2921. [CrossRef] [PubMed]

2.   Niess, H.; Kleespies, A.; Andrassy, J.; Pratschke, S.; Angele, M.K.; Guba, M.; Jauch, K.-W.; Bruns, C.J. Pancreatic cancer in the elderly: Guidelines and individualized therapy. *Der Chir.* **2013**, *84*, 291–295. [CrossRef]

3.   Oberstein, P.E.; Olive, K.P. Pancreatic cancer: Why is it so hard to treat? *Ther. Adv. Gastroenterol.* **2013**, *6*, 321–337. [CrossRef] [PubMed]

4.   Rebelo, A.; Molpeceres, J.; Rijo, P.; Reis, C.P. Pancreatic Cancer Therapy Review: From Classic Therapeutic Agents to Modern Nanotechnologies. *Curr. Drug Metab.* **2017**, *18*, 346–359. [CrossRef] [PubMed]

5.   Neoptolemos, J.P.; Stocken, D.D.; Friess, H.; Bassi, C.; Dunn, J.A.; Hickey, H.; Beger, H.; Fernandez-Cruz, L.; Dervenis, C.; Lacaine, F.; et al. A Randomized Trial of Chemoradiotherapy and Chemotherapy after Resection of Pancreatic Cancer. *N. Engl. J. Med.* **2004**, *350*, 1200–1210. [CrossRef] [PubMed]

6.   Gourav, L.; Deepak-K., S.; Pawan-K., S.; Chand, M.P. Anticancer, antimicrobial and antifertility activities of some medicinal plants: A review. *Med. Drug Res.* **2015**, *3*, 7–11.

7.   Nicolai, M.; Pereira, P.; Vitor, R.F.; Pinto, C.; Roberto, A.; Rijo, P. Antioxidant activity and rosmarinic acid content of ultrasound-assisted ethanolic extracts of medicinal plants. *Measurement* **2016**, *89*, 328–332. [CrossRef]

8.   Burmistrova, O.; Perdomo, J.; Simões, M.F.; Rijo, P.; Quintana, J.; Estévez, F. The abietane diterpenoid parvifloron D from *Plectranthus ecklonii* is a potent apoptotic inducer in human leukemia cells. *Phytomedicine* **2015**, *22*, 1009–1016. [CrossRef] [PubMed]

9.   Simões, M.F.; Rijo, P.; Duarte, A.; Matias, D.; Rodríguez, B. An easy and stereoselective rearrangement of an abietane diterpenoid into a bioactive microstegiol derivative. *Phytochem. Lett.* **2010**, *3*, 234–237. [CrossRef]

10. Burmistrova, O.; Simões, M.F.; Rijo, P.; Quintana, J.; Bermejo, J.; Estévez, F. Antiproliferative activity of abietane diterpenoids against human tumor cells. *J. Nat. Prod.* **2013**, *76*, 1413–1423. [CrossRef] [PubMed]

11. Rosa, S.; Correia, V.; Ribeiro, I.; Rijo, P.; Saraiva, N.; Fernandes, A. In vitro antioxidant properties of the diterpenes Parvifloron D and 7α-acetoxy-6β-hydroxyroyleanone. *Biomed. Biopharm. Res.* **2015**, *12*, 59–67. [CrossRef]

12. Bonifácio, B.V.; Silva, P.B.; Aparecido dos Santos Ramos, M.; Maria Silveira Negri, K.; Maria Bauab, T.; Chorilli, M. Nanotechnology-based drug delivery systems and herbal medicines: A review. *Int. J. Nanomed.* **2014**, *9*, 1–15. [CrossRef]

13. Reis, C.P.; Figueiredo, I.V.; Carvalho, R.A.; Jones, J.; Nunes, P.; Soares, A.F.; Silva, C.F.; Ribeiro, A.J.; Veiga, F.J.; Damgé, C.; et al. Toxicological assessment of orally delivered nanoparticulate insulin. *Nanotoxicology* **2008**, *2*, 205–217. [CrossRef]

14. Kouchakzadeh, H.; Shojaosadati, S.A.; Maghsoudi, A.; Farahani, E.V. Optimization of PEGylation Conditions for BSA Nanoparticles Using Response Surface Methodology. *AAPS PharmSciTech* **2010**, *11*, 1206–1211. [CrossRef] [PubMed]

15. Abrantes, G.; Duarte, D.; Reis, C.P. An Overview of Pharmaceutical Excipients: Safe or Not Safe? *J. Pharm. Sci.* **2016**, *105*, 2019–2026. [CrossRef] [PubMed]

16. Reis, C.P.; Damgé, C. Nanotechnology as a promising strategy for alternative routes of insulin delivery. *Methods Enzymol.* **2012**, *508*, 271–294. [CrossRef] [PubMed]

17. Pinto Reis, C.; Silva, C.; Martinho, N.; Rosado, C. Drug carriers for oral delivery of peptides and proteins: Accomplishments and future perspectives. *Ther. Deliv.* **2013**, *4*, 251–265. [CrossRef] [PubMed]

18. Harwood, L. "Dry-Column" Flash Chromatography. *Aldrichim. Acta* **1985**, *18*, 25.

19. Gaspar-Marques, C.; Simões, M.F.; Valdeira, M.L.; Rodríguez, B. Terpenoids and phenolics from *Plectranthus strigosus*, bioactivity screening. *Nat. Prod. Res.* **2008**, *22*, 167–177. [CrossRef] [PubMed]

20. Rijo, P.; Falé, P.L.; Serralheiro, M.L.; Simões, M.F.; Gomes, A.; Reis, C. Optimization of medicinal plant extraction methods and their encapsulation through extrusion technology. *Measurement* **2014**, *58*, 249–255. [CrossRef]

21. Coelho, S.C.; Almeida, G.M.; Santos-Silva, F.; Pereira, M.C.; Coelho, M.A.N. Enhancing the efficiency of bortezomib conjugated to pegylated gold nanoparticles: An in vitro study on human pancreatic cancer cells and adenocarcinoma human lung alveolar basal epithelial cells. *Expert Opin. Drug Deliv.* **2016**, *13*, 1075–1081. [CrossRef] [PubMed]

22. Hills, M.; Hudson, C.; Smith, P.G. Global monitoring of the resistance of malarial parasites to drugs: Statistical treatment of micro-test data. In *Working Paper No. 2.8. 5 for the Informal Consultation on the Epidemiology of Drug Resistance of Malaria Parasites*; World Health Organisation: Geneva, Switzerland, 1986.

23. Silva, C.O.; Molpeceres, J.; Batanero, B.; Fernandes, A.S.; Saraiva, N.; Costa, J.G.; Rijo, P.; Figueiredo, I.V.; Faísca, P.; Reis, C.P. Functionalized diterpene parvifloron D-loaded hybrid nanoparticles for targeted delivery in melanoma therapy. *Ther. Deliv.* **2016**, *7*, 521–544. [CrossRef] [PubMed]

24. Smith, R.; Tanford, C. Hydrophobicity of Long Chain n-Alkyl Carboxylic Acids, as Measured by Their Distribution Between Heptane and Aqueous Solutions. *Proc. Natl. Acad. Sci. USA* **1973**, *70*, 289–293. [CrossRef] [PubMed]

25. Silva, P.J. Inductive and resonance effects on the acidities of phenol, enols, and carbonyl α-hydrogens. *J. Org. Chem.* **2009**, *74*, 914–916. [CrossRef] [PubMed]

26. Bilia, A.R.; Piazzini, V.; Guccione, C.; Risaliti, L.; Asprea, M.; Capecchi, G.; Bergonzi, M.C. Improving on Nature: The Role of Nanomedicine in the Development of Clinical Natural Drugs. *Planta Med.* **2017**, *83*, 366–381. [CrossRef] [PubMed]

27. Pinto Reis, C.; Neufeld, R.J.; Ribeiro, A.J.; Veiga, F. Nanoencapsulation I. Methods for preparation of drug-loaded polymeric nanoparticles. *Nanomed. Nanotechnol. Biol. Med.* **2006**, *2*, 8–21. [CrossRef] [PubMed]

28. Weber, C.; Coester, C.; Kreuter, J.; Langer, K. Desolvation process and surface characterisation of protein nanoparticles. *Int. J. Pharm.* **2000**, *194*, 91–102. [CrossRef]

29. Figueiredo, N.L.; Falé, P.L.; Madeira, P.J.A.; Florêncio, M.H.; Ascensão, L.; Serralheiro, M.L.M.; Lino, A.R.L. Phytochemical Analysis of Plectranthus sp. Extracts and Application in Inhibition of Dental Bacteria, Streptococcus sobrinus and Streptococcus mutans. *Eur. J. Med. Plants* **2014**, *4*, 794–809. [CrossRef]

30. Yu, X.; Di, Y.; Xie, C.; Song, Y.; He, H.; Li, H.; Pu, X.; Lu, W.; Fu, D.; Jin, C. An in vitro and in vivo study of gemcitabine-loaded albumin nanoparticles in a pancreatic cancer cell line. *Int. J. Nanomed.* **2015**, *10*, 6825–6834. [CrossRef] [PubMed]

31. Singh, A.; Xu, J.; Mattheolabakis, G.; Amiji, M. EGFR-targeted gelatin nanoparticles for systemic administration of gemcitabine in an orthotopic pancreatic cancer model. *Nanomed. NBM* **2015**, *12*, 589–600. [CrossRef] [PubMed]

32. Acuna, A.; Jeffery, J.J.; Abril, E.R.; Nagle, R.B.; Guzman, R.; Pagel, M.D.; Meuillet, E.J. Nanoparticle delivery of an AKT/PDK1 inhibitor improves the therapeutic effect in pancreatic cancer. *Int. J. Nanomed.* **2014**, *9*, 5653–5665. [CrossRef]
33. Mukai, S.; Moriya, S.; Hiramoto, M.; Kazama, H.; Kokuba, H.; Che, X.F.; Yokoyama, T.; Sakamoto, S.; Sugawara, A.; Sunazuka, T.; et al. Macrolides sensitize EGFR-TKI-induced non-apoptotic cell death via blocking autophagy flux in pancreatic cancer cell lines. *Int. J. Oncol.* **2016**, *48*, 45–54. [CrossRef] [PubMed]
34. Wang, L.I.N.; Zhu, Z.; Zhang, W.; Zhang, W. Schedule-dependent cytotoxic synergism of pemetrexed and erlotinib in BXPC-3 and PANC-1 human pancreatic cancer cells. *Exp. Ther. Med.* **2011**, *2*, 969–975. [CrossRef] [PubMed]
35. Wright, A.E.; Roth, G.P.; Hoffman, J.K.; Divlianska, D.B.; Pechter, D.; Sennett, S.H.; Guzmán, E.A.; Linley, P.; McCarthy, P.J.; Pitts, T.P.; et al. Isolation, synthesis, and biological activity of aphrocallistin, an adenine-substituted bromotyramine metabolite from the hexactinellida sponge *Aphrocallistes beatrix*. *J. Nat. Prod.* **2009**, *72*, 1178–1183. [CrossRef] [PubMed]
36. Merlot, A.M.; Kalinowski, D.S.; Richardson, D.R. Unraveling the mysteries of serum albumin—More than just a serum protein. *Front. Physiol.* **2014**, *5*, 1–7. [CrossRef] [PubMed]
37. Yameen, B.; Choi, W.I.; Vilos, C.; Swami, A.; Shi, J.; Farokhzad, O.C. Insight into nanoparticle cellular uptake and intracellular targeting. *J. Control. Release* **2015**, *28*, 485–499. [CrossRef] [PubMed]
38. Marrese, M.; Guarino, V.; Ambrosio, L. Atomic Force Microscopy: A Powerful Tool to Address Scaffold Design in Tissue Engineering. *J. Funct. Biomater.* **2017**, *8*, 7. [CrossRef] [PubMed]
39. Kowoll, T.; Müller, E.; Fritsch-Decker, S.; Hettler, S.; Störmer, H.; Weiss, C.; Gerthsen, D. Contrast of backscattered electron SEM images of nanoparticles on substrates with complex structure. *Scanning* **2017**, *2017*. [CrossRef] [PubMed]

5

Nanolipid-Trehalose Conjugates and Nano-Assemblies as Putative Autophagy Inducers

Eleonora Colombo [1], Michele Biocotino [1], Giulia Frapporti [2], Pietro Randazzo [3],
Michael S. Christodoulou [4], Giovanni Piccoli [2], Laura Polito [5], Pierfausto Seneci [1,*]
and Daniele Passarella [1,*]

[1] Dipartimento di Chimica, Università degli Studi di Milano, Via Golgi 19, 20133 Milano, Italy
[2] CIBIO, Università di Trento, Via Sommarive 9, 38123 Povo (TN), Italy
[3] Promidis Srl, San Raffaele Scientific Research Park, Torre San Michele 1, Via Olgettina 60, 20132 Milan, Italy
[4] DISFARM, Sezione di Chimica Generale e Organica "A. Marchesini", Universitdegli Studi di Milano, via Venezian 21, 20133 Milano, Italy
[5] ISTM-CNR, via Fantoli 16/15, 20138 Milan, Italy
[*] Correspondence: pierfausto.seneci@unimi.it (P.S.); daniele.passarella@unimi.it (D.P.);

Abstract: The disaccharide trehalose is an autophagy inducer, but its pharmacological application is severely limited by its poor pharmacokinetics properties. Thus, trehalose was coupled via suitable spacers with squalene (in 1:2 and 1:1 stoichiometry) and with betulinic acid (1:2 stoichiometry), in order to yield the corresponding nanolipid-trehalose conjugates **1-Sq-mono**, **2-Sq-bis** and **3-Be-mono**. The conjugates were assembled to produce the corresponding nano-assemblies (NAs) **Sq-NA1**, **Sq-NA2** and **Be-NA3**. The synthetic and assembly protocols are described in detail. The resulting NAs were characterized in terms of loading and structure, and tested in vitro for their capability to induce autophagy. Our results are presented and thoroughly commented upon.

Keywords: nano-assemblies; trehalose; squalene; betulinic acid; autophagy induction

1. Introduction

Nano-vectors are used as therapeutics and diagnostics [1,2]. Iron-based [3], gold-based [4] and silica-based inorganic nano-vectors [5] were tested as being a diagnostic (magnetic resonance imaging reagents/MRIs [6]), or as therapeutics (hyperthermia against tumors [7], iron replacement therapies [8]). Liposome- [9], micelle- [10] and polymer-based nano-assemblies (NAs) [11] are marketed, mostly as anti-cancer agents [12]. Exploratory efforts [13] up to clinical trials [14] against diseases of the central nervous system (CNS) were reported.

Trehalose [15,16] is a non-reducing disaccharide made by a 1,1 linkage between two D-glucose molecules. It is bio-synthesized in lower organisms [16] to stabilize life processes and support survival in extreme conditions (freezing [17], heat and desiccation [18]). Trehalose induces autophagy in vitro and in vivo [19] and reduces protein misfolding and aggregation in vitro [20] by acting as a chemical chaperone and solvating them [20]. Reduction of aggregated huntingtin (Huntington Disease) [21], synuclein (Parkinson Disease) [20] and amyloid species (Alzheimer Disease) [22] was observed in vitro. Trehalose was tested as a safe, cheap, neuroprotective agent in preclinical and clinical studies [16]. Unfortunately, high mM trehalose concentrations are needed in vivo for efficacy, due to its high hydrophilicity and due to trehalase enzymes [23], that hydrolyze trehalose in the brush border cells of the small intestine and in the proximal tubules of the kidneys, preventing its oral absorption.

Nano lipid-drug conjugates [24], obtained by the covalent coupling of a drug to bio-compatible lipids, improve pharmacokinetics, decrease toxicity and increase the therapeutic index of the associated drugs. In particular, squalene-based amphiphilic conjugates have a proven track record for therapeutic applications [25]. They spontaneously assemble in water into nano-assemblies (NAs), encasing the bioactive payload, they do not show the drug on their surface, minimizing any side effect [26], they are internalized by cells via endocytic pathways [27] and release the free drug at its site of action, when a biologically labile linkage is used [28]. We also selected betulinic acid-based conjugates, a less studied but promising class of self-assembling NAs [29,30].

In recent years we worked on anticancer drug-containing self-assembling drug conjugates that spontaneously form NAs in aqueous media [31]. We reported NAs composed by conjugate releasable compounds [32]; by single and dual drug fluorescent hetero-NAs [33,34], by dual drug hetero-NAs (cyclopamine/taxol [34], cyclopamine/doxorubicin [35], ecdysteroid/doxorubicin [36]), and by self-assembling conjugate dual drug NAs [37]. We prepared compounds containing a squalene [31–35] or a 4-(1,2-diphenylbut-1-en-1-yl)aniline tail [37,38] that leads to NAs ability to self-assemble in water. We recently reported the assembly and characterization of squalene-thiocolchicine NAs that release cytotoxic, free thiocolchicine in cancer cells through a disulfide bond or a *p*-hydroxybenzyl moiety [38]. Here we describe the synthesis of two squalene-trehalose conjugates **1-Sq-mono** and **2-Sq-bis**, and of a betulinic acid-trehalose conjugate **3-Be-mono**, their assembly and characterization as NAs (respectively **mono-Sq-NA1**, **bis-Sq-NA2** and **mono-Be-NA3**, Figure 1), and their effects in biological assays. We measured cell viability to determine the safety of our NAs, while autophagy induction was selected as a validated neuroprotective mechanism of action in multiple neurodegenerative diseases [39]. Trehalose-containing NAs may significantly increase the weak, high mM effects of trehalose on autophagy induction [19], by facilitating its cellular internalization, and by releasing after NA disassembly/ester hydrolysis.

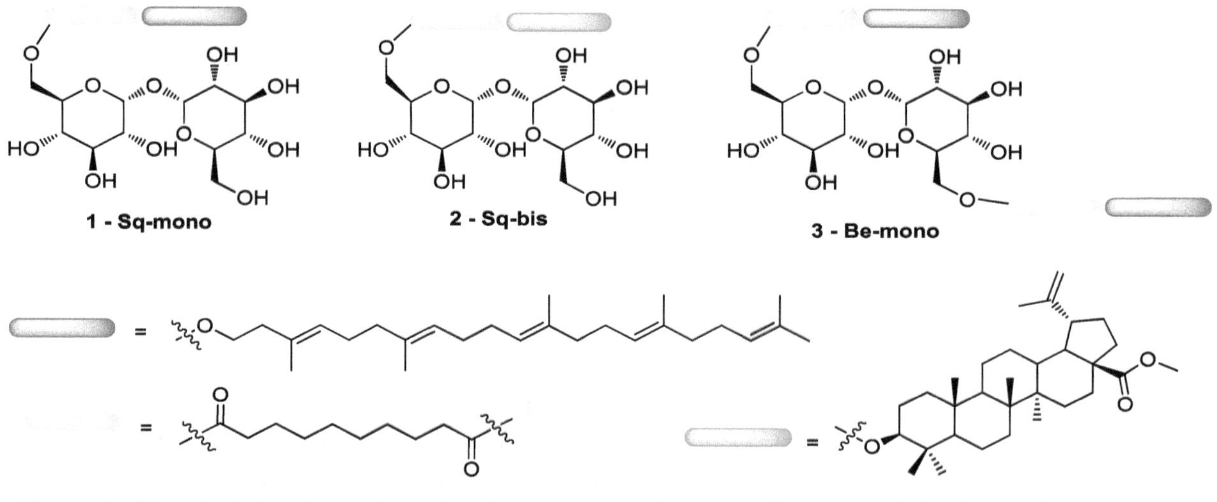

Figure 1. Chemical structure of nanolipid-trehalose conjugates **1-Sq-mono**, **2-Sq-bis**, and **3-Be-mono**.

2. Materials and Methods

2.1. Synthesis-General

Each reaction was carried out in oven-dried glassware, using dry solvents under a nitrogen atmosphere. Unless otherwise stated, these solvents were purchased from Sigma Aldrich Italy (Milan, Italy) and used without further purification. Chemical reagents were purchased from Sigma Aldrich, and used as such. Thin layer chromatography (TLC) was performed on Merck-pre-coated $60F_{254}$ plates. Reactions were monitored by TLC on silica gel, with detection by UV light (254 nm), or by charring either with a 1% permanganate solution or a 50% H_2SO_4 solution. Flash chromatography columns were run using silica gel (240–400 mesh, Merck Italy, Milan, Italy).

^{1}H-NMR spectra were recorded on Bruker DRX-400 and Bruker DRX-300 instruments (Billerica, MA, USA) in either $CDCl_3$, CD_3OD or DMSO-d6. ^{13}C-NMR spectra were recorded on the same

instrumentation (100 and 75 MHz) in either CDCl$_3$, CD$_3$OD or DMSO-d6. Chemical shifts (δ) for proton and carbon signals are quoted in parts per million (ppm) relative to tetramethylsilane (TMS), which was used as an internal standard. Electrospray ionization (ESI) MS spectra were recorded with a Waters Micromass Q-Tof micro mass spectrometer (Milford, MA, USA); HR-ESI mass spectra were recorded on a FT-ICR APEX$_{II}$ (Bruker, Billerica, MA, USA), while EI mass spectra were recorded at an ionizing voltage of 6 kEv on a VG 70-70 EQ. Specific rotations were measured with a P-1030-Jasco polarimeter with 10 cm optical path cells and 1 mL capacity (Na lamp, λ = 589 nm).

2.2. Synthesis-Squalene-Trehalose Conjugates 1-Sq-Mono and 2-Sq-Bis

1-[(2R,3R,4S,5R,6R)-6-{[(2R,3R,4S,5R,6R)-6-(hydroxymethyl)-3,4,5-tris[(trimethylsilyl)oxy]oxan-2-yl]oxy}-3,4,5-tris[(trimethylsilyl)oxy]oxan-2-yl]methyl10-(3E,7E,11E,15E)-3,7,12,16,20pentamethylhenicosa-3,7,11,15,19-pentaen-1-yl decanedioate/**15-mono** and 1-[(2R,3R,4S,5R,6R)-6-{[(2R,3R,4S,5R,6R)-6-{[(10-oxo-10-{[(3E,7E,11E,15E)-3,7,12,16,20-penta-methylhenicosa-3,7,11,15,19-pentaen-1-yl]oxy}-decanoyl)oxy]methyl}-3,4,5-tris[(trimethylsilyl)oxy]oxan-2-yl]oxy}-3,4,5-tris[(trimethylsilyl)oxy]-oxan-2-yl]methyl10-(3E,7E,11E,15E)-3,7,12,16,20-penta-methylhenicosa-3,7,11,15,19-pentaen-1-yl decanedioate/**16-bis**. EDC·HCl (223 mg, 1.161 mmol) and DMAP (5 mg, 0.039 mmol) were added under stirring at room temperature (RT) to a solution of hexaTMS-protected trehalose **5** [40] (300 mg, 0.387 mmol) in anhydrous toluene (8.3 mL). After 30 min, carboxylated squalene-linker adduct **6** [32] (221 mg, 0.387 mmol) was added, and the reaction mixture was stirred at 50 °C overnight. Reaction monitoring (TLC, eluant: 9:1 *n*-hexane/AcOEt) confirmed the disappearance of hexaTMS-protected trehalose **5**. The solvent was then removed under reduced pressure, and the crude oil was purified by flash chromatography (silicagel, eluant: 9:1 *n*-hexane/AcOEt) to obtain pure **15-mono** (232.9 mg, 0.175 mmol, 45% yield) and pure **16-bis** (101.2 mg, 0.054 mmol, 14% yield).

Analytical characterization. **15-mono**: ^1H-NMR (CDCl$_3$, 400 MHz): δ(ppm) = 5.21–5.05 (m, 5H), 4.94 (t, *J* = 2.8 Hz, 2H), 4.32 (dd, *J* = 11.8, 2.1 Hz, 1H), 4.12–3.98 (m, 4H), 3.98–3.82 (m, 3H), 3.71 (dd, *J* = 6.4, 3.4 Hz, 2H), 3.54–3.41 (m, 4H), 2.41–2.26 (m, 4H), 2.14–1.96 (m, 16H), 1.79–1.67 (m, 5H), 1.62–1.58 (m, 21H), 1.37–1.29 (m, 8H), 0.22–0.11 (m, 54H). ^{13}C-NMR (CDCl$_3$, 400 MHz): δ(ppm) = 173.33, 173.18, 134.88, 134.76, 134.07, 132.4, 132.00, 129.28, 129.17, 124.84, 124.57, 124.37, 93.83, 93.67, 73.77, 73.66, 73.03, 72.05, 71.94, 70.59, 70.10, 68.28, 63.61, 63.24, 61.27, 39.73 (2C), 35.72, 33.98, 33.87, 29.45, 29.04 (3C), 28.99, 28.86, 28.18, 26.68, 26.43 (2C), 25.95, 25.01, 24.91, 22.38 (2C), 17.95, 16.28, 16.22, 16.05, (1.35, 1.18, 0.36 = 18C). HR-ESI-MS: MW 1349.7973 calcd. for C$_{67}$H$_{130}$O$_{14}$Si$_6$Na, MW 1349.7982 found. Optical rotation, $[\alpha]_D^{20}$: −61.9°. **16-bis**: ^1H-NMR ((CDCl$_3$, 400 MHz): δ(ppm) = 5.16–5.10 (m, 10H), 4.94 (d, *J* = 3.0 Hz, 2H), 4.31–4.28 (m, 2H), 4.10–3.99 (d, *J* = 38.8 Hz, 8H), 3.95–3.90 (m, 2H), 3.52–3.44 (m, 4H), 2.38–2.28 (m, 8H), 2.13–1.98 (m, 36H), 1.77–1.68 (m, 10H), 1.66–1.59 (m, 38H), 1.36–1.28 (m, 16H), 0.21–0.11 (m, 54H). ^{13}C-NMR (CDCl$_3$, 400 MHz): δ(ppm) = 173.78 (2C), 173.62 (2C), 135.05 (2C), 134.90 (2C), 134.82 (2C), 133.65 (2C), 131.15 (2C), 125.07 (2C), 124.40 (4C), 124.29 (4C), 94.40 (2C), 73.48 (2C), 72.67 (2C), 71.94 (2C), 70.74 (2C), 63.94 (2C), 63.30 (2C), 39.73 (4C), 35.80 (2C), 34.33 (2C), 34.09 (2C), 29.68 (2C), 29.11 (6C), 28.77 (2C), 28.25 (4C), 26.91 (2C), 26.76 (2C), 26.65 (4C), 25.67 (4C), 24.96 (2C), 24.74 (2C), 17.66 (2C), 16.02 (4C), 15.85 (2C), (1.05, 0.87, 0.44, 0.17 = 18C). HR-ESI-MS: MW 1902.2516 calcd. for C$_{104}$H$_{190}$O$_{17}$Si$_6$Na, MW 1902.2524 found. Optical rotation, $[\alpha]_D^{20}$: −43.9°.

1-(3E,7E,11E,15E)-3,7,12,16,20-pentamethylhenicosa-3,7,11,15,19-pentaen-1-yl 10-[(2R,3S,4S,5R,6R)-3,4,5-trihydroxy-6-{[(2R,3R,4S,5S,6R)-3,4,5-trihydroxy-6-(hydroxymethyl)oxan-2-yl]oxy}oxan-2-yl]-methyl decanedioate/**1-Sq-mono**. Acetic acid (0.1 mL, 1.73 mmol) was added under stirring at RT to a solution of **15-mono** (230.0 mg, 0.173 mmol) in MeOH (3 mL), and the reaction mixture was stirred at 40 °C overnight. Reaction monitoring (TLC, eluant: 9:1 *n*-hexane/AcOEt) confirmed the disappearance of **15-mono**. The solvent was then removed under reduced pressure, and the crude solid was purified by flash chromatography (silicagel, eluant: 85:15 CH$_2$Cl$_2$/MeOH) to obtain pure target **1-Sq-mono** (153.2 mg, 0.171 mmol, quantitative yield).

Analytical characterization. ^1H-NMR (DMSO-d6, 400 MHz): δ(ppm) = 5.00–4.91 (m, 6H), 4.75 (d, *J* = 3.7 Hz, 2H), 4.72 (d, *J* = 3.6 Hz, 1H), 4.64 (t, *J* = 4.7 Hz, 2H), 4.55 (dd, *J* = 6.2, 1.8 Hz, 2H), 4.22

(t, J = 6.0 Hz, 1H), 4.13–4.10 (m, 1H), 3.92 (dd, J = 11.8, 5.4 Hz, 1H), 3.83 (t, J = 6.6 Hz, 2H), 3.80–3.76 (m, 1H), 3.55–3.51 (m, 1H), 3.46–3.40 (m, 3H), 3.38–3.32 (m, 1H), 3.16–3.10 (m, 2H), 3.04–2.98 (m, 2H), 2.1–2.12 (m, 4H), 1.95–1.79 (m, 18H), 1.56–1.49 (m, 5H), 1.44 (bs, 15H), 1.41–1.37 (m, 4H), 1.13 (bs, 8H). ^{13}C-NMR (DMSO-d6, 100 MHz): δ(ppm): δ 173.28, 173.22, 134.83, 134.77, 134.73, 133.97, 131.04, 124.82, 124.59, 124.52, 124.46, 124.35, 93.81, 93.71, 73.30, 73.26, 73.04, 72.05, 71.94, 70.59 (2C), 70.10, 63.63, 63.56, 61.27, 40.62, 39.64, 39.59, 39.37, 35.71, 33.98 (2C), 31.59, 30.28, 29.46, 29.06, 29.03, 28.91, 28.16, 26.82, 26.67, 26.42 (2C), 25.90, 24.96, 24.89, 17.94, 16.21, 16.06. *HR-ESI-MS*: MW 917.5602 calcd. for $C_{49}H_{82}O_{14}Na$, MW 917.5623 found. Optical rotation, $[\alpha]_D^{20}$: −59.4°.

1-(3E,7E,11E,15E)-3,7,12,16,20-pentamethylhenicosa-3,7,11,15,19-pentaen-1-yl   10-[(2R,3S,4S, 5R,6R)-3,4,5-trihydroxy-6-{[(2R,3R,4S,5S,6R)-3,4,5-trihydroxy-6-{[(10-oxo-10-{[(3E,7E,11E,15E)-3,7,12,16, 20-pentamethylhenicosa-3,7,11,15,19-pentaen-1-yl]oxy}decanoyl)oxy]methyl}oxan-2-yl]oxy}oxan-2-yl]-methyl decanedioate/**2-Sq-bis**. Acetic acid (30 μL, 0.53 mmol) was added under stirring at RT to a solution of **16-bis** (100.0 mg, 0.053 mmol) in MeOH (1 mL), and the reaction mixture was stirred at 40 °C overnight. Reaction monitoring (TLC, eluant: 9:1 *n*-hexane/AcOEt) confirmed the disappearance of **16-bis**. The solvent was then removed under reduced pressure, and the crude solid was purified by flash chromatography (silicagel, eluant: 85:15 CH_2Cl_2/MeOH) to obtain pure target **2-Sq-bis** (69.1 mg, 0.047 mmol, 90% yield). Analytical characterization. ^1H-NMR (DMSO-d6, 400 MHz): δ(ppm) = 5.12–5.04 (m, 12H), 4.88 (d, J = 4.9 Hz, 2H), 4.83 (d, J = 3.6 Hz, 2H), 4.75 (d, J = 6.1 Hz, 2H), 4.25–4.21 (m, 2H), 4.03 (dd, J = 11.7, 5.6 Hz, 2H), 3.95 (t, J = 6.6 Hz, 4H), 3.92–3.87 (m, 2H), 3.58–3.52 (m, 2H), 3.28–3.23 (m, 2H), 3.15–3.09 (m, 2H), 2.28–2.23 (m, 8H), 2.07–1.90 (m, 36H), 1.67–1.60 (m, 10H), 1.55–1.47 (m, 38H), 1.24 (s, 16H). ^{13}C-NMR (DMSO-d6, 100 MHz): δ(ppm): 173.90 (2C), 173.64 (2C), 134.81 (2C), 134.72 (2C), 134.64 (2C), 133.63 (2C), 131.08 (2C), 124.94 (2C), 124.57 (2C), 124.52 (2C), 124.47 (2C), 124.32 (2C), 93.75 (2C), 73.52 (2C), 72.56 (2C), 71.93 (2C), 70.71 (2C),63.99 (2C), 63.34 (2C), 39.74 (4C), 39.65 (2C), 35.86 (2C), 34.38 (2C), 34.12 (2C), 29.74 (2C), 29.17 (2C), 29.10 (4C), 28.28 (4C), 26.92 (2C), 26.81 (2C), 26.68 (2C), 26.65 (2C), 25.67 (4C), 24.98 (2C), 24.90 (2C), 17.94 (2C), 16.24 (4C), 16.06 (2C). *HR-ESI-MS*: MW 1470.0147 calcd. for $C_{86}H_{142}O_{17}Na$, MW 1470.0146 found. Optical rotation, $[\alpha]_D^{20}$: −33.7°.

2.3. Synthesis—Betulinic Acid-trehalose Conjugate 3–Be-mono

Methyl(1R,3aS,5aR,5bR,9S,11aR)-9-hydroxy-5a,5b,8,8,11a-pentamethyl-1-(prop-1-en-2-yl)-icosa-hydro-1H-cyclopenta[a]chrysene-3a-carboxylate/**18**. Trimethylsilyl diazomethane (2M in *n*-hexane, 0.66 mL, 1.312 mmol) was added to a solution of betulinic acid **17** (500 mg, 1.093 mmol) in dry MeOH (10 mL) and dry toluene (15 mL). The reaction was stirred overnight at RT, and reaction monitoring (TLC, eluant 7:3 *n*-hexane/AcOEt with 1% HCOOH) confirmed the disappearance of starting material **16**. The reaction mixture was diluted with diethyl ether (13 mL) and 10% AcOH (10 mL). The aqueous layer was extracted with diethyl ether (3 × 10 mL), and the collected organic phases were washed with sat. Na_2CO_3 (10 mL), dried with Na_2SO_4 and then evaporated under reduced pressure to obtain pure **18** as a white solid (486.1 mg, 1.032 mmol, 95% yield).

Analytical characterization. ^1H-NMR (CDCl_3, 400 MHz): δ(ppm) = 4.63 (bs, 1H), 4.49 (bs, 1H), 3.56 (s, 3H), 3.07 (dd, J = 11.2, 5.1 Hz, 1H), 2.89 (td, J = 10.9, 4.4 Hz, 1H), 2.20–2.02 (m, 2H), 1.77 (dt, J = 10.9, 5.9 Hz, 2H), 1.58 (s, 3H), 0.86 (s, 6H), 0.81 (s, 3H), 0.71 (s, 3H), 0.65 (s, 3H). *HR-ESI-MS*: MW 493.3658 calcd. for $C_{31}H_{50}O_3Na$, MW 493.3661 found. Optical rotation, $[\alpha]_D^{20}$: +5.1°.

10-oxo-10-[2-(trimethylsilyl)ethoxy]decanoic acid/**19**. Trimethylsilylethanol (313 mL, 2.181 mmol), EDC.HCl (559 mg, 2.909 mmol) and DMAP (89 mg, 0.727 mmol) were added under stirring at RT to a solution of sebacic acid **14** (1 g, 0.4942 mmol) in dry CH_2Cl_2 (25 mL) and pyridine (2.5 mL). The reaction mixture was stirred at RT overnight. The reaction mixture was then washed with 10% phosphoric acid (2 × 15 mL) and brine (20 mL).

The organic layer was dried with Na_2SO_4 and evaporated under reduced pressure, and the crude oil was purified by flash chromatography (silicagel, eluant: 8:2 *n*-hexane/AcOEt with 1% HCOOH) to obtain pure **19** (408 mg, 1.342 mmol, 27% yield).

Analytical characterization. ^1H-NMR (CDCl$_3$, 400 MHz): δ(ppm) = 4.21–4.12 (m, 2H), 2.38 (t, J = 4.5 Hz, 2H), 2.32 (t, J = 4.3 Hz, 2H), 1.73–1.59 (m, 4H), 1.41–1.28 (m, 8H), 1.01–0.97 (m, 2H), 0.04 (s, 9H). ^{13}C-NMR: (CDCl$_3$, 100 MHz): δ(ppm) = 177.93, 173.60, 62.58, 34.32, 34.22, 29.46, 29.48, 29.30, 29.10, 25.12, 25.07, 17.05, −1.53 (3C). HR-ESI-MS: MW 325.1811 calcd. for C$_{15}$H$_{30}$O$_4$SiNa, MW 325.1815 found.

(1R,3aS,5aR,5bR,9S,11aR)-3a-(methoxycarbonyl)-5a,5b,8,8,11a-pentamethyl-1-(prop-1-en-2-yl)-icosahydro-1H-cyclopenta[a]chrysen-9-yl 1-[2-(trimethylsilyl)ethyl] decanedioate/20. Dicyclohexylcarbodiimide (DCC, 201 mg, 0.973 mmol) and dimethylaminopyridine (DMAP, 30 mg, 0.243 mmol) were added under stirring to a solution of compound 18 (229 mg, 0.487 mmol) and compound 19 (221 mg, 0.731 mmol) in dry CH$_2$Cl$_2$ (5 mL) at 0 °C. The reaction was left stirring at RT overnight. Reaction monitoring (TLC, eluant: 9:1 n-hexane/AcOEt) confirmed the disappearance of starting material 18. The mixture was diluted with CH$_2$Cl$_2$ (10 mL) and was filtered on a plug of celite. The solvent was removed under reduced pressure, and the resulting crude oil was purified by flash chromatography (silicagel, eluant: 96:4 n-hexane/AcOEt) to obtain pure 20 (339 mg, 0.449 mmol, 92% yield).

Analytical characterization. ^1H-NMR (CDCl$_3$, 400 MHz): δ(ppm) = 4.74 (bs, 1H), 4.61 (bs, 1H), 4.48 (dd, J = 10.1, 6.2 Hz, 1H), 4.21–4.12 (m, 2H), 3.67 (s, 3H), 3.06–2.95 (m, 1H), 2.33–2.13 (m, 6H), 1.97–1.82 (m, 2H), 1.69 (s, 3H), 1.47–1.34 (m, 8H), 0.97 (s, 3H), 0.92 (s, 3H), 0.85 (s, 3H), 0.84 (s, 6H), 0.05 (s, 9H). ^{13}C-NMR: (CDCl$_3$, 100 MHz): δ(ppm) = 176.67, 174.00, 173.64, 150.57, 109.63, 80.61, 62.37, 56.57, 55.45 (2C), 51.25, 50.46, 49.48, 47.01, 42.40, 40.70, 38.40, 38.27, 37.85, 37.12, 36.98, 34.82, 34.52, 34.27, 32.18, 30.61, 29.68, 29.10 (3C), 27.97, 25.49, 25.12, 24.95, 23.75, 20.91, 19.36, 18.19, 17.33, 16.57, 16.18, 15.96, 14.69, −1.47 (3C). HR-ESI-MS: MW 777.5465 calcd. for C$_{46}$H$_{78}$O$_6$SiNa, MW 777.5469 found. Optical rotation, $[\alpha]_D^{20}$: +10.2°.

10-{[(1R,3aS,5aR,5bR,9S,11aR)-3a-(methoxycarbonyl)-5a,5b,8,8,11a-pentamethyl-1-(prop-1-en-2-yl)-icosahydro-1H-cyclopenta[a]chrysen-9-yl]oxy}-10-oxodecanoic acid/21. Tetrabutylammonium fluoride (TBAF, 0.61 mL, 2.11 mmol) was added under stirring to a solution of compound 19 (318 mg, 0.421 mmol) in dry THF (15 mL), and the reaction mixture was stirred at RT overnight. Reaction monitoring (TLC, eluant: 9:1 n-hexane/AcOEt with 1% HCOOH) confirmed the disappearance of starting material 20. The reaction was quenched by an addition of sat. NH$_4$Cl (10 mL). The aqueous phase was extracted with AcOEt (2 × 10 mL), the collected organic phases were dried with Na$_2$SO$_4$ and evaporated under reduced pressure to obtain pure 21 (258 mg, 0.393 mmol, 93% yield).

Analytical characterization. ^1H-NMR (CDCl$_3$, 400 MHz): δ(ppm) = 4.72 (bs, 1H), 4.58 (bs, 1H), 4.44 (dd, J = 10.1, 6.2 Hz, 1H), 3.65 (s, 3H), 3.03–2.94 (m, 1H), 2.23–2.16 (m, 6H), 1.92–1.82 (m, 2H), 1.67 (s, 3H), 1.47–1.34 (m, 8H), 0.95 (s, 3H), 0.90 (s, 3H), 0.84 (s, 3H), 0.82 (s, 6H). ^{13}C-NMR (CDCl$_3$, 100 MHz): δ(ppm) 180.32, 177.30, 174.33, 151.11, 110.29, 81.31, 57.20, 56.08 (2C), 51.89, 51.10, 50.12, 47.63, 43.04, 41.34, 39.04, 38.90, 38.47, 37.76, 37.60, 35.43, 34.92, 34.70, 32.81, 31.25, 30.32, 29.68 (3C), 28.61, 26.13, 25.73, 25.29, 24.38, 21.56, 20.00, 18.84, 17.21, 16.81, 16.59, 15.33. HR-ESI-MS: MW 677.4757 calcd. for C$_{41}$H$_{66}$O$_6$Na, MW 677.4761 found. Optical rotation, $[\alpha]_D^{20}$: +12.9°.

(1R,3aS,5aR,5bR,9S,11aR)-3a-(methoxycarbonyl)-5a,5b,8,8,11a-pentamethyl-1-(prop-1-en-2-yl)-icosahydro-1H-cyclopenta[a]chrysen-9-yl-1-[(2R,3R,4S,5R,6R)-6-{[(2R,3R,4S,5R,6R)-6-(hydroxy met-hyl)-3,4,5-tris[(trimethylsilyl)oxy]oxan-2-yl]oxy}-3,4,5-tris[(trimethylsilyl)oxy]oxan-2-yl]methyl decanedioate/22-mono and (1R,3aS,5aR,5bR,9S,11aR)-3a-(methoxycarbonyl)-5a,5b,8,8,11a-pentamethyl-1-(prop-1-en-2-yl)-icosahydro-1H-cyclopenta[a]chrysen-9-yl 1-[(2R,3R,4S,5R,6R)-6-{[(2R,3R,4S,5R,6R)-6-{[(10-{[(1R,3aS,5aR,5bR,9S,11aR)-3a-(methoxycarbonyl)-5a,5b,8,8,11a-penta-methyl-1-(prop-1-en-2-yl)-icosahydro-1H-cyclopenta[a]chrysen-9-yl]oxy}-10-oxodecanoyl)oxy]-methyl}-3,4,5-tris[(trimethylsilyl)oxy]oxan-2-yl]oxy}-3,4,5-tris[(trimethylsilyl)oxy]oxan-2-yl]methyl decanedioate/23-bis. EDC·HCl (15 mg, 0.0763 mmol) and DMAP (1 mg, 0.00763 mmol) were added under stirring at RT to a solution of hexaTMS-protected trehalose 5 [40]. (59 mg, 0.0763 mmol) in anhydrous toluene (4 mL). After 30 min, compound 21 (50 mg, 0.0763 mmol) was added, and the reaction mixture was stirred at 50 °C overnight. Reaction monitoring (TLC, eluant: 7:3 n-hexane/AcOEt) confirmed the disappearance of starting material 21. The solvent was then removed under reduced pressure, and the crude oil was purified by flash chromatography (silicagel, eluant: 85:15 n-hexane/AcOEt) to obtain pure **22-mono** (23 mg, 0.0163 mmol, 21% yield) and pure **23-bis** (24 mg, 0.0117 mmol, 15% yield).

Analytical characterization. **22-mono**: ^1H-NMR (CD$_3$OD, 400 MHz): δ(ppm) = 4.96 (dd, J = 3.0, 1.9 Hz, 2H), 4.74 (d, J = 2.1 Hz, 1H), 4.67–4.58 (m, 1H), 4.47 (dd, J = 10.6, 5.7 Hz, 1H), 4.43–4.34 (m, 1H), 4.12–4.02 (m, 2H), 3.99 (td, J = 9.0, 3.1 Hz, 2H), 3.87 (dt, J = 9.5, 3.0 Hz, 1H), 3.70–3.68 (m, 5H), 3.61–3.45 (m, 4H), 3.34–3.32 (m, 2H), 3.02 (td, J = 10.8, 4.7 Hz, 1H), 2.44–2.23 (m, 6H), 1.90 (tt, J = 11.7, 5.8 Hz, 2H), 1.78–1.70 (m, 6H), 1.36 (s, 3H), 1.04 (s, 3H), 0.97 (s, 3H), 0.92 (s, 3H), 0.89 (s, 3H), 0.88 (s, 3H), 0.25–0.14 (m, 54H). ^{13}C-NMR (CD$_3$OD, 400 MHz): δ (ppm) = 176.69, 173.89, 173.68, 150.33, 108.96, 94.45, 94.19, 80.81, 73.58, 73.54, 73.31, 72.66 (2C), 72.01, 71.21, 70.72, 62.91, 60.41, 56.48, 55.45 (2C), 50.44, 49.24, 47.09, 42.17, 40.53, 38.24, 38.19, 37.52, 36.91, 36.47, 34.16, 34.06, 33.62, 31.74, 30.24, 29.42, 28.78 (2C), 28.73, 28.62, 27.22, 25.38, 24.80, 24.58, 23.38, 20.72, 18.21, 17.90, 15.75, 15.42, 15.20, 13.83, (0.19, −0.25, −0.99, −1.07 = 18C). HR-ESI-MS: MW 1433.8185 calcd. for C$_{71}$H$_{134}$O$_{16}$Si$_6$Na, MW 1433.8191 found. Optical rotation, $[\alpha]_D^{20}$: +60.3°. **23-bis**: ^1H-NMR (CDCl$_3$, 400 MHz, detected signals): δ(ppm) = 4.94 (d, J = 3.0 Hz, 2H), 4.76 (d, J = 2.0 Hz, 2H), 4.62 (d, J = 3.2 Hz, 2H), 4.53–4.44 (m, 2H), 4.29 (dd, J = 11.8, 2.0 Hz, 2H), 4.07 (dd, J = 11.8, 4.3 Hz, 2H), 4.02 (ddd, J = 9.4, 4.2, 2.1 Hz, 2H), 3.92 (t, J = 9.0 Hz, 2H), 3.69 (s, 6H), 3.50 (t, J = 9.0 Hz, 2H), 3.46 (dd, J = 9.3, 3.1 Hz, 2H), 3.01 (td, J = 10.8, 4.2 Hz, 2H), 2.40–2.16 (m, 12H), 1.98–1.83 (m, 4H), 1.71 (s, 6H), 1.68–1.56 (m, 16H), 1.28 (s, 6H), 0.98 (s, 6H), 0.93 (s, 6H), 0.86 (s, 6H), 0.85 (s, 12H), 0.16 (m, 54H).

^{13}C-NMR (CDCl$_3$, 100 MHz): δ (ppm) = 176.66 (2C), 173.68 (2C), 173.60 (2C), 150.55 (2C), 109.62 (2C), 94.44 (2C), 80.61 (2C), 73.49 (2C), 72.67 (2C), 71.94 (2C), 70.75 (2C), 63.31 (2C), 56.57 (2C), 55.46 (2C), 51.23 (2C), 50.47 (2C), 49.49 (2C), 47.01 (2C), 42.40 (2C), 40.71 (2C), 38.40 (2C), 38.27 (2C), 37.84 (2C), 37.13 (2C), 36.97 (2C), 34.81 (2C), 34.28 (2C), 34.11 (2C), 32.18 (2C), 30.61 (2C), 29.68 (2C), 29.14 (2C), 29.11 (2C), 29.09 (2C), 27.97 (2C), 25.49 (2C), 25.12 (2C), 24.75 (2C), 23.75 (2C), 20.91 (2C), 19.35 (2C), 18.19 (2C), 16.56 (2C), 16.16 (2C), 15.96 (2C), 14.69 (2C), 14.10 (2C), (1.06, 0.88, 0.18 =18C). HR-ESI-MS: MW 2070.2939 calcd. for C$_{112}$H$_{198}$O$_{21}$Si$_6$Na, MW 2070.2949 found. Optical rotation, $[\alpha]_D^{20}$: +41.2°.

(1R,3aS,5aR,5bR,9S,11aR)-3a-(methoxycarbonyl)-5a,5b,8,8,11a-pentamethyl-1-(prop-1-en-2-yl)-icosahydro-1H-cyclopenta[a]chrysen-9-yl 1-[(2R,3S,4S,5R,6R)-3,4,5-trihydroxy-6-{[(2R,3R,4S,5S,6R)-3,4,5-trihydroxy-6-(hydroxymethyl)oxan-2-yl]oxy}oxan-2-yl]methyl decanedioate/**3-Be-mono**. Acetic acid (18 μL, 0.324 mmol) was added under stirring at RT to a solution of **22-mono** (23 mg, 0.0162 mmol) in MeOH (1 mL), and the reaction mixture was stirred at 40 °C for two days. Reaction monitoring (TLC, eluant: 98:2 CH$_2$Cl$_2$/MeOH) confirmed the disappearance of starting **22-mono**. The solvent was then removed under reduced pressure to obtain pure target **3-Be-mono** (13 mg, 0.0133 mmol, 82% yield).

Analytical characterization. ^1H-NMR (CDCl$_3$, 400 MHz): δ(ppm) = 4.98 (dd, J = 3.0, 1.9 Hz, 2H), 4.76 (d, J = 2.0 Hz, 1H), 4.65–4.59 (m, 1H), 4.52–4.42 (m, 1H), 4.45–4.37 (m, 1H), 4.11–4.02 (m, 2H), 3.97 (td, J = 8.9, 3.1 Hz, 2H), 3.84 (dt, J = 9.4, 3.1 Hz, 1H), 3.72–3.67 (m, 5H), 3.60–3.43 (m, 4H), 3.35–3.33 (m, 2H), 3.01 (td, J = 10.8, 4.7 Hz, 1H), 2.43–2.17 (m, 6H), 1.98–1.85 (m, 2H), 1.75–1.68 (m, 6H), 1.28 (s, 3H), 0.98 (s, 3H), 0.94 (s, 3H), 0.87 (s, 3H), 0.85 (s, 6H). ^{13}C-NMR (CDCl$_3$, 100 MHz): δ(ppm) = 176.64, 173.80, 173.72, 150.50, 109.65, 94.42, 94.15, 80.74, 73.59, 73.51, 73.30, 72.66, 72.62, 72.04, 71.25, 70.68, 62.90, 60.37, 56.56, 55.44, 51.24, 50.46, 49.49, 47.00, 42.40, 40.71, 38.40, 38.26, 37.85, 37.13, 36.96, 34.82, 34.28, 34.18, 34.12, 34.09, 32.18, 30.62, 29.69, 29.35, 29.17, 28.01, 25.48, 25.14, 24.81, 23.75, 20.92, 19.38, 18.21, 16.61, 16.18, 15.96, 14.71. HR-ESI-MS: MW 1001.5813 calcd. for C$_{53}$H$_{86}$O$_{16}$Na, MW 1001.5819 found. Optical rotation, $[\alpha]_D^{20}$: +70.6°.

Attempted synthesis of (1R,3aS,5aR,5bR,9S,11aR)-3a-(methoxycarbonyl)-5a,5b,8,8,11a-pentamethyl-1-(prop-1-en-2-yl)-icosahydro-1H-cyclopenta[a]chrysen-9-yl 1-[(2R,3S,4S,5R,6R)-6-{[(2R,3R,4S,5S,6R)-6-{[(10-{[(1R,3aS,5aR,5bR,9S,11aR)-3a-(methoxycarbonyl)-5a,5b,8,8,11a-pentamethyl-1-(prop-1-en-2-yl)-icosahydro-1H-cyclopenta[a]chrysen-9-yl]oxy}-10-oxodecanoyl)oxy]methyl}-3,4,5-trihydroxyoxan-2-yl]oxy}-3,4,5-trihydroxyoxan-2-yl]methyl decanedioate/**4-Be-bis**. Acetic acid (13 μL, 0.234 mmol) was added under stirring at RT to a solution of **23-bis** (24 mg, 0.0117 mmol) in MeOH (1 mL), and the reaction mixture was stirred at 40 °C for four days. Reaction monitoring (TLC, eluant: 98:2 CH$_2$Cl$_2$/MeOH) showed the formation of a series of uncharacterizable degradation products.

2.4. NA Assembly and Characterization

Mono-Sq-NA1. In accordance with standard solvent evaporation protocols [41] the squalene-trehalose conjugate **1-mono** (4.0 mg) was first dissolved in THF (1 mL) in a vial while stirring at RT. The resulting solution was added dropwise to a round bottom flask containing MilliQ grade distilled water (2 mL) under magnetic stirring (500 rpm). The resulting suspension was stirred for 5 min, then THF was thoroughly evaporated under reduced pressure, obtaining pure **mono-Sq-NA1** as an opalescent suspension (2 mL, 2 mg/mL).

Bis-Sq-NA2. In accordance with standard solvent evaporation protocols [41] the squalene-trehalose conjugate **2-bis** (4.0 mg) was first dissolved in THF (1 mL) in a vial while stirring at RT. The resulting solution was added dropwise to a round bottom flask containing MilliQ grade distilled water (2 mL) under magnetic stirring (500 rpm). The resulting suspension was stirred for 5 min, then THF was thoroughly evaporated under reduced pressure, obtaining pure **bis-Sq-NA2** as opalescent suspension (2 mL, 2 mg/mL).

Mono-Be-NA3. In accordance with standard solvent evaporation protocols [41] the betulinic acid-trehalose conjugate **3-mono** (4.0 mg) was first dissolved in THF (1 mL) in a vial while stirring at RT. The resulting solution was added dropwise to a round bottom flask containing MilliQ grade distilled water (2 mL) under magnetic stirring (500 rpm). The resulting suspension was stirred for 5 min, then THF was thoroughly evaporated under reduced pressure, obtaining pure **mono-Be-NA3** as opalescent suspension (2 mL, 2 mg/mL).

NA Characterization. NAs were characterized by dynamic light scattering (DLS), using a 90 Plus Particle Size Analyzer from Brookhaven Instrument Corporation (Holtsville, NY, USA) operating at 15 mW of a solid-state laser (λ = 661 nm), using a 90-degree scattering angle. The ζ-potential was determined at 25 °C using a 90 Plus Particle Size Analyzer from Brookhaven Instrument Corporation (Holtsville, NY, USA) equipped with an AQ-809 electrode, operating at an applied voltage of 120 V. Each sample was diluted to a concentration of 0.2 mg/mL and sonicated for 3 min before each experiment. Ten independent measurements of 60 s duration were performed for each sample. Hydrodynamic diameters were calculated using Mie theory, considering the absolute viscosity and refractive index values of the medium to be 0.890 cP and 1.33, respectively. The same aqueous samples at a concentration of 0.2 mg/mL were used for ζ-potential measurement, without any change for the ionic strength (no addition of KCl). The ζ-potential was calculated from the electrophoretic mobility of nanoparticles, by using the Smoluchowski theory [42].

2.5. Biology

Cell cultures. HeLa cells (ATCC: CCL-2) were cultured in DMEM with 10% FBS, 1% penicillin/streptomicin and 1% glutamine in a humidified atmosphere of 5% CO_2 at 37 °C (all reagents from Euroclone). Cultures were treated with lipid-trehalose conjugates or NAs for 2 or 48 h at 37 °C at the concentration indicated in the text.

Cytotoxicity assay. We performed the 3-(4,5-dimethylthiazol-2-yl)-2,5-diphenyltetrazolium bromide (MTT) assay to measure culture vitality. HeLa cells were cultured in a 96-well plate at a concentration of 5×10^3 cell/cm^2 and incubated at 37 °C for 24 h. MTT was added in cell medium at a final concentration of 0.25 mg/mL. Incubation lasted 30 min at 37 °C. Then, the medium was removed and formazan precipitates were collected in 200 μL of DMSO. The absorbance measured at 570 nm using a spectrophotometer reflects cell viability. Cell viability was expressed as fold over control condition set at 100%.

Autophagy assay. We assessed autophagy by monitoring LC3 conversion by western-blotting as previously described [43]. Briefly, upon a wash in PBS, cells were solubilized in RIPA buffer (150 mM NaCl, 50 mM HEPES, 0.5% NP40, 1% sodium-deoxycholate). After 1 h under mild agitation, the lysate was clarified by centrifugation for 20 min at 16,000 g. All experimental procedures were performed at 4 °C. Protein concentrations were evaluated via Bradford assay (Bio-Rad, Segrate, Italy). For Western blotting experiments, an equal amount of proteins was diluted with 0.25% 5X Laemmli buffer, separated onto 10% SDS-PAGE gels and transferred onto nitrocellulose membrane (Sigma-Aldrich Italy, Milan, Italy) at 80 V for 120 min at 4 °C.

Primary antibodies (source in parentheses) included: Mouse anti-LC3, 1:500 (Enzo Life Sciences AG, Lausen, Switzerland), and mouse anti β-actin 1:1000 (Sigma Aldrich Italy, Milan, Italy) which were applied overnight in blocking buffer (20 mM Tris, pH 7.4, 150 mM NaCl, 0.1% Tween 20, and 5% nonfat dry milk). Proteins were detected using the ECL prime detection system (GE Healthcare). Images were acquired with the imaging ChemiDoc Touch system (Bio Rad Laboratory Italy, Segrate, Italy), and the optical density of the specific bands was measured with ImageLab software (Bio Rad).

2.6. Statistical Analysis

All data are reported as mean ± standard error of the mean (SEM). The entire data-set was logged into GraphPad Prism and analyzed via unpaired Student's T-test (two classes) or ANOVA followed by Tukey's posthoc test (more than two classes). Number of experiments (n) and level of significance (p) are indicated throughout the text.

3. Results

3.1. Synthesis of Target 1-mono and 2-bis Squalene-Trehalose Conjugates

In order to obtain either a mono-(target compound **1-Sq-mono**, 1:1 squalene-trehalose conjugate) and a bis-squalenylated trehalose construct (target compound **2-Sq-bis**, 2:1 squalene-trehalose conjugate), we focused our attention onto the hexaTMS-protected trehalose derivative **5** [38] and the carboxylated squalene-linker adduct **6** [31] (Figure 2).

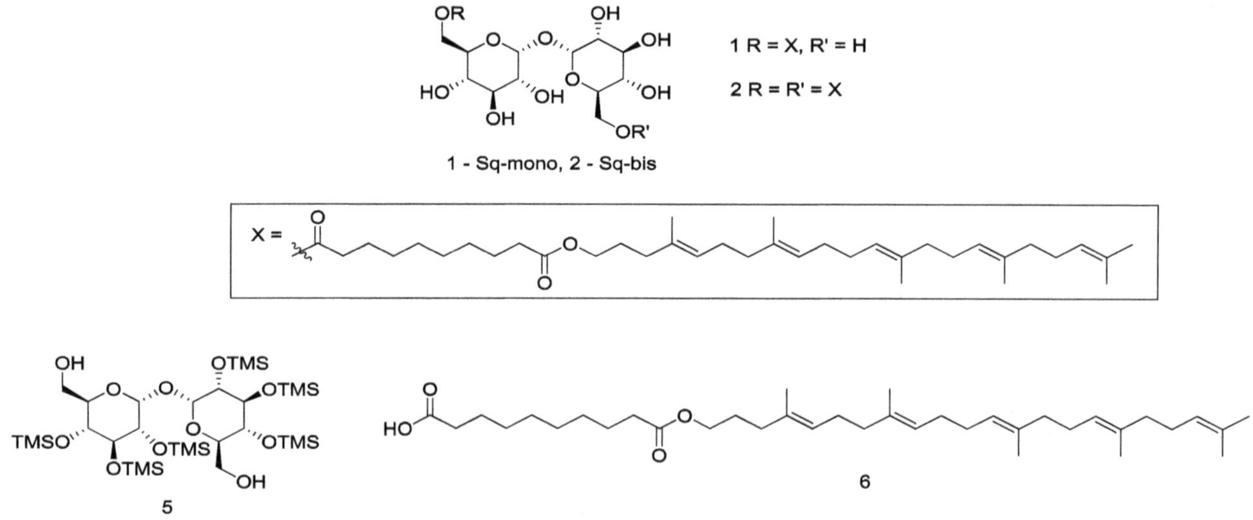

Figure 2. Chemical structure of target squalene-trehalose conjugates **1-Sq-mono** and **2-Sq-bis**, and of key synthetic intermediate hexaTMS-protected trehalose **5** and carboxylated squalene-linker adduct **6**.

The synthesis of key intermediates **5** [38] and **6** [31] is reported respectively in Schemes 1 and 2.

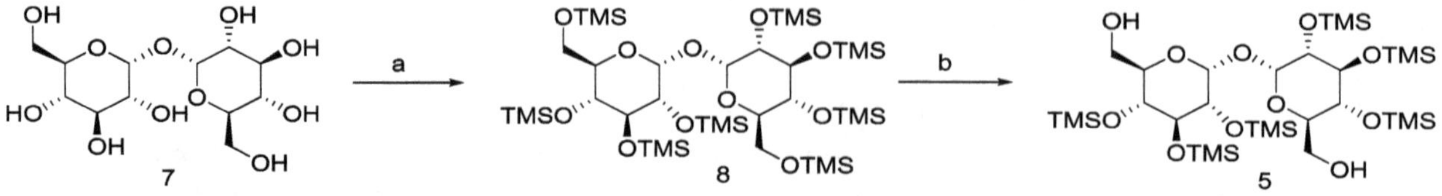

a: TMS-Cl, pyridine, 0°C to rt, overnight; b: K$_2$CO$_3$, 3:1 MeOH/CH$_2$Cl$_2$, 0°C to rt, 90 min, **75% yield** (2 steps)

Scheme 1. Synthesis of hexaTMS-protected trehalose **5**.

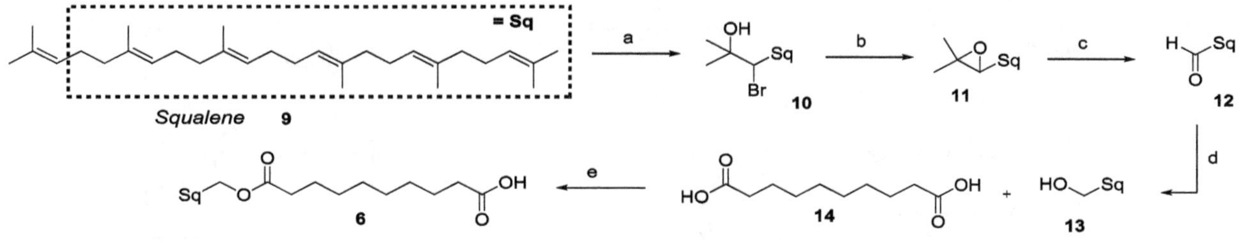

a: NBS, H$_2$O, THF, rt, 3h, **31%** yield; b: K$_2$CO$_3$, MeOH, rt, 2h, **quantitative** yield; c: H$_5$IO$_6$, dioxane, H$_2$O, rt, 2h, **86%** yield;
d: NaBH$_4$, MeOH, rt, 2h, **91%** yield; e: EDC.HCl, DMAP, CH$_2$Cl$_2$, rt, overnight, **60%** yield.

Scheme 2. Synthesis of carboxylated squalene-linker adduct **6**.

HexaTMS-protected trehalose **5** was obtained through per-silylation of commercially-available trehalose **7** with TMS-Cl (per-silylated **8**, step a), followed by a selective deprotection of primary, more easily accessible, hydroxyls (step b, Scheme 1).

Commercial squalene **9** was sequentially submitted to halohydration (bromohydrine **10**, step a), base-promoted elimination (epoxide **11**, step b), oxidative cleavage (aldehyde **12**), reduction (alcohol **13**) and mono-esterification with diacid **14**, to provide target carboxylated squalene adduct **6** (step e, Scheme 2).

Finally, key intermediates **5** and **6** were coupled in equimolar amounts in an esterification protocol, obtaining a ≈ 3:1 mixture of **15-mono** and **16-bis** hexaTMS-protected compounds (step a, Scheme 3).

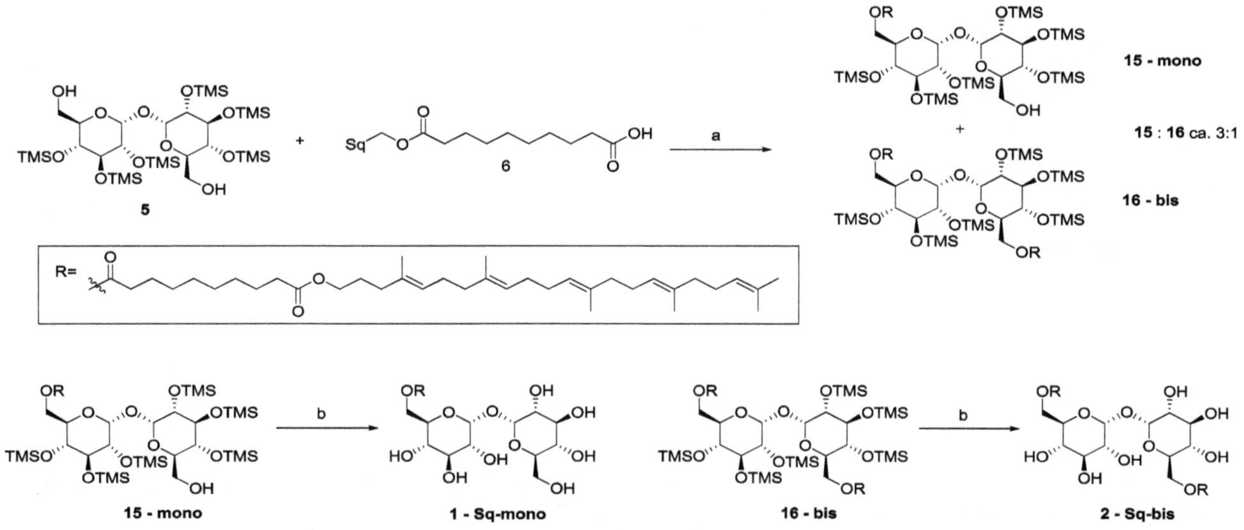

a: EDC.HCl, DMAP, CH$_2$Cl$_2$, rt, overnight, **45%** yield (**15-mono**), **14%** yield (**16 - bis**);
b: AcOH, MeOH, 40°C, overnight, **quantitative** yield (**1 - Sq-mono**), **90%** yield (**2 - Sq-bis**).

Scheme 3. Synthesis of target **1-Sq-mono** and **2-Sq-bis** squalene-trehalose conjugates.

After chromatographic separation, both hexaTMS protected compounds **15-mono** and **16-bis** were submitted to acidic deprotection, yielding respectively **1-Sq-mono** and **2-Sq-bis** targets, respectively in **45%** and **13%** overall yields from **5** and **6** (step b, Scheme 3).

*3.2. Synthesis of Target **3-Be-mono** Betulinic Acid-Trehalose Conjugate, Attempted Synthesis of Target **4-Be bis** Betulinic Acid-Trehalose Conjugate*

In order to obtain the target **3-Be-mono** betulinic acid-trehalose conjugate we adopted a similar strategy, focusing our attention onto the same hexaTMS-protected trehalose derivative **5** [38] and the carboxylated betulinic-linker adduct **21** (Figure 3).

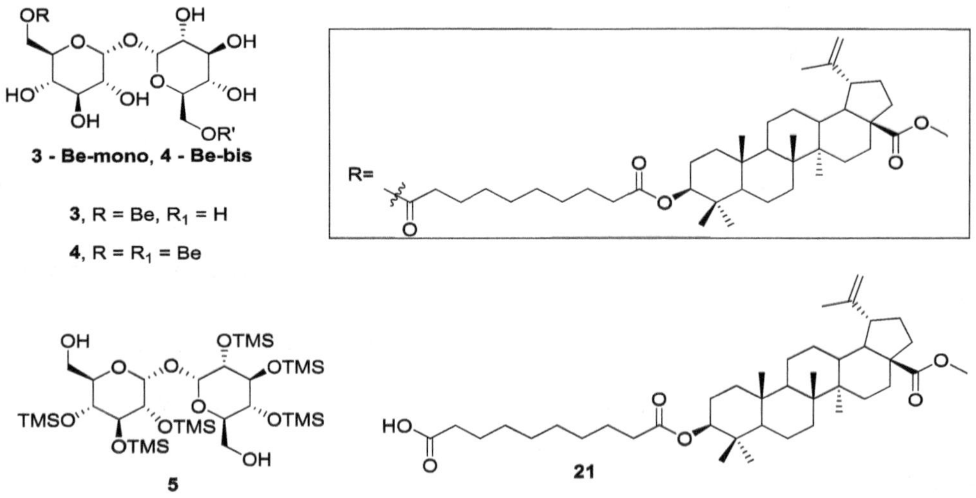

Figure 3. Chemical structure of target betulinic-trehalose conjugates **3-Be-mono** and **4-Be-bis**, of key synthetic intermediate hexaTMS-protected trehalose **5** and carboxylated betulinic-linker adduct **21**.

The synthesis of key intermediate **21** is reported in Scheme 4.

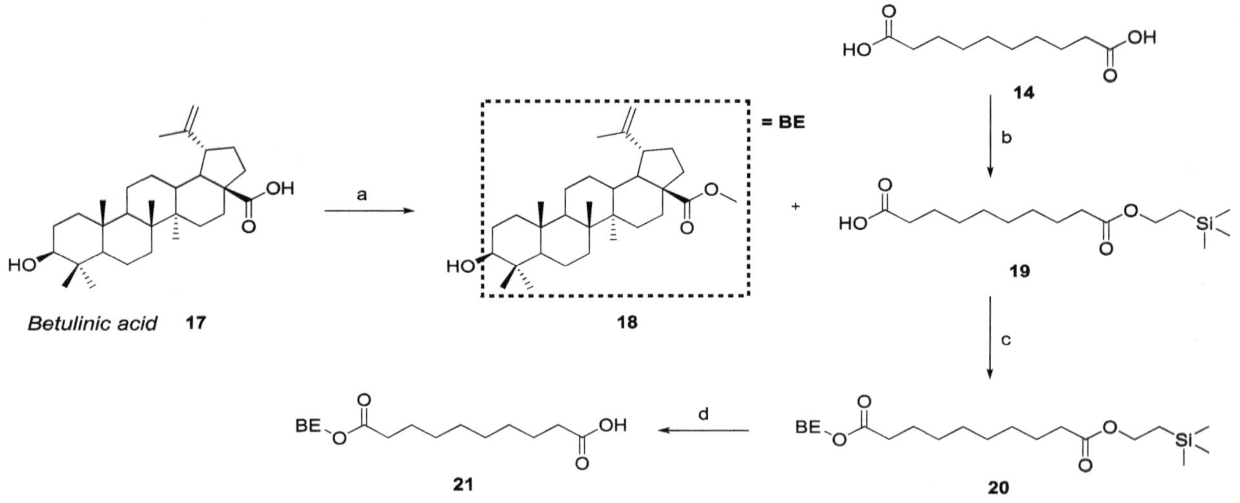

a: Me₃SiCH=N₂, MeOH, toluene, rt, overnight, **95%** yield; b: trimethylsilyl ethanol, EDC·HCl, DMAP, CH₂Cl₂, Py, rt, overnight, **40%** yield; c: DCC, DMAP, CH₂Cl₂, rt,overnight, **92%** yield; d: TBAF, THF, rt, overnight, **93%** yield.

Scheme 4. Synthesis of carboxylated betulinic-linker adduct **21**.

Betulinic acid **17** was first esterified (methyl ester **18**, step a), then coupled with mono-protected diacid **19** (prepared by a controlled esterification of sebacic acid **14**, step b) to provide silyl-protected construct **20** (step c). Carboxylic acid deprotection finally provided target carboxylated betulinic-linker adduct **21** (step d, Scheme 4).

Finally, key intermediates **5** and **21** were coupled in equimolar amounts in an esterification protocol, obtaining a ≈ 1.5:1 mixture of **22-mono** and **23-bis** hexaTMS-protected compounds (step a, Scheme 5).

After chromatographic separation, hexaTMS protected compound **22-mono** was submitted to acidic deprotection, yielding target **3-Be-mono** betulinic acid–trehalose conjugate, in 21% overall yield from **5** and **21** (step b, Scheme 5). The same reaction, targeting **4-Be-bis** from **23-bis**, leads to uncharacterizable degradation products.

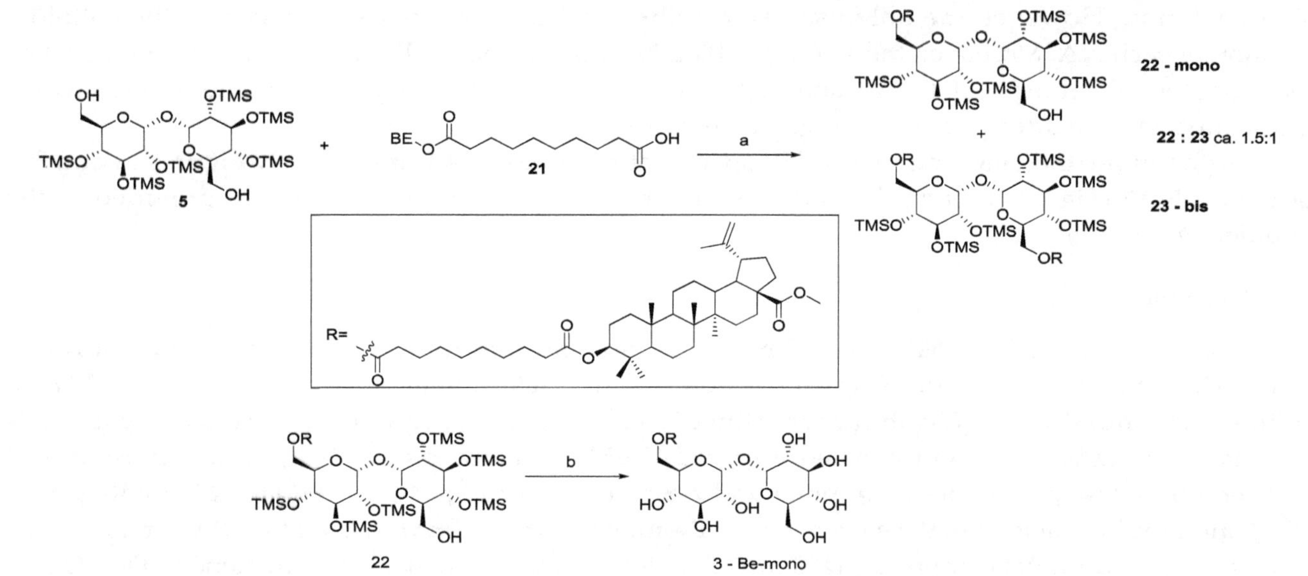

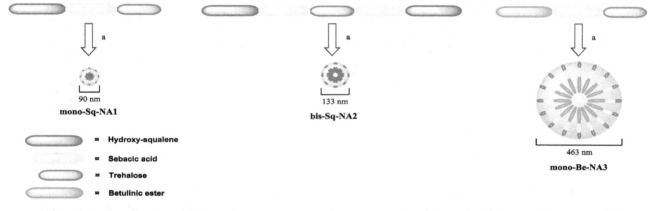

a: EDC·HCl, DMAP, toluene, 50°C, overnight, **21%** yield (**22-mono**), **15%** yield (**23 - bis**); b: AcOH, MeOH, 40°C, overnight, **quantitative** yield (**3 - Be-mono**), degradation (attempted synthesis of **4 - Be-bis**).

Scheme 5. Synthesis of target **3-Be-mono** betulinic-trehalose conjugate.

3.3. NA Assembly and Structural Characterization

Both **1-Sq-mono** and **2-Sq-bis** squalene-trehalose conjugates, and **3-Be-mono** betulinic acid-trehalose conjugate were assembled into their corresponding NAs (**mono-Sq-NA1**, left, **bis-Sq-NA2**, middle, and **mono-Be-NA3**, right, Scheme 6) following a standard experimental protocol [38].

90 nm
mono-Sq-NA1

133 nm
bis-Sq-NA2

463 nm
mono-Be-NA3

= **Hydroxy-squalene**

= **Sebacic acid**

= **Trehalose**

= **Betulinic ester**

a: 1. THF, rt; 2. MilliQ water, rt, 5 min; 3. Solvent evaporation.

Scheme 6. Assembly and graphic representation of **mono-Sq-NA1**, **bis-Sq-NA2** and **mono-Be-NA3**.

Self-assembled **mono-Sq-NA1**, **bis-Sq-NA2** and **mono-Be-NA3** were characterized in terms of hydrodynamic diameter and ζ-potential, as shown in Table 1.

Table 1. Mono-Sq-NA1, mono-Be-NA3 and **bis-Sq-NA2**: characterization.

Nanovector/Test	Hydrodynamic Diameter (HD, nm)	ζ-Potential (mV)	Polydispersity Index
mono-Sq-NA1	90.4 ± 0.7	−25.12 ± 0.79	0.121 ± 0.019
bis-Sq-NA2	132.8 ± 0.9	−25.43 ± 0.69	0.072 ± 0.010
mono-Be-NA3	463 ±29	−23.53± 0.29	0.126 ± 0.010

The size of the hydrodynamic diameters shows an increase from **mono-Sq-NA1** to **bis-Sq-NA2**, while the self-assembly of **mono-Be-NA3** results in much larger NAs with a mean HD centered at about 460 nm. However, the polydispersity index confirms the mono-dispersion of the colloidal solution of each NA. Moreover, the self-assembled NAs show good colloidal stability as confirmed by their ζ-potential value (<-20.0 mV), and by the stability of their hydrodynamic diameter (HD) which is not affected even after 10 days' storage in aqueous solution.

Furthermore, the TEM images and UV spectra of **mono-Sq-NA1** (respectively Figures S1 and S2), of **bis-Sq-NA2** (Figures S3 and S4) and of **mono-Be-NA3** (Figures S5 and S6) are provided in the Supplementary Materials.

3.4. Biological Profiling

Finally, the set of three NAs was submitted to biological profiling in HeLa cells for cytotoxicity (safety determination) and autophagy induction (activity determination). Namely, we treated HeLa cultures for 2 and 48 h at 37 °C with either the three NAs (either estimated, adjusted 20 µM concentrations of trehalose in water for 2 h, or estimated, adjusted 40 µM concentrations for 48 h), their non-assembled squalene-trehalose precursors **1-Sq-mono** and **2-Sq-bis** (either 20 µM in DMSO for 2 h, or 40 µM for 48 h) and betulinic acid-trehalose precursor **3-Be-mono** (either 20 µM in EtOH for 2 h, or 40 µM for 48 h), or each individual component (100 mM trehalose in water, either 20 µM squalene in DMSO and 20 µM betulinic acid in EtOH for 2 h, or 40 µM with both for 48 h), and relative vehicle (DMSO or EtOH). Assays were carried out at 48 h to ensure the release of free trehalose from NAs.

At first, we determined the in vitro safety profile of each sample via the MTT cytotoxicity assay (Figure 4).

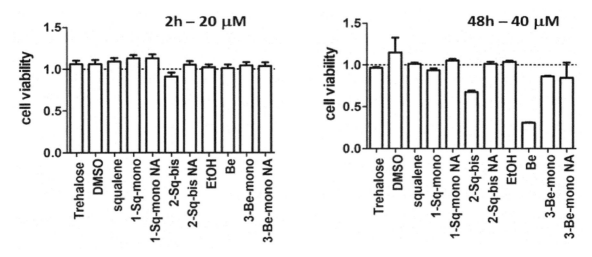

Figure 4. Cytotoxicity assay on betulinic acid, squalene, **1-Sq-mono**, **2-Sq-bis**, **3-Be-mono**, **mono-Sq-NA1**, **bis-Sq-NA2** and **mono-Be-NA3**. MTT assay, 2 h/20 µM (**left**) and 48 h/40 µM (**right**), trehalose = 100 mM.

The tested samples do not elicit an overt toxicity upon 2 hours of treatment. Instead, while the set of three NAs confirmed lack of cytotoxicity at 48 h, both the **2-Sq-bis** construct ($\approx$65% viable cells at 48 h) and free betulinic acid ($\approx$25% viable cells at 48 h) show significant cytotoxicity ($p < 0.001$ versus not treated, $n = 4$).

Next, we assessed if NAs, non-assembled precursors and individual components, could induce autophagy by western-blotting. In accordance with cytotox results, we tested NAs at both timelines (2 h/Figure 5, and 48 h/Figure 6), while non-assembled precursors and individual components were tested only at 2 h. Autophagy can be monitored by tracking the mobility shift from LC3I to LC3II (Figures 5 and 6, right), that is a bona fide reporter of the induction of autophagy; and by the amount of LC3II, that correlates with the formation of autophagosomes (Figures 5 and 6, left). α-Tubulin was used as an internal control in the assays.

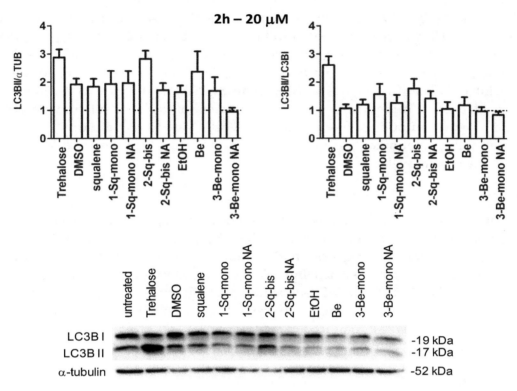

Figure 5. Autophagy induction on betulinic acid, squalene, **1-Sq-mono**, **2-Sq-bis**, **3-Be-mono**, **mono-Sq-NA1**, **bis-Sq-NA2** and **mono-Be-NA3**. LC3BII amount (**left**), LC3BII/LC3BI ratio (**right**), 2 h/20 μM, trehalose = 100 mM.

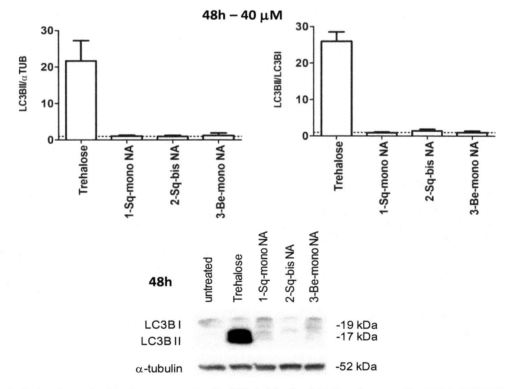

Figure 6. Autophagy induction on **mono-Sq-NA1**, **bis-Sq-NA2** and **mono-Be-NA3**. LC3BII amount (**left**), LC3BII/LC3BI ratio (**right**), 48 h/40 μM, trehalose = 100 mM.

At 2 h, we only observed a moderate effect by the **2-Sq-bis** construct that did not reach statistical significance (Figure 5, left and right). At 48 h, surprisingly, the three NAs did not show any effect on autophagy induction/progress (Figure 6).

We investigated the fate of our NAs in the biological medium, to rationalize their lack of biological effects. Thus, HeLa cell lysates were treated following a published procedure [44], obtaining two protein-free aqueous (≈4:3 MeOH:water) and organic (≈3:1 MeOH:chloroform) layers. Their LC-MS analysis could neither detect trehalose as such at the expected μM concentration, nor the most likely lipid-trehalose intermediates (see Figures S7–S10, **mono-Sq-NA1**; and Figures S11–S14 **mono-Be-NA3**, Supplementary Materials). We could not rule out the presence of trehalose at lower, nM concentrations that would not elicit an autophagy-inducing effect in cells, due to its detection LC-MS limits; and we suggest that highly lipophilic lipid-trehalose intermediates **1-Sq-mono** and **3-Be-mono** remain trapped within the protein pellet.

4. Discussion

Accumulating evidence indicates that induction of autophagy can be clinically relevant in the context of neurodegenerative disorders characterized by protein aggregation [39]. Pre-clinically, trehalose alleviates protein aggregation and cellular toxicity in pathological deposition of amyloid/Alzheimer [22] and alpha synuclein/Parkinson [20]. It may act by binding to extra-cellular GLUT transporters and by inducing AMPK-dependent autophagy [19], and/or by cytosolic activation of the TFEP pathway [45]. Trehalose is highly hydrophilic, preventing its passive cell permeation [46]. Moreover, trehalases hydrolyze it to glucose at the GI barrier [23]. Thus, trehalose PK in humans is challenging. By conjugating trehalose with squalene and betulinic acid, and self-assembling three constructs into NAs, we generated entities with a putatively higher permeability profile, hopefully leading to higher effects on autophagy at lower dosages.

The 2:1 **2-Sq-bis** construct showed per se an indication of higher potency than trehalose on autophagy induction at much lower, ≈40 μM, concentrations. We hypothesize that its higher lipophilicity, compared to its 1:1 **1-Sq-mono** and **3-Be-mono** counterparts, may yield better cell permeability after 2 hours of incubation, with a significant effect on autophagy induction.

The three NAs did not show any cytotoxicity, supporting their testing in the autophagy induction assay. The three **mono-Sq-NA1**, **bis-Sq-NA2** and **mono-Be-NA3** NAs did not show any effect upon autophagy induction; their inactivity could be justified by the absence of μM-free trehalose in cell lysates (LC-MS determination), possibly due to limited degradation of NAs in 48 h.

Our next efforts will include the design and execution of modified assays to measure autophagy induction at longer times and/or more NA degradation-prone conditions, and the synthesis of modified self-assembly trehalose-nanolipid conjugates to fine-tune their properties.

Supplementary Materials:
Figure S1: TEM images of **mono-Sq-NA1**, Figure S2: UV-vis spectrum of **mono-Sq-NA1**, Figure S3: TEM images of **bis-Sq-NA2**, Figure S4: UV-vis spectrum of **bis-Sq-NA2**, Figure S5: TEM images of **mono-Be-NA3**, Figure S6: UV-vis spectrum of **mono-Be-NA3**, Figure S7: HPLC (220 nm, top) and TIC spectrum (ESI+, bottom) of the aqueous methanolic phase from the treatment of HeLa cells with **mono-Sq-NA1/EC-37**, Figure S8: MS analysis / compound searching for **2-Sq-bis** (MW = 1448, first lane), **1-Sq-mono** (MW=895, second lane), squalene alcohol (MW = 386, third lane) and trehalose (MW = 342 Da, fourth lane) in the aqueous methanolic phase from the treatment of HeLa cells with **mono-Sq-NA1/EC-37**, Figure S9: HPLC (220 nm, top) and TIC spectrum (ESI+, bottom) of the lipophilic methanol-chloroform phase from the treatment of HeLa cells with **mono-Sq-NA1/EC-37**, Figure S10: MS analysis / compound searching for **2-Sq-bis** (MW = 1448, first lane), **1-Sq-mono** (MW = 895, second lane), squalene alcohol (MW = 386, third lane) and trehalose (MW = 342 Da, fourth lane) in the lipophilic methanol-chloroform phase from the treatment of HeLa cells with **mono-Sq-NA1/EC-37**, Figure S11: HPLC (220 nm, top) and TIC spectrum (ESI+, bottom) of the aqueous methanolic phase from the treatment of HeLa cells with **mono–Be-NA3/MIC-17**, Figure S12: MS analysis / compound searching for **3-Be-mono** (MW = 979, first lane), betulinic acid (MW = 456, second lane), betulinic acid methyl ester (MW = 470, third lane) and trehalose (MW = 342 Da, fourth lane) in the aqueous methanolic phase from the treatment of HeLa cells with **mono-Be-NA3/MIC-17**, Figure S13: HPLC (220 nm, top) and TIC spectrum (ESI+, bottom) of the lipophilic methanol-chloroform phase from the treatment of HeLa cells with **mono-Be-NA3/MIC-17**, Figure S14: MS analysis / compound searching for **3-Be-mono** (MW = 979, first lane), betulinic acid (MW = 456, second lane), betulinic acid methyl ester (MW = 470, third lane) and trehalose (MW = 342 Da, fourth lane) in the lipophilic methanol-chloroform phase from the treatment of HeLa cells with **mono-Be-NA3/MIC-17**.

Author Contributions: Conceptualization, P.S., G.P. and D.P.; chemistry, M.B. and E.C.; structural characterization, L.P.; biology, G.F.; bioanalytical studies, P.R.; writing—original draft preparation, E.C. and P.S.; HPLC-MS analysis, P.R.; structure elucidation, M.S.C.; writing—review and editing, P.S., G.P. and D.P.

Acknowledgments: D.P. expresses his gratitude to MAECI Italia-India Strategic Projects 2017–2019.

References

1. Farjadian, F.; Ghasemi, A.; Gohari, O.; Roointan, A.; Karimi, M.; Hamblin, M.R. Nanopharmaceuticals and nanomedicines currently on the market: Challenges and opportunities. *Nanomedicine* **2019**, *14*, 93–126. [CrossRef] [PubMed]
2. Ventola, C.L. Progress in nanomedicine: Approved and investigational nanodrugs. *Pharm. Ther.* **2017**, *42*, 742–755.
3. Bobo, D.; Robinson, K.J.; Islam, J.; Thurecht, K.J.; Corrie, S.R. Nanoparticle-based medicines: A review of FDA-approved materials and clinical trials to date. *Pharm. Res.* **2016**, *33*, 2373–2387. [CrossRef] [PubMed]
4. Jain, S.; Hirst, D.; O'Sullivan, J. Gold nanoparticles as novel agents for cancer therapy. *Br. J. Radiol.* **2012**, *85*, 101–113. [CrossRef] [PubMed]
5. Bharti, C.; Nagaich, U.; Pal, A.K.; Gulati, N. Mesoporous silica nanoparticles in target drug-delivery system: A review. *Int. J. Pharm. Investig.* **2015**, *5*, 124–133. [CrossRef] [PubMed]
6. Farjadian, F.; Moradi, S.; Hosseini, M. Thin chitosan films containing super-paramagnetic nanoparticles with contrasting capability in magnetic resonance imaging. *J. Mater. Sci. Mater. Med.* **2017**, *28*, 47. [CrossRef] [PubMed]
7. Maier-Hauff, K.; Ulrich, F.; Nestler, D.; Niehoff, H.; Wust, P.; Thiesen, B.; Orawa, H.; Budach, V.; Jordan, A. Efficacy and safety of intratumoral thermotherapy using magnetic iron-oxide nanoparticles combined with external beam radiotherapy on patients with recurrent glioblastoma multiforme. *J. Neuro-Oncol.* **2011**, *103*, 317–324. [CrossRef] [PubMed]
8. Schwenk, M.H. Ferumoxytol: A new intravenous iron preparation for the treatment of iron deficiency anemia in patients with chronic kidney disease. *Pharmacotherapy* **2010**, *33*, 70–79. [CrossRef] [PubMed]
9. Lasic, D.D. Doxorubicin in sterically stabilized liposomes. *Nature* **1996**, *380*, 561–562. [CrossRef] [PubMed]
10. Buster, J.E. Transdermal menopausal hormone therapy: Delivery through skin changes the rules. *Expert Opin. Pharmacother.* **2010**, *11*, 1489–1499. [CrossRef] [PubMed]
11. Turecek, P.L.; Bossard, M.J.; Schoetens, F.; Ivens, I.A. PEGylation of biopharmaceuticals: A review of chemistry and nonclinical safety information of approved drugs. *J. Pharm. Sci.* **2016**, *105*, 460–475. [CrossRef] [PubMed]
12. Awasthi, R.; Roseblade, A.; Hansbro, P.M.; Rathbone, M.J.; Dua, K.; Bebawy, M. Nanoparticles in cancer treatment: Opportunities and obstacles. *Curr. Drug Targets* **2018**, *69*, 1696–1709. [CrossRef] [PubMed]
13. Saeedi, M.; Eslamifar, M.; Khezri, K.; Dizaj, S.M. Applications of nanotechnology in drug delivery to the central nervous system. *Biomed. Pharmacother.* **2019**, *111*, 666–675. [CrossRef] [PubMed]
14. Hu, X.; Miller, L.; Richman, S.; Hitchman, S.; Glick, G.; Liu, S.; Zhu, Y.; Crossman, M.; Nestorov, I.; Gronke, R.S.; et al. A novel PEGylated interferon beta- 1a for multiple sclerosis: Safety, pharmacology, and biology. *J. Clin. Pharmacol.* **2012**, *52*, 798–808. [CrossRef] [PubMed]
15. Birch, G.G. Trehaloses. *Adv. Carbohydr. Chem.* **1963**, *18*, 201–225. [PubMed]
16. Richards, A.B.; Krakowka, S.; Dexter, L.B.; Schmid, H.; Wolterbeek, A.P.; Waalkens-Berendsen, D.H.; Shigoyuki, A.; Kurimoto, M. Trehalose: A review of properties, history of use and human tolerance, and results of multiple safety studies. *Food Chem. Toxicol.* **2003**, *40*, 871–898. [CrossRef]
17. Sussman, A.S.; Lingappa, B.T. Role of trehalose in ascaspores of Neurospora tetrasperma. *Science* **1959**, *130*, 1343. [CrossRef] [PubMed]
18. Van Dijck, P.; Colavizza, D.; Smet, P.; Thevelein, J.M. Differential importance of trehalose in stress resistance in fermenting and nonfermenting Saccharomyces cerevisiae cells. *Appl. Environ. Microbiol.* **1995**, *61*, 109–115. [PubMed]
19. Mardones, P.; Rubinsztein, D.C.; Hetz, C. Mystery solved: Trehalose kickstarts autophagy by blocking glucose transport. *Sci. Signal.* **2016**, *9*, fs2. [CrossRef]

20. Tanaka, M.; Machida, Y.; Niu, S.; Ikeda, T.; Jana, N.R.; Doi, H.; Kurosawa, M.; Nekooki, M.; Nukina, N. Trehalose alleviates polyglutamine-mediated pathology in a mouse model of Huntington disease. *Nat. Med.* **2004**, *10*, 148–154. [CrossRef]

21. Jain, N.K.; Roy, I. Effect of trehalose on protein structure. *Protein Sci.* **2009**, *18*, 24–36. [CrossRef] [PubMed]

22. Liu, R.; Barkhordarian, H.; Emadi, S.; Park, C.B.; Sierks, M.R. Trehalose differentially inhibits aggregation and neurotoxicity of beta-amyloid 40 and 42. *Neurobiol. Dis.* **2005**, *20*, 74–81. [CrossRef] [PubMed]

23. Kalf, G.F.; Rieder, S.V. The purification and properties of trehalase. *J. Biol. Chem.* **1958**, *230*, 691–698. [PubMed]

24. Adhikari, P.; Pal, P.; Das, A.K.; Ray, S.; Bhattacharjee, A.; Mazumder, B. Nano lipid-drug conjugate: An integrated review. *Int. J. Pharm.* **2017**, *529*, 629–641. [CrossRef] [PubMed]

25. Couvreur, P.; Stella, B.; Reddy, L.H.; Mangenot, S.; Poupaert, J.H.; Desmaele, D.; Lepetre-Mouelhi, S.; Rocco, F.; Dereuddre-Bosquet, N.; Clayette, P.; et al. Squalenoyl nanomedicines as potential therapeutics. *Nano Lett.* **2006**, *6*, 2544–2548. [CrossRef] [PubMed]

26. Desmaele, D.; Gref, R.; Couvreur, P. Squalenoylation: A generic platform for nanoparticular drug delivery. *J. Control. Release* **2012**, *161*, 609–618. [CrossRef]

27. Semiramoth, N.; Di Meo, C.; Zouhiri, F.; Said-Hassane, F.; Valetti, S.; Gorges, R.; Nicolas, V.; Poupaert, J.H.; Chollet-Martin, S.; Desmaele, D.; et al. Selfassembled squalenoylated penicillin bioconjugates: An original approach for the treatment of intracellular infections. *ACS Nano* **2012**, *6*, 3820–3831. [CrossRef]

28. Buchy, E.; Valetti, S.; Mura, S.; Mougin, J.; Troufflard, C.; Couvreur, P.; Desmaële, D. Synthesis and cytotoxic activity of self-assembling squalene conjugates of 3-[(pyrrol-2-yl)methylidene]-2,3-dihydro-1H-indol-2-one anticancer agents. *Eur. J. Org. Chem.* **2015**. [CrossRef]

29. Dash, S.K.; Giri, B. Self-assembled betulinic acid: A better alternative form of betulinic acid for anticancer therapy. *J. Exp. Med. Biol.* **2019**, *1*, 1–2.

30. Dash, S.K.; Dash, S.S.; Chattopadhyay, S.; Ghosh, T.; Tripathy, S.; Mahapatra, S.K.; Bag, B.G.; Das, D.; Roy, S. Folate decorated delivery of self-assembled betulinic acid nano fibers: A biocompatible antileukemic therapy. *RCS Adv.* **2015**, *5*, 24144. [CrossRef]

31. Fumagalli, G.; Marucci, C.; Christodoulou, M.S.; Stella, B.; Dosio, F.; Passarella, D. Self-assembly drug conjugates for anticancer treatment. *Drug Discov. Today* **2016**, *21*, 1321–1329. [CrossRef] [PubMed]

32. Borrelli, S.; Christodoulou, M.S.; Ficarra, I.; Silvani, A.; Cappelletti, G.; Cartelli, D.; Damia, G.; Ricci, F.; Zucchetti, M.; Dosio, F.; et al. New class of squalene-based releasable nanoassemblies of paclitaxel, podophyllotoxin, camptothecin and epothilone A. *Eur. J. Med. Chem.* **2014**, *85*, 179–190. [CrossRef] [PubMed]

33. Borrelli, S.; Cartelli, D.; Secundo, F.; Fumagalli, G.; Christodoulou, M.S.; Borroni, A.; Perdicchia, D.; Dosio, F.; Milla, P.; Cappelletti, G.; et al. Self-Assembled Squalene-based Fluorescent Heteronanoparticles. *ChemPlusChem* **2015**, *80*, 47–49. [CrossRef]

34. Fumagalli, G.; Mazza, D.; Christodoulou, M.S.; Damia, G.; Ricci, F.; Perdicchia, D.; Stella, B.; Dosio, F.; Sotiropoulou, P.A.; Passarella, D. Cyclopamine-paclitaxel-containing nanoparticles: Internalization in cells detected by confocal and super-resolution microscopy. *ChemPlusChem* **2015**, *80*, 1380–1383. [CrossRef]

35. Fumagalli, G.; Stella, B.; Pastushenko, I.; Ricci, F.; Christodoulou, M.S.; Damia, G.; Mazza, D.; Arpicco, S.; Giannini, C.; Morosi, L.; et al. Heteronanoparticles by self-assembly of doxorubicin and cyclopamine conjugates. *ACS Med. Chem. Lett.* **2017**, *8*, 953–957. [CrossRef] [PubMed]

36. Fumagalli, G.; Giorgi, G.; Vágvölgyi, M.; Colombo, E.; Christodoulou, M.S.; Collico, V.; Prosperi, D.; Dosio, F.; Hunyadi, A.; Montopoli, M.; et al. Hetero-nanoparticles by self-assembly of ecdysteroid and doxorubicin conjugates to overcome cancer resistance. *ACS Med. Chem. Lett.* **2018**, *9*, 468–471. [CrossRef] [PubMed]

37. Fumagalli, G.; Christodoulou, M.S.; Riva, B.; Revuelta, I.; Marucci, C.; Collico, V.; Prosperi, D.; Riva, S.; Perdicchia, D.; Bassanini, I.; et al. Self-assembled 4-(1,2-diphenylbut-1-en-1-yl)aniline based nanoparticles: Podophyllotoxin and aloin as building blocks. *Org. Biomol. Chem.* **2017**, *15*, 1106–1109. [CrossRef] [PubMed]

38. Fumagalli, G.; Polito, L.; Colombo, E.; Foschi, F.; Christodoulou, M.S.; Galeotti, F.; Perdicchia, D.; Bassanini, I.; Riva, S.; Seneci, P.; et al. Self-assembling releasable thiocolchicine-diphenylbutenylaniline conjugates. *ACS Med. Chem. Lett.* **2019**, *10*, 611–614. [CrossRef]

39. Guo, F.; Liu, X.; Cai, H.; Le, W. Autophagy in neurodegenerative diseases: Pathogenesis and therapy. *Brain Pathol.* **2018**, *28*, 3–13. [CrossRef] [PubMed]

40. Sarpe, A.V.; Kulkarni, S.S. Synthesis of maradolipid. *J. Org. Chem.* **2011**, *76*, 6866–6870. [CrossRef] [PubMed]

41. Battaglia, L.; Gallarate, M. Lipid nanoparticles: State of the art, new preparation methods and challenges in drug delivery. *Expert Opin. Drug Deliv.* **2012**, *9*, 497–508. [CrossRef] [PubMed]

42. Von Smoluchowski, M. Contribution à la théorie de l'endosmose électrique et de quelques phenomènes. *Pisma Mariana Smoluchowskiego* **1924**, *1*, 403.

43. Klionski, D.J.; Abdelmohsen, K.; Abe, A.; Abedin, M.J.; Abeliovich, H.; Acevedo Arozena, A.; Adachi, H.; Adams, C.M.; Adams, P.D.; Adeli, K.; et al. Guidelines for the use and interpretation of assays for monitoring autophagy (3rd edition). *Autophagy* **2016**, *12*, 1–222. [CrossRef] [PubMed]

44. Fic, E.; Kedracka-Krok, S.; Jankowska, U.; Pirog, A.; Dziedzicka-Wasylewska, M. Comparison of protein precipitation methods for various rat brain structures prior of proteomic analysis. *Electrophoresis* **2010**, *31*, 3573–3579. [CrossRef] [PubMed]

45. Emanuele, E. Can trehalose prevent neurodegeneration? Insights from experimental studies. *Curr. Drug Targets* **2014**, *15*, 551–557. [CrossRef] [PubMed]

46. Rusmini, P.; Cortese, K.; Crippa, V.; Cristofani, R.; Cicardi, M.E.; Ferrari, V.; Vezzoli, G.; Tedesco, B.; Meroni, M.; Messi, E.; et al. Trehalose induces autophagy via lysosomal-mediated TFEB activation in models of motoneuron degeneration. *Autophagy* **2019**, *15*, 631–651. [CrossRef] [PubMed]

Fluorescence and Cytotoxicity of Cadmium Sulfide Quantum Dots Stabilized on Clay Nanotubes

Anna V. Stavitskaya [1], Andrei A. Novikov [1,*], Mikhail S. Kotelev [1], Dmitry S. Kopitsyn [1], Elvira V. Rozhina [2], Ilnur R. Ishmukhametov [2], Rawil F. Fakhrullin [2], Evgenii V. Ivanov [1], Yuri M. Lvov [1,3,*] and Vladimir A. Vinokurov [1]

[1] Functional Aluminosilicate Nanomaterials Lab, Gubkin University, Moscow 119991, Russia; stavitsko@mail.ru (A.V.S.); kain@inbox.ru (M.S.K.); kopicin.d@inbox.ru (D.S.K.); ivanov166@list.ru (E.V.I.); vinok_ac@mail.ru (V.A.V.)

[2] Bionanotechnology Lab, Institute of Fundamental Medicine and Biology, Kazan Federal University, Kazan, Republic of Tatarstan, Russian Federation, 420008; rozhinaelvira@gmail.com (E.V.R.); sal.ilnur@gmail.com (I.R.I.); kazanbio@gmail.com (R.F.F.)

[3] Institute for Micromanufacturing, Louisiana Tech University, Ruston, LA 71272, USA

[*] Correspondence: novikov.a@gubkin.ru (A.A.N.); ylvov@latech.edu (Y.M.L.);

Abstract: Quantum dots (QD) are widely used for cellular labeling due to enhanced brightness, resistance to photobleaching, and multicolor light emissions. CdS and $Cd_xZn_{1-x}S$ nanoparticles with sizes of 6–8 nm were synthesized via a ligand assisted technique inside and outside of 50 nm diameter halloysite clay nanotubes (QD were immobilized on the tube's surface). The halloysite–QD composites were tested by labeling human skin fibroblasts and prostate cancer cells. In human cell cultures, halloysite–QD systems were internalized by living cells, and demonstrated intense and stable fluorescence combined with pronounced nanotube light scattering. The best signal stability was observed for QD that were synthesized externally on the amino-grafted halloysite. The best cell viability was observed for $Cd_xZn_{1-x}S$ QD immobilized onto the azine-grafted halloysite. The possibility to use QD clay nanotube core-shell nanoarchitectures for the intracellular labeling was demonstrated. A pronounced scattering and fluorescence by halloysite–QD systems allows for their promising usage as markers for biomedical applications.

Keywords: bioimaging; nanoarchitectures; halloysite; intracellular labeling

1. Introduction

Nanomaterials show great promise when it comes to targeted drug delivery, diagnostics, and controlled-release drug treatment. In recent years, formulations based on halloysite clay nanotubes have attracted attention in biology and medicine as a drug delivery vehicle [1–6], in implants and tissue engineering [7], and in chemical- and bio-sensing [8,9]. Halloysite nanotubes can be employed as encapsulation containers due to their tubular structure, mesoporous 10–15 nm diameter lumen, and site-dependent chemistry with positively (Al_2O_3) and negatively (SiO_2) charged inner and outer tube surfaces [10–13].

Halloysite has been proposed as a template for synthesis and stabilization of various nanoparticles following a core–shell nanoarchitecture strategy. Halloysite–metal nanoparticle composites have been employed in heterogeneous catalysis [14,15]. Antibacterial Ag [16,17], as well as plasmonic Au nanoparticles [18], were synthesized into and onto halloysite tubes to form new nanosystems with enhanced biological activity. Metal chalcogenide halloysite-based formulations have already been tested in photocatalysis and bioimaging [19,20]. Metal chalcogenide quantum dots (QD) are semiconductor nanoparticles with a size of up to 10 nm that emit light with a wavelength that can be finely tuned from ultraviolet to infrared, depending on sizes, structure, and composition; among them, cadmium containing QDs are one of the most useable [21]. QDs are favorable for intracellular labeling because of the easily tunable light emission, wide absorption band, high resistance to photobleaching, and possibilities of surface modification by conjugation with proteins [22].

One of the main problems with nanomaterial applications in living organisms is the toxicity of such tiny objects. For example, QD for bioimaging are often synthesized using complicated stabilization techniques to make them less cytotoxic and better dispersible in water, and this is especially important for cadmium-containing QDs [23]. Halloysite clay encapsulation could help dispersing the quantum dots in water, as well as decrease the toxicity of QD via the tube surface immobilization and decreasing amounts of free CdSe or CdS. These natural alumosilicate clay rolled structures, named halloysite, are known to be biocompatible [24]. One of the first reports on halloysite exposition for HeLa and MCF-7 mammal cell lines demonstrated that halloysite has low toxicity at concentrations up to 100 μg/mL. Although halloysite can be easily taken up by the cultured cells, its toxicity was reported to be very low, both for cell cultures and in vivo for animals [25]. Even at higher concentrations (up to 1500 μg/mL), halloysite nanotubes conjugated with noble metal nanoparticles, which have low toxicity for plants, as was reported for radish seeds [26].

Here, we report that site-selective immobilization of cadmium-containing QDs on halloysite nanotubes opens the way to obtain new fluorescent materials with broad emission spectra, good stability, and low in vitro toxicity. To reduce the cadmium content, a solid solution of cadmium-zinc sulfide was also used as fluorescent nanoparticle shells on core clay nanotubes.

2. Materials and Methods

Halloysite nanotubes (HNT), (3-Aminopropyl)triethoxysilane (APTES), furfural, hydrazine hydrate, cadmium nitrate tetrahydrate ($Cd(NO_3)_2 \cdot 4H_2O$), zinc nitrate hexahydrate ($Zn(NO_3)_2 \cdot 6H_2O$), thioacetamide (TAA), ethylenediaminetetraacetic acid (EDTA), ammonium hydroxide solution (NH_4OH), and ethanol 96% were all purchased from Sigma-Aldrich (Rushim, Moscow, Russia).

2.1. QDs Stabilization on Halloysite

Cadmium sulfide and cadmium-zinc sulfide QDs were stabilized on halloysite using the two following synthesis strategies.

In first case, APTES was used as a grafting agent. The halloysite salinization was performed using 0.2 g of APTES per 1 g of halloysite dispersed in ethanol and stirred at 60 °C for 24 h (modified from [27]). After the reaction, the dispersion was washed several times with ethanol. The resulting precipitate was dried for 12 h at 60 °C. Afterwards, the resulting $HNT-NH_2$ was dispersed in a $Cd(NO_3)_2$ solution and stirred for 30 min using sonication. Then a TAA solution was added in the cadmium-containing mixture, and pH was adjusted to 10 using NH_4OH. After 5 min, the yellow precipitate was centrifuged, washed with ethanol several times, and dried at 60 °C for 24 h. The obtained sample was labeled as $HNT-NH_2-CdS$ (see Scheme 1).

In second case, azine produced from furfural and hydrazine hydrate was used as a ligand to form stable CdS and Cd_xZn_yS QD on halloysite nanotubes. The procedure for HNT-Azine synthesis is described elsewhere [20,28]. The synthesis of CdS QDs was performed according to the same procedure described above. The obtained sample was labeled as HNT-Azine-CdS. The same HNT-Azine was used to stabilize $Cd_{0.7}Zn_{0.3}S$ QD, where a solution of $Cd(NO_3)_2$ and $Zn(NO_3)_2$ with Cd:Zn molar ratio of 0.7:0.3 was taken as a metal precursor solution. The procedure of QD synthesis was the same as for $HNT-NH_2-CdS$ and HNT-Azine-CdS. The sample was labeled as $HNT-Azine-Cd_{0.7}Zn_{0.3}S$.

To compare the photostability of synthesized HNT-QD materials with commonly used fluorescent dyes, we prepared rhodamine 6G (R6G) and fluorescein (Fluor) dyes that were adsorbed onto the halloysite nanotubes. Dyes were adsorbed on the halloysite surfaces from concentrated ethanol solutions, using a vacuum for better loading. After soaking the halloysite in dye solution for 30 min, the ethanol was evaporated under vacuum, and obtained composites (HNT-R6G and HNT-Fluor) were washed with ethanol and dried overnight.

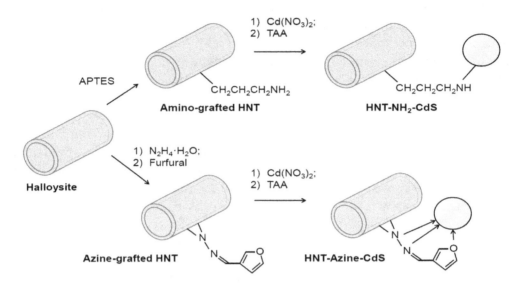

Scheme 1. Synthesis of halloysite-CdS composites.

2.2. Cell Cultures

Epithelial human prostate cell line (PC-3) was obtained from the American Type Culture Collection (ATCC, Manassas, VA, USA). The cells were seeded in a sterile culture flask with a growth area of 75 cm^2 (Corning Inc., Corning, NY, USA), and contained 12 mL of Dulbecco's Modified Eagle's Medium (DMEM), supplemented with 10% fetal bovine serum (PAA laboratories, Dartmouth, MA, USA), 100 IU/mL of penicillin, and 100 ng/mL of streptomycin. The cells were cultivated at 37 °C in a humidified atmosphere containing 5% CO_2, and sub-cultured by trypsinization every three days at 80% confluency.

2.3. Characterization

Fluorescent materials' morphology evaluation and elemental analysis were performed with a JEM-2100 transmission electron microscope (Jeol, Tokyo, Japan), equipped with a JED-2300 X-ray fluorescence spectrometer (Jeol, Tokyo, Japan). Size distributions of QD were estimated by measuring the diameters of electron-dense particles in transmission electron microscopy (TEM) images with ImageJ v1.50i suite (National Institutes of Health, Bethesda, MD, USA). Reflectance spectra of the synthesized materials were registered in 45°/45° geometry using a 150 W xenon arc lamp (LOT Oriel, Darmstadt, Germany) and QE65000 spectrometer (Ocean Optics, Dunedin, FL, USA). Elemental analysis was performed using an ARL™ PERFORM'X Sequential X-ray Fluorescence Spectrometer (Thermo Scientific, Waltham, MA, USA).

For the study of cells' morphology and cytoskeleton structure, 1×10^5 cells were added to the six-well plate re-suspended in medium (1 mL) on coverslips (10 mm), where the plate was previously at the bottom of each well. The cells were grown for 24 h, the HNT-QD (100 mg/mL) was added, and cells were cultured for 24 h (37 °C and 5% CO_2). Then, the cells were washed with phosphate-buffered saline (PBS) and stained with 4′,6-diamidino-2-phenylindole (DAPI) solution (1 mg/mL) and Phalloidin Alexa Fluor® 488 (Thermo Fisher Scientific Inc., Waltham, MA, USA), according to the standard protocols. The slides were observed with laser scanning microscope Carl Zeiss LSM-780 (Jena City, Germany) with 543 nm, 488 nm, and 405 nm lasers, and images were processed using ZEN Black software (Carl Zeiss MicroImaging GmbH, Göttingen, Germany). Enhanced dark-field microscopy images were obtained using an Olympus BX51 upright microscope (Tokyo, Japan) equipped with a CytoViva® oil immersion dark-field condenser (Auburn, AL, USA).

2.4. Cell Viability

To measure the cell viability while incubated with HNT-QD, they were seeded in a sterile culture flask with growth area of 75 cm^2 (Corning Inc., Corning, NY, USA) until the confluence reached ~80%. Cells were rinsed with PBS and then were detached from the substrate by trypsinization. Then, the cells were grown in a six-well plate for 24 h and HNT-QD were added. After 24 h of incubation in standard conditions, we assessed cell death induction using ReadyProbes® Cell Viability Imaging Kit (Blue/Green) (Thermo Fisher Scientific Inc., Waltham, MA, USA) according to the standard protocol. The nuclei of all cells were analyzed with a standard DAPI filter (excitation/emission maxima: 360/460 nm), and the nuclei of dead cells with compromised plasma membranes were detected with standard FITC/GFP (green) filter set (excitation/emission maxima: 504/523 nm) on a flow cytometer FACS (BD Biosciences, San Jose, CA, USA).

3. Results

3.1. Fluorescent Materials Morphology and Composition

Halloysite nanotubes (HNT) that were used varied in length from 300 nm to 1 μm, with an average length of 600 nm, inner diameter of 15–20 nm, and their chemical formula is similar to kaolinite ($Al_2Si_2O_5(OH)_4 \cdot nH_2O$). The outer surface of halloysite is negatively charged at pH above 4 and was comprised of silica [29]. Surface modification of halloysite with silane is a common method that allows nanoparticles to bind to halloysite surface and to prevent their detachment from the tubes and aggregate [30–32]. In the case of cadmium containing QD (CdS or $Cd_{0.7}Zn_{0.3}S$), it is preferable to have complexation agents that cover QD to prevent cadmium release. Therefore, we have chosen an organic azine as a ligand for chalcogenide nanoparticle formation. This technique makes it possible to load nanoparticles inside the lumen of halloysite nanotubes [15], preventing QD nanoparticles from aggregating.

Figure 1 shows TEM images of halloysite nanotubes before modification (A), and after synthesis of fluorescent nanomaterials (B–D). The content of CdS in the samples, as evaluated by X-ray fluorescence elemental analysis, was 3.2, 3.5, and 2.9 wt% for cadmium sulfide quantum dots immobilized onto the amino-grafted halloysite HNT-NH$_2$-CdS (Figure 1B), cadmium sulfide quantum dots immobilized onto the azine-grafted halloysite HNT-Azine-CdS (Figure 1C), and cadmium-zinc sulfide quantum dots immobilized onto the azine-grafted halloysite HNT-Azine-$Cd_{0.7}Zn_{0.3}S$ (Figure 1D), respectively.

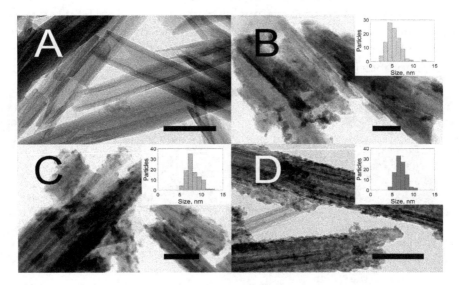

Figure 1. TEM images of pristine HNT (**A**); HNT-NH$_2$-CdS (**B**); HNT-Azine-CdS (**C**); and HNT-Azine-$Cd_{0.7}Zn_{0.3}S$ (**D**). Particle size distributions derived from measurements of 100 particles for each sample are shown in insets (**B–D**), (see also Table S1 in Supplementary Materials).

As shown above, the particle location on the tubes was different in every case. In the case of amino-grafted halloysite, the clusters were distributed all over the nanotubes. The particle size varied in a wide range from 2 to 13 nm (Figure 1B, inset). The concentration of nanoparticles in case of amino-grafted halloysite (Figure 1B) was lower than that of azine-grafted QD (Figure 1C,D). HNTs-Azine-CdS materials contained QD with better monodispersity; the majority of QD have size within 6 to 8 nm (Figure 1C,D, insets). There were no large Cd-clusters observed separate from the nanotubes. HNTs-Azine-Cd$_{0.7}$Zn$_{0.3}$S had densely located particles with size from 5 to 10 nm. Such a difference in the nanoparticle size distributions caused a variation in the material's spectral properties.

The synthesized cadmium QD materials had a bright yellow color, which is associated with their strong light absorption in blue spectral range (Figure 2). The positions of absorption peaks imply that these nanomaterials might demonstrate fluorescence when excited by a laser in the 400–500 nm range.

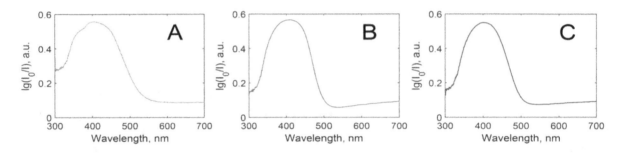

Figure 2. Diffusive reflectance spectra of HNT-NH$_2$-CdS (**A**); HNT-Azine-CdS (**B**); and HNT-Azine-Cd$_{0.7}$Zn$_{0.3}$S (**C**). Spectra were registered using pristine halloysite as a reference.

3.2. Laser Scanning and Dark Field Microscopy

We applied the halloysite-QD composites to label human cells in vitro to demonstrate the optical effects of these materials within live cells. Figure 3 presents the laser scanning microscopy (LSM) images of different Cd-composites with QD stabilized on halloysite nanotubes. Bright and well-resolved fluorescence was observed in all cases. It can be seen that every material had different emission spectra ranging from green (HNTs-Azine-CdS), to yellow-red (HNTs-Azine-Cd$_{0.7}$Zn$_{0.3}$S), to red (HNT-NH$_2$-CdS). Figure 3C shows the confocal microscopy image of the sample that had been stored for nine months. Cell nuclei were stained with DAPI, and were visible as large blue spots. Smaller red, yellow-red, and green spots around the nuclei correspond to HNT-QD composites, and imply that these composites are well-distributed on the cells' surfaces or inside them. These images confirm the effective uptake of QD-modified halloysite; apparently the uptake occurs in the same way as with dextrin-coated clay nanotubes [6].

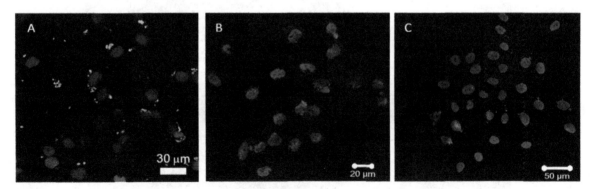

Figure 3. Laser scanning microscopy (LSM) images of PC-3 cells that were QD-labeled with HNTs-Azine-CdS (**A**), HNTs-NH$_2$-CdS (**B**), and HNTs-Azine-Cd$_{0.7}$Zn$_{0.3}$S (**C**). The nuclei were stained with DAPI (blue channel, 405-nm laser), QD are shown in green (488-nm laser) and red channel (543-nm laser).

More detailed distributions of the QD-nanotubes within the PC-3 cell are presented in Figure 4, demonstrating the correlative microscopy images taken using dark-field and epifluorescence microscopy. When observed using enhanced darkfield microscopy (Figure 4A), halloysite nanotubes appear as bright spots due to their good light-scattering properties. The cell membrane and cytoplasm can also be seen; however, at the same illumination intensity, the halloysite-lacking regions of the cell appeared to be faint. The corresponding fluorescence image of the same cell (Figure 4B) was stained with ReadyProbes® viability dye, while HNT-NH$_2$-CdS appeared as red spots, and their locations correspond to the brightest spots in Figure 4A, allowing us to correlate the QD fluorescence with halloysite light scattering.

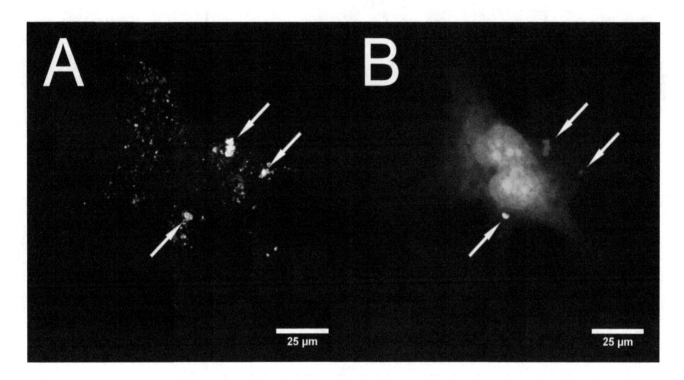

Figure 4. Visualization of PC-3 cell labeled with HNT-NH$_2$-CdS: dark-field microscopy image of PC-3 with HNT-NH$_2$-CdS (**A**) and fluorescence image of cells stained with ReadyProbes® Cell Viability Imaging Kit (Blue/Green) (ThermoFisher) (**B**). HNT-NH$_2$-CdS appeared as bright white spots (A, marked by arrows), or yellow and red spots (B), (marked by arrows).

3.3. Luminescence Stability

Time-dependent change of the intensity of QD fluorescence was observed using a laser confocal microscope equipped with a 405-nm diode laser in time-series mode. The signal intensity was recorded every 30 min for 4 h, and is shown in Figure 5. In Figure 5, the photostability of synthesized materials is shown, along with the photostability of fluorescent dyes rhodamine 6G and fluorescein immobilized onto the halloysite (HNT-R6G and HNT-Fluor, respectively). It is known that photobleaching of fluorescent dyes follows pseudo-first-order kinetics [33,34], so experimental points (circles and crosses in Figure 5) were approximated by first-order kinetics fits (lines in Figure 5). The highest luminescence signal stability was observed for the HNTs-NH$_2$-CdS (k = 0.00086 min^{-1}), which is comparable with the photostability of rhodamine 6G (k = 0.0012 min^{-1}). Azine-grafted materials (HNT-Azine-CdS and HNT-Azine-Cd$_{0.7}$Zn$_{0.3}$S) and halloysite-fluorescein composite (HNT-Fluor) showed a decreasing fluorescence intensity with time (k = 0.0139, 0.0057, and 0.0045 min^{-1}, respectively).

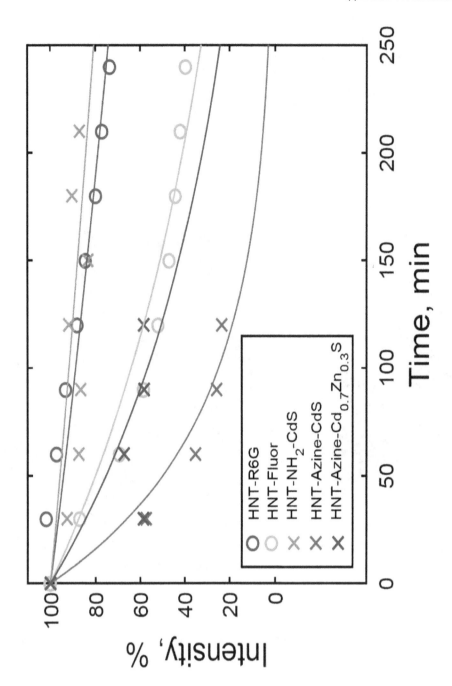

Figure 5. Time-dependent luminescence intensity of the synthesized materials (lines are first-order kinetics fits; see also Table S2 in Supplementary Materials).

3.4. Cytotoxicity

Earlier, we have shown the lack of toxic effects of halloysite-QD on cells with colorimetric assays and flow cytometry [20]. The toxicity of quantum dots depends on their size, chemical structure, and coating used [35,36]. We developed QDs that have a wide range of fluorescence, which is crucial for in vivo visualization. The toxicity of quantum dots was measured using the flow cytometry method. As one can see, viability of the cell is high in all cases as compared to the control (Figure 6). The percentage of live cells is higher when the HNT-Azine-$Cd_{0.7}Zn_{0.3}$S was used in cell cultivation.

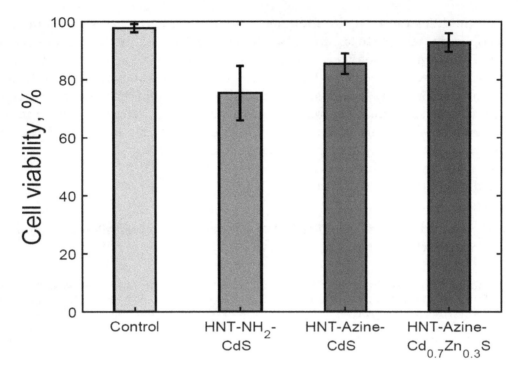

Figure 6. Flow cytometry data on viability of PC-3 cells exposed to halloysite-QD composites. Error bars are sample standard deviations (see also Figures S5–S8 in Supplementary Materials).

4. Discussion

The synthesis of halloysite with grafted nitrogen-containing electron donating groups leads to the formation of fluorescent core-shell materials, which are comprised of QDs immobilized onto the surface of the clay nanotubes. The nature of the grafted groups affects the particle organization, size distribution, and spectral properties of the formed QD systems. Generally, azine-grafted materials provide a higher surface coverage of halloysite nanotubes with QDs and a narrower cadmium-containing nanoparticle size distribution. The immobilization of QDs onto the halloysite nanotubes prevents the aggregation of QD and ensures their good dispersibility in water. This immobilization approach is suitable even for nanoparticles without hydrophilic ligands or an amphiphilic polymer coating employed for the surfactant-stabilized nanoparticles [37].

One of the known problems of QD bioimaging applications is their blinking behavior, namely the transition between a photoluminescent "on" state and the Auger-recombination "off" state [38]. The halloysite-QD composites with high surface QD coverage provide a simple and robust workaround of the blinking problem because the luminescence is provided by many QD, thus making the blinking by individual QD negligible.

The produced halloysite-QD tubular nanocomposites demonstrate the affinity towards living cells; PC-3 cells were contrasted by the designed nanosystems, and no free fluorescent particles were detected. The remarkable differences in the fluorescence signal stability show that better particle size distribution and higher concentration of QD do not guarantee the stability of composites. HNTs-NH$_2$-CdS formulations show higher photobleaching resistance, probably because of more sparsely distributed particles that are resistant to aggregation. The high photobleaching stability is crucial for real-life applications, such as study of the dynamics of intracellular processes, or prolonged diagnostics of organism malfunctions.

As one can see in Figures 3 and 4, halloysite-QD composites are either taken up by human cells or adsorbed onto the cell membranes. The underlying mechanism is not clear yet, but based on earlier observations [39], we assume that uptake of halloysite occurs via endocytosis, and depends on proliferation rate of different cell cultures.

The surface modification of halloysite affects not only the synthesis and immobilization of cadmium chalcogenide nanoparticles, but also the cytotoxicity of the halloysite-QD composites. The HNTs-NH$_2$-CdS formulations were most resistant to photobleaching, but at the same time demonstrated the highest cytotoxicity. Cadmium-containing QD are known to be cytotoxic because of Cd^{2+} ion emissions and direct interaction of QD with cell surface [40]. Thus, the immobilization of QD onto the surface of halloysite nanotubes may lower the cytotoxicity induced by the latter mechanism. Interestingly, among the azine-grafted halloysite composites, HNTs-Azine-Cd$_{0.7}$Zn$_{0.3}$S showed the lowest cytotoxicity together with moderate photobleaching resistance. The lower cytotoxicity of HNTs-Azine-Cd$_{0.7}$Zn$_{0.3}$S is probably due to the lower emission of Cd^{2+} ions from mixed cadmium-zinc sulfide, combined with the immobilization of QD.

We conclude that cadmium-zinc sulfide QD azine-grafted onto the halloysite clay nanotubes are the most promising materials for bioimaging.

Author Contributions: Conceptualization, Y.M.L. and V.A.V.; Data curation, A.V.S., A.A.N., M.S.K., D.S.K., E.V.R., and I.R.I.; Funding acquisition, Y.M.L. and V.A.V.; Investigation, A.V.S., M.S.K., D.S.K., and E.V.R.; Project administration, Y.M.L.; Resources, R.F.F., E.V.I., Y.M.L., and V.A.V.; Supervision, R.F.F., Y.M.L., and V.A.V.; Visualization, A.V.S., A.A.N., M.S.K., E.V.R., and I.R.I.; Writing—original draft, A.V.S.; Writing—review and editing, A.V.S., A.A.N., E.V.R., R.F.F., Y.M.L., and V.A.V.

Acknowledgments: Authors thank Sergey Egorov (A.V. Topchiev Institute of Petrochemical Synthesis, RAS) for elemental analysis of fluorescent nanomaterials.

References

1. Yendluri, R.; Otto, D.P.; De Villiers, M.M.; Vinokurov, V.; Lvov, Y.M. Application of halloysite clay nanotubes as a pharmaceutical excipient. *Int. J. Pharm.* **2017**, *521*, 267–273. [CrossRef] [PubMed]

2. Lvov, Y.M.; DeVilliers, M.M.; Fakhrullin, R.F. The application of halloysite tubule nanoclay in drug delivery. *Expert Opin. Drug Deliv.* **2016**, *13*, 977–986. [CrossRef] [PubMed]

3. Cavallaro, G.; Lazzara, G.; Milioto, S.; Parisi, F.; Evtugyn, V.; Rozhina, E.; Fakhrullin, R. Nanohydrogel Formation within the Halloysite Lumen for Triggered and Sustained Release. *ACS Appl. Mater. Interfaces* **2018**, *10*, 8265–8273. [CrossRef] [PubMed]

4. Cavallaro, G.; Danilushkina, A.; Evtugyn, V.; Lazzara, G.; Milioto, S.; Parisi, F.; Rozhina, E.; Fakhrullin, R. Halloysite Nanotubes: Controlled Access and Release by Smart Gates. *Nanomaterials* **2017**, *7*, 199. [CrossRef] [PubMed]

5. Lazzara, G.; Riela, S.; Fakhrullin, R.F. Clay-based drug-delivery systems: What does the future hold? *Ther. Deliv.* **2017**, *8*, 633–646. [CrossRef]

6. Yendluri, R.; Lvov, Y.; de Villiers, M.M.; Vinokurov, V.; Naumenko, E.; Tarasova, E.; Fakhrullin, R. Paclitaxel encapsulated in halloysite clay nanotubes for intestinal and intracellular delivery. *J. Pharm. Sci.* **2017**, *106*, 3131–3139. [CrossRef] [PubMed]

7. Abdullayev, E.; Lvov, Y. Halloysite clay nanotubes as a ceramic "skeleton" for functional biopolymer composites with sustained drug release. *J. Mater. Chem. B* **2013**, *1*, 2894–2903. [CrossRef]

8. Ghanei-Motlagh, M.; Taher, M.A. A novel electrochemical sensor based on silver/halloysite nanotube/molybdenum disulfide nanocomposite for efficient nitrite sensing. *Biosens. Bioelectron.* **2018**, *109*, 279–285. [CrossRef] [PubMed]

9. Yang, M.; Xiong, X.; He, R.; Luo, Y.; Tang, J.; Dong, J.; Lu, H.; Yu, J.; Guan, H.; Zhang, J.; et al. Halloysite Nanotube-Modified Plasmonic Interface for Highly Sensitive Refractive Index Sensing. *ACS Appl. Mater. Interfaces* **2018**, *10*, 5933–5940. [CrossRef] [PubMed]

10. Prishchenko, D.A.; Zenkov, E.V.; Mazurenko, V.V.; Fakhrullin, R.F.; Lvov, Y.M.; Mazurenko, V.G. Molecular dynamics of the halloysite nanotubes. *Phys. Chem. Chem. Phys.* **2018**, *20*, 5841–5849. [CrossRef] [PubMed]

11. Cavallaro, G.; Lazzara, G.; Konnova, S.; Fakhrullin, R.; Lvov, Y. Composite films of natural clay nanotubes with cellulose and chitosan. *Green Mater.* **2014**, *2*, 232–242. [CrossRef]

12. Hillier, S.; Brydson, R.; Delbos, E.; Fraser, T.; Gray, N.; Pendlowski, H.; Phillips, I.; Robertson, J.; Wilson, I. Correlations among the mineralogical and physical properties of halloysite nanotubes (HNTs). *Clay Miner.* **2016**, *51*, 325–350. [CrossRef]

13. Massaro, M.; Cavallaro, G.; Colletti, C.G.; D'Azzo, G.; Guernelli, S.; Lazzara, G.; Pieraccini, S.; Riela, S. Halloysite nanotubes for efficient loading, stabilization and controlled release of insulin. *J. Colloid Interface Sci.* **2018**, *524*, 156–164. [CrossRef] [PubMed]

14. Massaro, M.; Colletti, C.G.; Lazzara, G.; Milioto, S.; Noto, R.; Riela, S. Halloysite nanotubes as support for metal-based catalysts. *J. Mater. Chem. A* **2017**, *5*, 13276–13293. [CrossRef]

15. Vinokurov, V.A.; Stavitskaya, A.V.; Glotov, A.P.; Novikov, A.A.; Zolotukhina, A.V.; Kotelev, M.S.; Gushchin, P.A.; Ivanov, E.V.; Darrat, Y.; Lvov, Y.M. Nanoparticles Formed Onto/Into Halloysite Clay Tubules: Architectural Synthesis and Applications. *Chem. Rec.* **2018**. [CrossRef] [PubMed]

16. Jana, S.; Kondakova, A.V.; Shevchenko, S.N.; Sheval, E.V.; Gonchar, K.A.; Timoshenko, V.Y.; Vasiliev, A.N. Halloysite nanotubes with immobilized silver nanoparticles for anti-bacterial application. *Colloids Surf. B* **2017**, *151*, 249–254. [CrossRef] [PubMed]

17. Shu, Z.; Zhang, Y.; Yang, Q.; Yang, H. Halloysite nanotubes supported Ag and ZnO nanoparticles with synergistically enhanced antibacterial activity. *Nanoscale Res. Lett.* **2017**, *12*, 135. [CrossRef] [PubMed]

18. Zieba, M.; Hueso, J.L.; Arruebo, M.; Martínez, G.; Santamaría, J. Gold-coated halloysite nanotubes as tunable plasmonic platforms. *New J. Chem.* **2014**, *38*, 2037–2042. [CrossRef]

19. Vinokurov, V.A.; Stavitskaya, A.V.; Ivanov, E.V.; Gushchin, P.A.; Kozlov, D.V.; Kurenkova, A.Y.; Kolinko, P.A.; Kozlova, E.A.; Lvov, Y.M. Halloysite nanoclay based CdS formulations with high catalytic activity in hydrogen evolution reaction under visible light irradiation. *ACS Sustain. Chem. Eng.* **2017**, *5*, 11316–11323. [CrossRef]

20. Micó-Vicent, B.; Martínez-Verdú, F.M.; Novikov, A.; Stavitskaya, A.; Vinokurov, V.; Rozhina, E.; Fakhrullin, R.; Yendluri, R.; Lvov, Y. Stabilized Dye-Pigment Formulations with Platy and Tubular Nanoclays. *Adv. Funct. Mater.* **2017**. [CrossRef]

21. Hoshino, A.; Hanada, S.; Yamamoto, K. Toxicity of nanocrystal quantum dots: The relevance of surface modifications. *Arch. Toxicol.* **2011**, *85*, 707–720. [CrossRef] [PubMed]

22. Mal, J.; Nancharaiah, Y.V.; van Hullebusch, E.D.; Lens, P.N.L. Metal chalcogenide quantum dots: Biotechnological synthesis and applications. *RSC Adv.* **2016**, *6*, 41477–41495. [CrossRef]

23. Li, J.; Zhu, J.-J. Quantum dots for fluorescent biosensing and bio-imaging applications. *Analyst* **2013**, *138*, 2506–2015. [CrossRef] [PubMed]

24. Lvov, Y.M.; Shchukin, D.G.; Möhwald, H.; Price, R.R. Halloysite clay nanotubes for controlled release of protective agents. *ACS Nano* **2008**, *2*, 814–820. [CrossRef] [PubMed]

25. Vergaro, V.; Abdullayev, E.; Lvov, Y.M.; Zeitoun, A.; Cingolani, R.; Rinaldi, R.; Leporatti, S. Cytocompatibility and uptake of halloysite clay nanotubes. *Biomacromolecules* **2010**, *11*, 820–826. [CrossRef] [PubMed]

26. Bellani, L.; Giorgetti, L.; Riela, S.; Lazzara, G.; Scialabba, A.; Massaro, M. Ecotoxicity of halloysite nanotube–supported palladium nanoparticles in *Raphanus sativus* L. *Environ. Toxicol. Chem.* **2016**, *35*, 2503–2510. [CrossRef] [PubMed]

27. Carli, L.N.; Daitx, T.S.; Soares, G.V.; Crespo, J.S.; Mauler, R.S. The effects of silane coupling agents on the properties of PHBV/halloysite nanocomposites. *Appl. Clay Sci.* **2014**, *87*, 311–319. [CrossRef]

28. Vinokurov, V.A.; Stavitskaya, A.V.; Chudakov, Y.A.; Ivanov, E.V.; Shrestha, L.K.; Ariga, K.; Darrat, Y.A.; Lvov, Y.M. Formation of metal clusters in halloysite clay nanotubes. *Sci. Technol. Adv. Mater.* **2017**, *18*, 147–151. [CrossRef] [PubMed]

29. Lvov, Y.; Wang, W.; Zhang, L.; Fakhrullin, R. Halloysite Clay Nanotubes for Loading and Sustained Release of Functional Compounds. *Adv. Mater.* **2016**, *28*, 1227–1250. [CrossRef] [PubMed]

30. Kumar-Krishnan, S.; Hernandez-Rangel, A.; Pal, U.; Ceballos-Sanchez, O.; Flores-Ruiz, F.J.; Prokhorov, E.; Arias de Fuentes, O.; Esparza, R.; Meyyappan, M. Surface functionalized halloysite nanotubes decorated with silver nanoparticles for enzyme immobilization and biosensing. *J. Mater. Chem. B* **2016**, *4*, 2553–2560. [CrossRef]

31. Zhang, H.; Ren, T.; Ji, Y.; Han, L.; Wu, Y.; Song, H.; Bai, L.; Ba, X. Selective modification of halloysite nanotubes with 1-pyrenylboronic acid: A novel fluorescence probe with highly selective and sensitive response to hyperoxide. *ACS Appl. Mater. Interfaces* **2015**, *7*, 23805–23811. [CrossRef] [PubMed]

32. Zhang, H. Selective modification of inner surface of halloysite nanotubes: A review. *Nanotechnol. Rev.* **2017**, *6*, 573–581. [CrossRef]

33. Eggeling, C.; Volkmer, A.; Seidel, C.A.M. Molecular photobleaching kinetics of Rhodamine 6G by one- and two-photon induced confocal fluorescence microscopy. *ChemPhysChem* **2005**, *6*, 791–804. [CrossRef] [PubMed]

34. Song, L.; Hennink, E.J.; Young, I.T.; Tanke, H.J. Photobleaching kinetics of fluorescein in quantitative fluorescence microscopy. *Biophys. J.* **1995**, *68*, 2588–2600. [CrossRef]

35. Guo, G.; Liu, W.; Liang, J.; He, Z.; Xu, H.; Yang, X. Probing the cytotoxicity of CdSe quantum dots with surface modification. *Mater. Lett.* **2007**, *61*, 1641–1644. [CrossRef]

36. Cho, S.J.; Maysinger, D.; Jain, M.; Röder, B.; Hackbarth, S.; Winnik, F.M. Long-term exposure to CdTe quantum dots causes functional impairments in live cells. *Langmuir* **2007**, *23*, 1974–1980. [CrossRef] [PubMed]

37. Pellegrino, T.; Manna, L.; Kudera, S.; Liedl, T.; Koktysh, D.; Rogach, A.L.; Keller, S.; Rädler, J.; Natile, G.; Parak, W.J. Hydrophobic nanocrystals coated with an amphiphilic polymer shell: A general route to water soluble nanocrystals. *Nano Lett.* **2004**, *4*, 703–707. [CrossRef]

38. Efros, A.L.; Nesbitt, D.J. Origin and control of blinking in quantum dots. *Nat. Nanotechnol.* **2016**, *11*, 661–671. [CrossRef] [PubMed]

39. Dzamukova, M.R.; Naumenko, E.A.; Lvov, Y.M.; Fakhrullin, R.F. Enzyme-activated intracellular drug delivery with tubule clay nanoformulation. *Sci. Rep.* **2015**, *5*, 10560. [CrossRef] [PubMed]

40. Kirchner, C.; Liedl, T.; Kudera, S.; Pellegrino, T.; Javier, A.M.; Gaub, H.E.; Stölzle, S.; Fertig, N.; Parak, W.J. Cytotoxicity of colloidal CdSe and CdSe/ZnS nanoparticles. *Nano Lett.* **2005**, *5*, 331–338. [CrossRef] [PubMed]

Protein Corona Fingerprints of Liposomes: New Opportunities for Targeted Drug Delivery and Early Detection in Pancreatic Cancer

Sara Palchetti [1], Damiano Caputo [2], Luca Digiacomo [1], Anna Laura Capriotti [3], Roberto Coppola [2], Daniela Pozzi [1,4,*] and Giulio Caracciolo [1,*]

[1] Department of Molecular Medicine, Sapienza University of Rome, Viale Regina Elena 291, 00161 Rome, Italy; sara.palchetti@uniroma1.it (S.P.); luca.digiacomo@uniroma1.it (L.D.)

[2] Department of General Surgery, University Campus-Biomedico di Roma, Via Alvaro del Portillo 200, 00128 Rome, Italy; d.caputo@unicampus.it (D.C.); r.coppola@unicampus.it (R.C.)

[3] Department of Chemistry, Sapienza University of Rome, P.le Aldo Moro 5, 00185 Rome, Italy; annalaura.capriotti@uniroma1.it

[4] Istituti Fisioterapici Ospitalieri, Istituto Regina Elena, Via Elio Chianesi 53, 00144 Rome, Italy

* Correspondence: daniela.pozzi@uniroma1.it (D.P.); giulio.caracciolo@uniroma1.it (G.C.);

Abstract: Pancreatic ductal adenocarcinoma (PDAC) is the fourth cause of cancer-related mortality in the Western world and is envisaged to become the second cause by 2030. Although our knowledge about the molecular biology of PDAC is continuously increasing, this progress has not been translated into better patients' outcome. Liposomes have been used to circumvent concerns associated with the low efficiency of anticancer drugs such as severe side effects and damage of healthy tissues, but they have not resulted in improved efficacy as yet. Recently, the concept is emerging that the limited success of liposomal drugs in clinical practice is due to our poor knowledge of the nano–bio interactions experienced by liposomes in vivo. After systemic administration, lipid vesicles are covered by plasma proteins forming a biomolecular coating, referred to as the protein corona (PC). Recent studies have clarified that just a minor fraction of the hundreds of bound plasma proteins, referred to as "PC fingerprints" (PCFs), enhance liposome association with cancer cells, triggering efficient particle internalization. In this study, we synthesized a library of 10 liposomal formulations with systematic changes in lipid composition and exposed them to human plasma (HP). Size, zeta-potential, and corona composition of the resulting liposome–protein complexes were thoroughly characterized by dynamic light scattering (DLS), micro-electrophoresis, and nano-liquid chromatography tandem mass spectrometry (nano-LC MS/MS). According to the recent literature, enrichment in PCFs was used to predict the targeting ability of synthesized liposomal formulations. Here we show that the predicted targeting capability of liposome–protein complexes clearly correlate with cellular uptake in pancreatic adenocarcinoma (PANC-1) and insulinoma (INS-1) cells as quantified by flow-assisted cell sorting (FACS). Of note, cellular uptake of the liposomal formulation with the highest abundance of PCFs was much larger than that of Onivyde®, an Irinotecan liposomal drug approved by the Food and Drug Administration in 2015 for the treatment of metastatic PDAC. Given the urgent need of efficient nanocarriers for the treatment of PDAC, we envision that our results will pave the way for the development of more efficient PC-based targeted nanomaterials. Here we also show that some BCs are enriched with plasma proteins that are associated with the onset and progression of PDAC (e.g., sex hormone-binding globulin, Ficolin-3, plasma protease C1 inhibitor, etc.). This could open the intriguing possibility to identify novel biomarkers.

Keywords: pancreatic ductal adenocarcinoma; liposomes; protein corona

1. Introduction

With a one-year survival rate of 12% that declines to 1% at five years, pancreatic ductal adenocarcinoma (PDAC) is one of the most lethal tumors worldwide [1]. It is currently the fourth leading cause of cancer-associated mortality and it is predicted to become the second leading cause in the next decade in Western countries [2]. When PDAC is diagnosed, surgery remains the only treatment chance, while chemotherapeutic agents are often inefficacious. To tackle this issue, numerous drugs have been tested. Gemcitabine (GEM) was the first drug to be approved for pancreatic cancer, but it is currently used only as a palliative agent [3]. Cisplatin and 5-Fluorouracile can extend life for a few months but both have collateral toxic properties [4]. Irinotecan is an antitumor drug belonging to the camptothecin family that targets DNA topoisomerase-1, a nuclear enzyme able to prevent torsional stress during DNA replication and transcription [5]. Nanotechnology has recently gained attention for its ability to treat numerous tumors, with nanocarriers being used to circumvent the problems associated with anticancer drugs, including high toxicity and irreversible damage of normal cells [6]. Recently, Onivyde®, an Irinotecan liposomal formulation, has been approved by the Food and Drug Administration (FDA) for the treatment of metastatic pancreatic cancer resistant to gemcitabine chemotherapy [7]. As a matter of fact, encapsulated liposomal drugs exhibit better pharmacokinetics and therapeutic index, as well as reduce the collateral toxic effects of free drugs. However, the adsorption of plasma opsonins (e.g., complement proteins, immunoglobulins, etc.) to the liposomal surface results in the clearance of liposomes from the blood circulation [8]. For a couple of decades, researchers have tried to prevent protein binding by grafting polymers to the liposome surface and, in this regard, polyethylene glycol (PEG) has been the gold standard for stealth polymers in drug delivery [9]. Conjugating PEG terminals to tissue-recognition ligands (e.g., peptides, antibodies, etc.) has long been supposed to provide such "long-circulating" liposomes with selective targeting ability [10]. However, recent findings have demonstrated that grafting polymers to a liposome surface can only reduce protein binding, but cannot fully prevent it [11]. Moreover, Schöttler et al. showed that PEG promotes the recruitment of specific plasma proteins [12], thus contributing to explain the accelerated blood clearance ("ABC phenomenon") of PEGylated nanosystems [13]. The main implication is that active targeting usually fails in vivo with the result that no targeted liposomal drug has been approved so far. While protein binding to a liposome surface is a well-established paradigm in drug delivery [14–16], the emerging field of nano–bio interactions between nanosized objects and biological systems is putting earlier findings in context, providing the liposome field with new perspectives [17–20].

When liposomes are introduced into a biological fluid, they are covered by a dynamic layer of biomolecules, in particular proteins, forming the so-called "protein corona" (PC) [21,22]. This complex interface is formed in seconds and, over time, it changes prevalently in the amount of bound protein and slightly in protein composition [23]. With respect to other kinds of nanoparticles, the liposome–PC evolves significantly during the first hour of exposure to biological fluids [24] and is the reason why exposure time is typically fixed at 1 h [24–26]. As a consequence of PC formation, liposomes lose their synthetic identity and attain a new one that is usually referred to as their "biological identity". It is this newly acquired biological identity that controls undesirable side effects of liposomal drug delivery, such as off-target interactions, toxicity, size-dependent particle recognition by immune cells [27], and clearance from the bloodstream [28,29]. On the other side, it is increasingly accepted that even particle accumulation at the target site is controlled by the biological identity acquired in biological environments [17]. For instance, non-specific interactions between liposomes and target cells are controlled by physical-chemical properties (i.e., size and zeta-potential) of liposome–protein complexes and not by those of pristine liposomes. Moreover, the PC may act as an endogenous trigger, promoting association with receptors of target cells and leading to efficient internalization. In a couple of recent investigations [26,30], we demonstrated that liposomes possessing specific size and zeta-potential are efficiently internalized within cancer cells [26,30]. Moreover, a minor fraction of identified "corona proteins" (typically 1–2%), referred to as "protein corona fingerprints" (PCFs), promote favorable cellular association. Globally, liposome physical-chemical properties, PC composition, and cellular uptake can be combined in a general strategy to predict the interaction of liposomes with cancer cells (Figure 1).

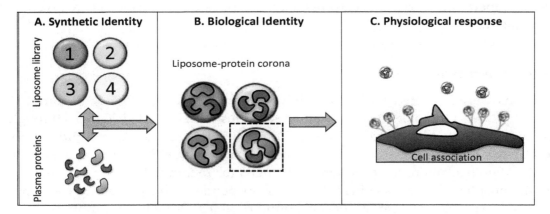

Figure 1. Schematic illustrating the protein corona fingerprinting strategy. (**A**) A library of liposomes is mixed with plasma proteins; (**B**) plasma proteins adsorb to the particle surface, forming liposome–protein complexes that are ranked for enrichment in protein corona 'fingerprints', i.e., plasma proteins that promote association with cancer cells; (**C**) selected formulations are incubated with cells in culture and cell association is measured by flow-assisted flow cytometry.

This work was therefore aimed at exploiting the liposome–PC to target human pancreatic carcinoma (PANC-1) cells. To this end, a library of 10 liposomal formulations was synthesized and liposome–protein complexes were thoroughly characterized by dynamic light scattering (DLS), micro-electrophoresis (ME), and nano-liquid chromatography tandem mass spectrometry (nano-LC MS/MS). Next, liposomes were screened for their particle properties and corona composition. Of note, cellular uptake by PANC-1 cells was found to correlate with physical-chemical properties of liposome–protein complexes and enrichment in PCFs. A second aim of the study was the complete identification of the protein patterns adsorbed to synthesized liposomes. Indeed, the recently introduced concept of the "disease-specific PC" [31] states that the PC composition is affected by changes in human proteome as those induced by numerous diseases such as cancer. Thus, identifying proteins that are related to pancreatic tumor onset and progression could pave the way to identify cancer in the early stages by differential analysis of the PC.

2. Materials and Methods

2.1. Liposomes Preparation

Cationic lipids 1,2-dioleoyl-3-trimethylammonium-propane (DOTAP) and (3β-[N-(N′,N′-dimethylaminoethane)carbamoyl])cholesterol; neutral lipids dioleoylphosphatidylethanolamine (DOPE), 1,2-dipalmitoyl-sn-glycero-3-phosphocholine (DPPC), and 1,2-diarachidoyl-sn-glycero-3-phosphocholine (20:0 PC); the zwitterionic lipid dioleoylphosphocholine (DOPC); and the anionic lipid 1,2-dioleoyl-sn-glycero-3-phospho-(1′-rac-glycerol) (DOPG) were purchased from Avanti Polar Lipids (Alabaster, AL, USA), while sphingosine and cholesterol were from Sigma-Aldrich (St. Louis, MO, USA). All lipids were used without further refinement and were prepared at desired molar ratios. Each lipid was dissolved in chloroform and the solvent was evaporated under a vacuum for at least 2 h. Lipid films were hydrated in ultrapure water to obtain a final lipid concentration of 1 mg/mL. The obtained liposome solutions were extruded 20 times through a 0.1-μm polycarbonate carbonate filter with the Avanti Mini-Extruder (Avanti Polar Lipids, Alabaster, AL, USA). Liposomes were incubated with human plasma (HP) (1:1 v/v) for 1 h at 37 °C. Incubation time was chosen according to previous findings as it represents a typical plateau of the temporal evolution of the liposome–PC [24].

2.2. Size and Zeta-Potential Experiments

For size and zeta-potential experiments, bare liposomes and liposome–HP complexes were diluted 1:100 with ddH$_2$O. All the measurements were performed using a Zetasizer Nano ZS90 (Malvern, UK) at room temperature. Experiments were made in triplicate and the results are given as means ± standard deviation.

2.3. Proteomics Experiments

Lipid films were hydrated with a dissolving buffer (Tris-HCl, pH 7.4, 10 mmol L^{-1}; NaCl, 150 mmol L^{-1}; EDTA, 1 mmol L^{-1}). The obtained solutions were extruded 20 times through a 0.1-μm polycarbonate carbonate filter with the Avanti Mini-Extruder (Avanti Polar Lipids, Alabaster, AL, USA) and stored at 4 °C until use. Liposomes were incubated with HP (1:1 v/v) and then incubated at 37 °C for 1 h. After incubation, samples were centrifuged for 15 min at 14,000 rpm. Pellet was robustly washed with phosphate-buffered saline (PBS) and resuspended. This procedure was repeated three times to wash the sample and remove loosely bound proteins. Protein denaturation, digestion, and desalting were carried out by a robust methodology that is commonly used to separate liposome−PC complexes from unbound and loosely bound proteins [11]. In brief, samples were lyophilized by a Speed-Vac apparatus (mod. SC 250 Express; Thermo Savant, Holbrook, NY, USA). Samples were reconstituted with 0.1% HCOOH solution (final concentration 0.32 mg/mL) and stored at −80 °C until LC MS/MS was carried out. Tryptic peptides were investigated by a nano-LC system (Dionex Ultimate 3000, Sunnyvale, CA, USA) connected to a hybrid mass spectrometer (Thermo Fisher Scientific, Bremen, Germany), equipped with a nanoelectrospray ion source. Xcalibur (v.2.07, Thermo Fisher Scientific) raw data files were submitted to Proteome Discover (1.2 version, Thermo Scientific) for a database search using Mascot (version 2.3.2 Matrix Science). Data was searched against the SwissProt database (v 57.15, 20,266 sequences) using the decoy search option of Mascot and protein quantification was made by Scaffold software. For each identified protein, the mean value of the normalized spectral countings (NSCs) was normalized to the protein molecular weight (MWNSC) to obtain the relative protein abundance (RPA) [32]. For each identified protein, the reported RPA is the mean of three independent replicates ± standard deviation.

2.4. Cell Culture

Human pancreatic carcinoma cell line (PANC-1) was purchased from Sigma-Aldrich (St. Louis, MO, USA) and maintained in DMEM medium. Rat insulinoma cell line (INS-1) was purchased from Thermo Fisher (Waltham, MA, USA) and was maintained in RPMI. Both mediums were supplemented with 2 mM L-glutamine, 100 IU/mL penicillin-streptomycin, 1 mM sodium pyruvate, 10 mM Hepes, 1.5 mg/L sodium bicarbonate, and 10% fetal bovine serum. Cell lines were cultured at 37 °C in a humidified atmosphere with 5% CO$_2$.

2.5. Flow-Assisted Cell Sorting Experiments

For cellular uptake experiments, Lip-1 and Lip-5 liposomes were synthesized using Texas Red® 1,2-dihexadecanoyl-*sn*-glycero-3-phosphoethanolamine, triethylammonium salt (TX-DHPE) (Thermo Fisher, Waltham, MA, USA). Onyvide-like liposomes were prepared using DSPC, Chol, MPEG-2000-DSPE, and TX-DHPE at the molar ratios 215:143:1:1. Cells were seeded on 12-well plates (150,000 cells/well) in complete medium and, after 2 h, cells were treated with liposomes incubated with human plasma for 1 h using Optimem medium. After 3 h, cells were detached with trypsine/EDTA, washed two times with cold PBS, and run on a BD LSR Fortessa™ (BD Bioscience, San Jose, CA, USA).

3. Results and Discussion

First, we synthesized a combinatorial library of 10 liposomal formulations. According to previous findings [33,34], liposomes were prepared by mixing cholesterol, DC-Chol, DOPC, DOPE, DOTAP, DPPC, PC (20:0), and sphingosine in specific molar ratios (Table 1).

Table 1. The molar ratios of lipids used for synthesized a library of 10 liposomal formulations.

Samples	CHOLESTEROL	DC-CHOL	DOPC	DOPE	DOTAP	DPPC	PC (20:0)	SPHINGOSINE
Lip-1	0	0	0	0.5	0.5	0	0	0
Lip-2	0	0.5	0	0.5	0	0	0	0
Lip-3	0	0.25	0.25	0.25	0.25	0	0	0
Lip-4	0	1	0	0	0	0	0	0
Lip-5	0.2	0	0	0	0	0	0.8	0
Lip-6	0.25	0	0	0	0.5	0	0.25	0
Lip-7	0.25	0	0	0	0.5	0.25	0	0
Lip-8	0.33	0	0	0	0	0	0.33	0.33
Lip-9	0.5	0	0	0	0.5	0	0	0
Lip-10	0.5	0.5	0	0	0	0	0	0

Next, the synthetic identity of liposomes (i.e., size, zeta-potential, and aggregation state post-synthesis) was characterized by DLS and ME (Figure 2). Pristine vesicles were small in size with a hydrodynamic diameter (D_H) ranging from ~100 nm to 150 nm (Figure 2A, blue points). Moreover, the polydispersity index (PDI) indicated that all liposomal formulations were monodisperse (Table 2).

Zeta-potential of liposomes varied between ~0 mV (Lip-5) and ~65 mV (Lip-10) depending on liposomal lipid composition (Figure 2B, blue points). One-hour exposure to HP lead to the formation of liposome–protein complexes that were characterized in terms of size, zeta-potential, and homogeneity of dispersion. The size of liposome–protein complexes (Figure 2A, red points) was larger than that of pristine vesicles and varied appreciably among formulations. This is in full agreement with previous findings showing that lipid composition plays a key role in protein binding to a lipid surface [35]. According to the literature [22], a size increase of a few nanometers is likely due to the formation of a PC on the liposome surface, while an enlargement of a few tenths of a nanometer reflects the clustering of single liposomes coated by plasma proteins [25,32].

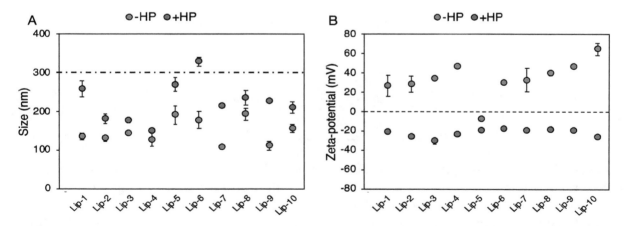

Figure 2. (A) Hydrodynamic diameter of liposomes before (blue points, "− human plasma (HP)") and after (red points, "+ HP") 1-h incubation with human plasma (HP) of pancreatic cancer patients. Values are means ± standard deviation from three independent experiments. The dashed line indicates a typical size threshold for particle removal from bloodstream by macrophages. (B) Zeta-potential of liposomes before (blue points, "− HP") and after (red points, "+ HP") 1-h incubation with human plasma (HP) of pancreatic cancer patients.

Table 2. Polydispersity index (PDI) of bare liposomal formulations and after 1-h incubation with HP.

Samples	PDI	
	−HP	+HP
Lip-1	0.14 ± 0.04	0.12 ± 0.04
Lip-2	0.11 ± 0.01	0.17 ± 0.05
Lip-3	0.08 ± 0.01	0.13 ± 0.01
Lip-4	0.12 ± 0.02	0.14 ± 0.01
Lip-5	0.10 ± 0.02	0.16 ± 0.05
Lip-6	0.10 ± 0.02	0.17 ± 0.01
Lip-7	0.12 ± 0.02	0.20 ± 0.04
Lip-8	0.11 ± 0.02	0.18 ± 0.03
Lip-9	0.15 ± 0.01	0.22 ± 0.02
Lip-10	0.14 ± 0.01	0.20 ± 0.01

Liposome aggregation is confirmed by an increase in PDI values (Table 2). On the other side, "normalization" in zeta-potential around −20 mV (Figure 2B, red points), regardless of pristine surface charge, has been reported for many classes of nanomaterials and is caused by the fact that most plasma proteins have a negative charge at physiological pH. Besides the size and zeta-potential of liposome–protein complexes, the biological identity of liposomes is also controlled by the composition of the PC. When in the blood, the liposome–PC could hamper the ability of the pristine vesicle to bind to target receptors [36] and may induce activation of the immune system, leading to particle clearance [21,37].

On the other hand, molecular recognition between endogenous plasma proteins (i.e., recruited from the blood) and cancer cell receptors [38] could promote selective accumulation at the tumor site. A crucial step towards the exploitation of the PC for targeted drug delivery is therefore the identification and quantification of corona proteins. Bradford assay results showed that the amount of bound protein is dependent on both the zeta-potential and lipid composition (Table 3).

Table 3. Micrograms of proteins bound to liposomal formulations after 1-h incubation with HP.

Samples	Protein (μg/μL)
	+HP
Lip-1	4.9 ± 0.4
Lip-2	5.3 ± 0.6
Lip-3	4.8 ± 0.5
Lip-4	9.0 ± 0.9
Lip-5	3.1 ± 0.4
Lip-6	4.6 ± 0.3
Lip-7	4.1 ± 0.4
Lip-8	3.7 ± 0.4
Lip-9	9.5 ± 0.9
Lip-10	6.6 ± 0.5

Generally, it was observed that cationic liposomes adsorb more proteins than neutrally charged vesicles. Likewise, nano-LC MS/MS showed that the liposome–PCs were highly complex entities containing between 140 and 222 proteins (Table 4).

The identified number of proteins in Table 4 is larger than that accommodated on the liposome surface. This apparent discrepancy was clarified by recent models that describe the corona as a coating made of several layers held together by protein–protein interactions [39,40]. To facilitate their rational identification, corona proteins were grouped according to physiological functions of the blood system. The relative protein abundance (RPA) of biologically relevant proteins such as complement proteins, coagulation proteins, immunoglobulins, acute phase proteins, tissue leakage, and lipoproteins are displayed in Figure 3.

Table 4. Number of proteins adsorbed on liposomal formulations after 1-h incubation with HP.

Samples	#Identified Proteins
Lip-1	220
Lip-2	140
Lip-3	205
Lip-4	170
Lip-5	174
Lip-6	202
Lip-7	206
Lip-8	180
Lip-9	222
Lip-10	190

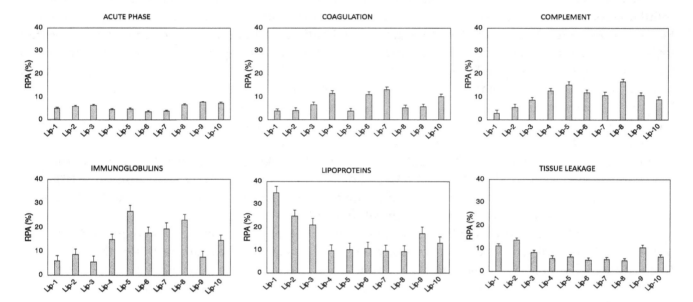

Figure 3. Bioinformatic classification of proteins identified in the corona of Lip-1–Lip-10 after 1-h exposure to HP. The relative protein abundances (RPAs) of total proteins are shown.

Our findings confirmed that each liposome exhibits a specific protein pattern dictated by its specific lipid composition. Over the last decade, numerous studies have tried to relate the cellular uptake of nanoparticle–protein complexes to PC composition by an oversimplified picture of particle–cell interaction; the more abundant a corona protein, the more probable the molecular recognition by cell receptors and, in turn, the more significant its role in promoting nanoparticle–cell association. However, to understand the link between a nanoparticle–corona complex and specific uptake pathways, mapping the exact location of protein binding sites is a necessary step [41,42]. To date, mapping protein epitopes at the liposome surface is challenging. To overcome this issue, computational methods such as quantitative structure–activity relation (QSAR) allow the identification of the most appropriate set of descriptors to predict the interactions between liposomes and cells at the nano–bio interface [43,44]. Correlations between the RPA of individual proteins and cellular uptake allowed us to identify eight "protein fingerprints" (Vitronectin, APOA1, APOA2, APOB, APOC2, Ig heavy chain V-III region BRO, vitamin K-dependent protein, and Integrin beta3) that promote the association of liposomes with cancer cells [26,30]. Among PCFs, a key role is played by Vitronectin, a glycoprotein of the hemopexin family containing an RGD motif (Arg-Gly-Asp) in the Somatomedin B domain (20−63 region) that is specifically recognized by $\alpha_v \beta_3$ integrins [38]. This class of integrins is overexpressed on many solid tumors and in tumor neovasculature [45,46]. This could be extremely relevant in pancreatic cancer, where roughly half of patients show elevated expression of $\alpha v \beta 3$, and this is positively correlated with lymph node metastasis [47]. Most chemotherapeutics given in the clinic today damage healthy tissues, leading to unwanted side effects. According to our present understanding, this could likely be related to off-target interactions between corona proteins and cell receptors of healthy cells. This means that receptors targeted by corona proteins should be overexpressed in cancer but not in normal cells. In this regard, it is known that $\alpha_v \beta_3$ integrin is expressed by normal (i.e., not-cancer) cells in a latent state characterized by its inability to stimulate cell adhesion to extra-cellular matrix ligands [48]. We also observed that, of eight PCFs, four are Apolipoproteins. It is well known that Apolipoproteins bind certain receptors such as scavenger receptor class B, type I (SR-BI), and low-density lipoprotein receptors (LDLR) that are overexpressed in several diseases. Recent studies showed that SR-BI and LDLR are overexpressed in pancreatic cancer, thus representing good targets of Apolipoprotein-enriched coronas [49,50]. Liposomal formulations were ranked for their PC-based targeting ability by calculating the total abundance of PCFs [51].

According to Figure 4, Lip-1 was identified as the most promising formulation to promote cellular association within PANC-1 and INS-1 cells. On the other side, Lip-5, being highly defective in PCFs, was expected to promote low cellular internalization. To support our conclusions, we treated PANC-1 cells with fluorescently labeled Lip-1- and Lip-5-protein complexes. Onivyde®, the liposomal formulation approved by the FDA for the treatment of metastatic pancreatic cancer [7,52], was used as a control. In order to obtain a quantitative view on this process, we performed FACS analysis. Figure 5A shows that about 95% of PANC-1 and INS-1 cells treated with Lip-1-protein complexes were fluorescence-positive. On the other hand, Lip-5-protein complexes were poorly internalized by PANC-1 cells, as demonstrated by the fact that less than 20% were positive for the fluorescence signal. This percentage was slightly higher in INS-1 cells (<30%). FACS results also show that the internalization of Onivyde® in both PANC-1 and INS-1 cells is extremely low, with only 10% and 20% of fluorescence-positive cells, respectively. The mean fluorescence intensity reported in Figure 5B shows the same trends as those observed for cellular uptake.

Lastly, our MS/MS results indicate that the composition of the PC (in terms of types and amounts of the constituent proteins) depends strongly on the physical-chemical properties of the liposomes. In particular, we observed that the coronas of Lip-1 and Lip-5 were particularly enriched with plasma proteins and were associated with the onset and progression of pancreatic cancer (e.g., sex hormone-binding globulin, Ficolin-3, plasma protease C1 inhibitor, etc.). Recently, some authors introduced the concept of the disease-specific PC [31], wherein alterations in human proteome of patients with various diseases produce appreciable changes in the PC protein pattern. Consequently, we envision that the manipulation of liposome surface chemistry can dictate the selective binding of plasma proteins with the possibility of identifying cancer at the early stages.

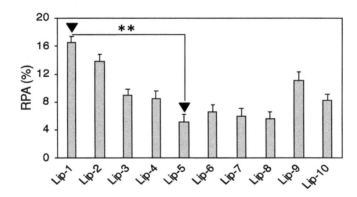

Figure 4. Relative protein abundance of biomolecular corona fingerprints. Lip-1 and Lip-5 were the liposomal formulations with the highest and lowest enrichment in PCFs (Vitronectin, APOA1, APOA2, APOB, APOC2, Ig heavy chain V-III region BRO, vitamin K-dependent protein, and Integrin beta3). Significance was statistically evaluated by Student's t-test (** $p < 0.05$).

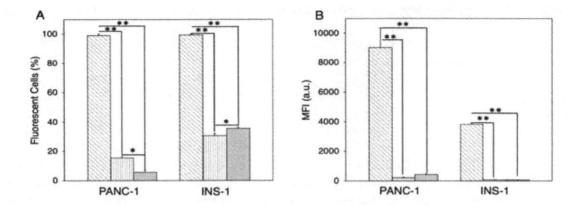

Figure 5. (**A**) Cellular uptake of Lip-1 (grey diagonal hatched lines), Lip-5 (grey vertical hatched lines), and Onivyde® (grey bar) in PANC-1 and INS-1 cells after 1-h incubation with human plasma (HP). (**B**) Mean fluorescence intensity of Lip-1 (grey diagonal hatched lines), Lip-5 (grey vertical hatched lines), and Onivyde® (grey bar) in PANC-1 and INS-1 cells after 1-h incubation with human plasma (HP). Statistical significance was evaluated using Student's *t*-test: * $p < 0.01$; ** $p < 0.005$ (no asterisk means lack of significance).

4. Conclusions

In conclusion, we have synthesized a library of 10 liposomal formulations that exhibit peculiar biological identities when exposed to HP. We found that the formulation exhibiting the highest levels of targeting fingerprints also had major cellular uptake in PANC-1 and INS-1 cells. Our results indicate that the exploitation of PCs could be a valuable means to develop targeted nanomedicine for PDAC treatment. Moreover, we found that the PCs of some liposome formulations were enriched with plasma proteins that are related to PDAC onset and progression. This possibility could pave the way for the identification of novel biomarkers and will be explored in future investigations.

Author Contributions: Conceptualization, D.C., R.C., G.C., and D.P.; methodology, G.C and D.P.; software, L.D.; validation, S.P., formal analysis, L.D.; investigation, S.P., L.D., and A.L.C.; resources, D.C., R.C., G.C., and D.P.; data curation, L.D.; writing—original draft preparation, G.C.; writing—review and editing, S.P, D.C., R.C., G.C., and D.P.; visualization, S.P. and L.D.; supervision, D.C., R.C., G.C., and D.P.; project administration, G.C. and D.P.; funding acquisition, D.C., G.C., and D.P.

References

1. Kamisawa, T.; Wood, L.D.; Itoi, T.; Takaori, K. Pancreatic cancer. *Lancet* **2016**, *388*, 73–85. [CrossRef]
2. Rahib, L.; Smith, B.D.; Aizenberg, R.; Rosenzweig, A.B.; Fleshman, J.M.; Matrisian, L.M. Projecting cancer incidence and deaths to 2030: The unexpected burden of thyroid, liver, and pancreas cancers in the united states. *Cancer Res.* **2014**, *74*, 2913–2921. [CrossRef] [PubMed]
3. Hidalgo, M. Pancreatic cancer. *N. Engl. J. Med.* **2010**, *362*, 1605–1617. [CrossRef]
4. Kundranda, M.N.; Niu, J. Albumin-bound paclitaxel in solid tumors: Clinical development and future directions. *Drug Des. Dev. Ther.* **2015**, *9*, 3767–3777. [CrossRef] [PubMed]
5. Pommier, Y. DNA topoisomerase i inhibitors: Chemistry, biology, and interfacial inhibition. *Chem. Rev.* **2009**, *109*, 2894–2902. [CrossRef] [PubMed]
6. Ud Din, F.; Aman, W.; Ullah, I.; Qureshi, O.S.; Mustapha, O.; Shafique, S.; Zeb, A. Effective use of nanocarriers as drug delivery systems for the treatment of selected tumors. *Int. J. Nanomed.* **2017**, *12*, 7291–7309. [CrossRef] [PubMed]

7. DiGiulio, S. FDA approves onivyde combo regimen for advanced pancreatic cancer. *Oncol. Times* **2015**, *37*, 8. [CrossRef]

8. Liu, D.; Liu, F.; Song, Y.K. Recognition and clearance of liposomes containing phosphatidylserine are mediated by serum opsonin. *Biochim. Biophys. Acta (BBA)-Biomembr.* **1995**, *1235*, 140–146. [CrossRef]

9. Knop, K.; Hoogenboom, R.; Fischer, D.; Schubert, U.S. Poly(ethylene glycol) in drug delivery: Pros and cons as well as potential alternatives. *Angew. Chem. Int. Edit.* **2010**, *49*, 6288–6308. [CrossRef]

10. Prencipe, G.; Tabakman, S.M.; Welsher, K.; Liu, Z.; Goodwin, A.P.; Zhang, L.; Henry, J.; Dai, H. Peg branched polymer for functionalization of nanomaterials with ultralong blood circulation. *J. Am. Chem. Soc.* **2009**, *131*, 4783–4787. [CrossRef]

11. Pozzi, D.; Colapicchioni, V.; Caracciolo, G.; Piovesana, S.; Capriotti, A.L.; Palchetti, S.; De Grossi, S.; Riccioli, A.; Amenitsch, H.; Laganà, A. Effect of polyethyleneglycol (PEG) chain length on the bio-nano-interactions between pegylated lipid nanoparticles and biological fluids: From nanostructure to uptake in cancer cells. *Nanoscale* **2014**, *6*, 2782–2792. [CrossRef] [PubMed]

12. Schöttler, S.; Becker, G.; Winzen, S.; Steinbach, T.; Mohr, K.; Landfester, K.; Mailänder, V.; Wurm, F.R. Protein adsorption is required for stealth effect of poly(ethylene glycol)-and poly(phosphoester)-coated nanocarriers. *Nat. Nanotechnol.* **2016**, *11*, 372–377. [CrossRef] [PubMed]

13. Ishida, T.; Harada, M.; Wang, X.Y.; Ichihara, M.; Irimura, K.; Kiwada, H. Accelerated blood clearance of pegylated liposomes following preceding liposome injection: Effects of lipid dose and peg surface-density and chain length of the first-dose liposomes. *J. Control. Release* **2005**, *105*, 305–317. [CrossRef] [PubMed]

14. Moghimi, S.M.; Hunter, A.C. Recognition by macrophages and liver cells of opsonized phospholipid vesicles and phospholipid headgroups. *Pharm. Res.* **2001**, *18*, 1–8. [CrossRef]

15. Moghimi, S.M.; Hunter, A.C.; Murray, J.C. Long-circulating and target-specific nanoparticles: Theory to practice. *Pharmacol. Rev.* **2001**, *53*, 283–318. [PubMed]

16. Moghimi, S.M.; Szebeni, J. Stealth liposomes and long circulating nanoparticles: Critical issues in pharmacokinetics, opsonization and protein-binding properties. *Prog. Lipid Res.* **2003**, *42*, 463–478. [CrossRef]

17. Caracciolo, G. Liposome-protein corona in a physiological environment: Challenges and opportunities for targeted delivery of nanomedicines. *Nanomed. Nanotechnol. Biol. Med.* **2015**, *11*, 543–557. [CrossRef] [PubMed]

18. Caracciolo, G.; Farokhzad, O.C.; Mahmoudi, M. Biological identity of nanoparticles in vivo: Clinical implications of the protein corona. *Trends Biotechnol.* **2017**, *35*, 257–264. [CrossRef] [PubMed]

19. Caracciolo, G. Clinically approved liposomal nanomedicines: Lessons learned from the biomolecular corona. *Nanoscale* **2018**, *10*, 4167–4172. [CrossRef]

20. Caracciolo, G.; Pozzi, D.; Capriotti, A.L.; Cavaliere, C.; Piovesana, S.; La Barbera, G.; Amici, A.; Laganà, A. The liposome-protein corona in mice and humans and its implications for in vivo delivery. *J. Mater. Chem. B* **2014**, *2*, 7419–7428. [CrossRef]

21. Monopoli, M.P.; Aberg, C.; Salvati, A.; Dawson, K.A. Biomolecular coronas provide the biological identity of nanosized materials. *Nat. Nanotechnol.* **2012**, *7*, 779–786. [CrossRef] [PubMed]

22. Walkey, C.D.; Chan, W.C. Understanding and controlling the interaction of nanomaterials with proteins in a physiological environment. *Chem. Soc. Rev.* **2012**, *41*, 2780–2799. [CrossRef] [PubMed]

23. Tenzer, S.; Docter, D.; Kuharev, J.; Musyanovych, A.; Fetz, V.; Hecht, R.; Schlenk, F.; Fischer, D.; Kiouptsi, K.; Reinhardt, C. Rapid formation of plasma protein corona critically affects nanoparticle pathophysiology. *Nat. Nanotechnol.* **2013**, *8*, 772–781. [CrossRef] [PubMed]

24. Barrán-Berdón, A.L.; Pozzi, D.; Caracciolo, G.; Capriotti, A.L.; Caruso, G.; Cavaliere, C.; Riccioli, A.; Palchetti, S.; Laganaì, A. Time evolution of nanoparticle-protein corona in human plasma: Relevance for targeted drug delivery. *Langmuir* **2013**, *29*, 6485–6494. [CrossRef] [PubMed]

25. Pozzi, D.; Caracciolo, G.; Digiacomo, L.; Colapicchioni, V.; Palchetti, S.; Capriotti, A.L.; Cavaliere, C.; Zenezini Chiozzi, R.; Puglisi, A.; Laganà, A. The biomolecular corona of nanoparticles in circulating biological media. *Nanoscale* **2015**, *7*, 13958–13966. [CrossRef] [PubMed]

26. Palchetti, S.; Digiacomo, L.; Pozzi, D.; Peruzzi, G.; Micarelli, E.; Mahmoudi, M.; Caracciolo, G. Nanoparticles-cell association predicted by protein corona fingerprints. *Nanoscale* **2016**, *8*, 12755–12763. [CrossRef] [PubMed]

27. Mirshafiee, V.; Mahmoudi, M.; Lou, K.; Cheng, J.; Kraft, M.L. Protein corona significantly reduces active targeting yield. *Chem. Commun.* **2013**, *49*, 2557–2559. [CrossRef]

28. Harashima, H.; Hiraiwa, T.; Ochi, Y.; Kiwada, H. Size dependent liposome degradation in blood: in vivo/in vitro correlation by kinetic modeling. *J. Drug Target.* **1995**, *3*, 253–261. [CrossRef]

29. Jiang, W.; Kim, B.Y.; Rutka, J.T.; Chan, W.C. Nanoparticle-mediated cellular response is size-dependent. *Nat. Nanotechnol.* **2008**, *3*, 145–150. [CrossRef]

30. Bigdeli, A.; Palchetti, S.; Pozzi, D.; Hormozi-Nezhad, M.R.; Baldelli Bombelli, F.; Caracciolo, G.; Mahmoudi, M. Exploring cellular interactions of liposomes using protein corona fingerprints and physicochemical properties. *ACS Nano* **2016**, *10*, 3723–3737. [CrossRef]

31. Hajipour, M.J.; Laurent, S.; Aghaie, A.; Rezaee, F.; Mahmoudi, M. Personalized protein coronas: A "key" factor at the nanobiointerface. *Biomater. Sci.* **2014**, *2*, 1210–1221. [CrossRef]

32. Monopoli, M.P.; Walczyk, D.; Campbell, A.; Elia, G.; Lynch, I.; Baldelli Bombelli, F.; Dawson, K.A. Physical—Chemical aspects of protein corona: Relevance to in vitro and in vivo biological impacts of nanoparticles. *J. Am. Chem. Soc.* **2011**, *133*, 2525–2534. [CrossRef] [PubMed]

33. Caracciolo, G.; Pozzi, D.; Caminiti, R.; Marchini, C.; Montani, M.; Amici, A.; Amenitsch, H. Transfection efficiency boost by designer multicomponent lipoplexes. *Biochim. Biophys. Acta Biomembr.* **2007**, *1768*, 2280–2292. [CrossRef] [PubMed]

34. Pozzi, D.; Marchini, C.; Cardarelli, F.; Rossetta, A.; Colapicchioni, V.; Amici, A.; Montani, M.; Motta, S.; Brocca, P.; Cantù, L.; et al. Mechanistic understanding of gene delivery mediated by highly efficient multicomponent envelope-type nanoparticle systems. *Mol. Pharm.* **2013**, *10*, 4654–4665. [CrossRef]

35. Caracciolo, G.; Pozzi, D.; Capriotti, A.L.; Cavaliere, C.; Piovesana, S.; Amenitsch, H.; Laganà, A. Lipid composition: A "key factor" for the rational manipulation of the liposome-protein corona by liposome design. *RSC Adv.* **2015**, *5*, 5967–5975. [CrossRef]

36. Salvati, A.; Pitek, A.S.; Monopoli, M.P.; Prapainop, K.; Bombelli, F.B.; Hristov, D.R.; Kelly, P.M.; Åberg, C.; Mahon, E.; Dawson, K.A. Transferrin-functionalized nanoparticles lose their targeting capabilities when a biomolecule corona adsorbs on the surface. *Nat. Nanotechnol.* **2013**, *8*, 137–143. [CrossRef] [PubMed]

37. Mahon, E.; Salvati, A.; Baldelli Bombelli, F.; Lynch, I.; Dawson, K.A. Designing the nanoparticle–biomolecule interface for "targeting and therapeutic delivery". *J. Control. Release* **2012**, *161*, 164–174. [CrossRef]

38. Caracciolo, G.; Cardarelli, F.; Pozzi, D.; Salomone, F.; Maccari, G.; Bardi, G.; Capriotti, A.L.; Cavaliere, C.; Papi, M.; Laganà, A. Selective targeting capability acquired with a protein corona adsorbed on the surface of 1,2-dioleoyl-3-trimethylammonium propane/dna nanoparticles. *ACS Appl. Mater. Interfaces* **2013**, *5*, 13171–13179. [CrossRef]

39. Docter, D.; Westmeier, D.; Markiewicz, M.; Stolte, S.; Knauer, S.; Stauber, R. The nanoparticle biomolecule corona: Lessons learned–challenge accepted? *Chem. Soc. Rev.* **2015**, *44*, 6094–6121. [CrossRef]

40. Treuel, L.; Docter, D.; Maskos, M.; Stauber, R.H. Protein corona–from molecular adsorption to physiological complexity. *Beil. J. Nanotechnol.* **2015**, *6*, 857–873. [CrossRef]

41. Kelly, P.M.; Åberg, C.; Polo, E.; O'Connell, A.; Cookman, J.; Fallon, J.; Krpetić, Ž.; Dawson, K.A. Mapping protein binding sites on the biomolecular corona of nanoparticles. *Nat. Nanotechnol.* **2015**, *10*, 472–479. [CrossRef] [PubMed]

42. Gianneli, M.; Polo, E.; Lopez, H.; Castagnola, V.; Aastrup, T.; Dawson, K. Label-free in-flow detection of receptor recognition motifs on the biomolecular corona of nanoparticles. *Nanoscale* **2018**, *10*, 5474–5481. [CrossRef] [PubMed]

43. Walkey, C.D.; Olsen, J.B.; Song, F.; Liu, R.; Guo, H.; Olsen, D.W.H.; Cohen, Y.; Emili, A.; Chan, W.C. Protein corona fingerprinting predicts the cellular interaction of gold and silver nanoparticles. *ACS Nano* **2014**, *8*, 2439–2455. [CrossRef] [PubMed]

44. Liu, R.; Jiang, W.; Walkey, C.D.; Chan, W.C.; Cohen, Y. Prediction of nanoparticles-cell association based on corona proteins and physicochemical properties. *Nanoscale* **2015**, *7*, 9664–9675. [CrossRef] [PubMed]

45. Lorger, M.; Krueger, J.S.; O'Neal, M.; Staflin, K.; Felding-Habermann, B. Activation of tumor cell integrin αVβ3 controls angiogenesis and metastatic growth in the brain. *Proc. Natl. Acad. Sci. USA* **2009**, *106*, 10666–10671. [CrossRef]

46. Weis, S.M.; Cheresh, D.A. αV integrins in angiogenesis and cancer. *Cold Spring Harb. Perspect. Med.* **2011**, *1*, a006478. [CrossRef]

47. Hosotani, R.; Kawaguchi, M.; Masui, T.; Koshiba, T.; Ida, J.; Fujimoto, K.; Wada, M.; Doi, R.; Imamura, M. Expression of integrin αvβ3 in pancreatic carcinoma: Relation to MMP-2 activation and lymph node metastasis. *Pancreas* **2002**, *25*, e30–e35. [CrossRef]

48. Trusolino, L.; Serini, G.; Cecchini, G.; Besati, C.; Ambesi-Impiombato, F.S.; Marchisio, P.C.; De Filippi, R. Growth factor–dependent activation of αvβ3 integrin in normal epithelial cells: Implications for tumor invasion. *J. Cell Biol.* **1998**, *142*, 1145–1156. [CrossRef]

49. Neyen, C.; Plüddemann, A.; Mukhopadhyay, S.; Maniati, E.; Bossard, M.; Gordon, S.; Hagemann, T. Macrophage scavenger receptor a promotes tumor progression in murine models of ovarian and pancreatic cancer. *J. Immunol.* **2013**, *190*, 3798–3805. [CrossRef]

50. Vasseur, S.; Guillaumond, F. LDL receptor: An open route to feed pancreatic tumor cells. *Mol. Cell. Oncol.* **2016**, *3*, e1033586. [CrossRef]

51. Arcella, A.; Palchetti, S.; Digiacomo, L.; Pozzi, D.; Capriotti, A.L.; Frati, L.; Oliva, M.A.; Tsaouli, G.; Rota, R.; Screpanti, I. Brain targeting by liposome–biomolecular corona boosts anticancer efficacy of temozolomide in glioblastoma cells. *ACS Chem. Neurosci.* **2018**. [CrossRef] [PubMed]

52. Papi, M.; Caputo, D.; Palmieri, V.; Coppola, R.; Palchetti, S.; Bugli, F.; Martini, C.; Digiacomo, L.; Pozzi, D.; Caracciolo, G. Clinically approved pegylated nanoparticles are covered by a protein corona that boosts the uptake by cancer cells. *Nanoscale* **2017**, *9*, 10327–10334. [CrossRef] [PubMed]

Chitosan-Based Polyelectrolyte Complexes for Doxorubicin and Zoledronic Acid Combined Therapy to Overcome Multidrug Resistance

Simona Giarra [1,†], Silvia Zappavigna [2,†], Virginia Campani [1], Marianna Abate [2], Alessia Maria Cossu [2], Carlo Leonetti [3], Manuela Porru [3], Laura Mayol [1], Michele Caraglia [2] and Giuseppe De Rosa [1,*]

[1] Department of Pharmacy, University of Naples Federico II, D. Montesano 49, 80131 Naples, Italy; simona.giarra@unina.it (S.G.); virginia.campani@unina.it (V.C.); laumayol@unina.it (L.M.)

[2] Department of Biochemistry, Biophysics and General Pathology, Second University of Naples, L. De Crecchio 7, 80138 Naples, Italy; silvia.zappavigna@unicampania.it (S.Z.); marianna.abate1991@gmail.com (M.A.); alessiacossu@libero.it (A.M.C.); michele.caraglia@unina2.it (M.C.)

[3] UOSD SAFU, IRCCS Regina Elena National Cancer Institute, E. Chianesi 53, 00144 Rome, Italy; carlo.leonetti@ifo.gov.it (C.L.); manuela.porru@ifo.gov.it (M.P.)

* Correspondence: gderosa@unina.it;

† These authors contributed equally to this work.

Abstract: This study aimed to develop nanovectors co-encapsulating doxorubicin (Doxo) and zoledronic acid (Zol) for a combined therapy against Doxo-resistant tumors. Chitosan (CHI)-based polyelectrolyte complexes (PECs) prepared by ionotropic gelation technique were proposed. The influence of some experimental parameters was evaluated in order to optimize the PECs in terms of size and polydispersity index (PI). PEC stability was studied by monitoring size and zeta potential over time. In vitro studies were carried out on wild-type and Doxo-resistant cell lines, to assess both the synergism between Doxo and Zol, as well as the restoring of Doxo sensitivity. Polymer concentration, incubation time, and use of a surfactant were found to be crucial to achieving small size and monodisperse PECs. Doxo and Zol, only when encapsulated in PECs, showed a synergistic antiproliferative effect in all the tested cell lines. Importantly, the incubation of Doxo-resistant cell lines with Doxo/Zol co-encapsulating PECs resulted in the restoration of Doxo sensitivity.

Keywords: chitosan; polyelectrolyte complexes; doxorubicin; zoledronic acid; multidrug resistance

1. Introduction

One of the main limitations of conventional chemotherapy is the development of a malignant cell's resistance to one or more anticancer drugs. This process is known as "multidrug resistance" (MDR) which inevitably leads to a reduction of therapy effectiveness [1–4]. Generally, hydrophobic and amphipathic natural molecules, such as anthracyclines (e.g., doxorubicin (Doxo)) are more prone to developing resistance compared to other substances [5,6]. It is well known that the over-expression of some proteins of the efflux pumps ATP-binding cassette (ABC) family is one of the major causes of the MDR phenomenon [7–9]. One of the main components of the ABC family is represented by P-glycoprotein (P-gp), also known as MDR protein 1 (MDR1). P-gp is normally expressed in different normal tissues, such as the kidney, liver, pancreas, colon, and bone, where it is involved in the extrusion of neutral or weakly basic amphiphilic substances penetrated into the cells [10,11]. Therefore, tumors derived from these tissues have a greater expression of P-gp compared to others [12]. The function, as well as the ATPase activity of the P-gp, seems to be affected by intracellular cholesterol levels because very high levels of cholesterol have been found in the plasma membranes of MDR$^+$ tumor cells [13–16]. The most frequent bone tumor observed clinically is osteosarcoma. The standard treatment for conventional osteosarcoma is based on pre- and post-operative chemotherapy, including Doxo, cisplatin, and methotrexate. Despite numerous attempts to find new therapeutic approaches for osteosarcoma, the patients' prognosis has not improved in the last decades. Because Doxo is a substrate of P-gp, its cytotoxicity is highly limited. Both natural and synthetic inhibitors of P-gp have been tested to reverse Doxo resistance in osteosarcoma cell lines in vitro. The specific silencing of P-gp or the inhibition of pathways involved in MDR—such as the hypoxia inducible factor-1—appear to be promising strategies. Bisphosphonates, such as zoledronic acid (Zol), have been shown to reduce osteolysis induced by bone metastasis and exhibit highly selective localization and retention in bone, thus making them attractive agents in the treatment of bone metastasis. Studies have shown that Zol exerts pleiotropic anti-tumor effects against osteosarcoma cells in vitro, including antiproliferative and immunomodulatory effects. In previous studies, the authors demonstrated that Zol is a multi-target chemo-immuno-sensitizing agent, acting on both tumor cell and tumor microenvironment. In particular, nanomedicine loaded with Zol reversed the MDR phenotype by inhibiting the mevalonate pathway and the HIF-1α-dependent signaling, two events that impair the energy metabolism and the activity of ABC transporters [17–19]. Free Zol showed a limited in vivo antitumor effect, probably associated with its rapid clearance from the circulation with a preferential bone accumulation. These observations represent the rationale for the use of Zol, in combination with the cytotoxic drug Doxo, as the first not toxic metabolic modifier effective against MDR tumors, such as osteosarcoma. Loading of Zol into conventional liposomes resulted in low drug encapsulation efficiency (EE) (around 5%), presumably due to its hydrophilic nature associated with poor water solubility [20]. On the contrary, high Zol loading into nanovectors can be achieved by exploiting the interaction of its negative charges with a positive counterpart, for example, by using hybrid self-assembling nanoparticles [21]. However, the latter should be not suitable to also guarantee a high Doxo loading.

In recent years, polyelectrolyte complexes (PECs) have attracted a great deal of attention thanks to their low manufacturing costs, together with an easy scale-up and the absence of organic solvents [22,23]. In particular, the ionotropic gelation process leads to the spontaneous formation of PECs, as a result of the electrostatic interactions between oppositely charged components. One of the main polymers suitable for gelation process is represented by chitosan (CHI), a natural cationic polysaccharide composed of D-glucosamine and N-acetyl-D-glucosamine units, with well-known biodegradability, biocompatibility, and bioadhesiveness properties [24]. In an acidic environment, CHI positive charges make it suitable for electrostatic interactions with an anionic counterpart, such as sodium tripolyphosphate (TPP) [25–29].

In this context, the authors hypothesized that CHI could be used to prepare nanomedicine-based formulations for combined delivery of both highly loaded Zol and Doxo to overcome multidrug resistance in Doxo-resistant tumors. Thus, PECs co-loaded with Doxo and Zol were developed by means of ionotropic gelation process. Specifically, the authors investigated experimental parameters crucial to achieve PECs with a low mean diameter, narrow size distribution, stability during storage, and high Doxo/Zol encapsulation efficiency. Finally, in vitro studies to assess the possibility of a combined therapy to overcome resistance in Doxo-resistant tumor cells were carried out on wild-type and MDR variants of the two human osteosarcoma cell lines, which were selected by continuous exposure to Doxo [30]. Resistant variants showed an overexpression of P-gp (referred to as p170). The level of expression of this protein in the different cell lines was directly related to the degree of resistance.

2. Materials and Methods

2.1. Materials

CHI with a Mn and Mw equal to $1.07 \pm 0.09 \times 10^6$ Da and $1.43 \pm 0.11 \times 10^5$ Da, respectively, inherent viscosity >400 mPa·s, and a degree of deacetylation ranges from 82 to 88%, and TPP were obtained from Sigma-Aldrich (St.Louis, Missouri, MO, USA). CHI molecular weight was measured by gel permeation chromatography (GPC) [24]. Poloxamer F127, an amphiphilic triblock polymer made up of hydrophilic polyethylene oxide (PEO) and hydrophobic polypropylene oxide (PPO) units (number of PEO units = 100, number of PPO units = 65), was purchased from Lutrol (Basf, Ludwigshafen, Germany). Doxo hydrochloride from 3V Chimica (Rome, Italy) and Zol monohydrate (1-Hydroxy-2-imidazol-1-ylethylidene) from U.S. Pharmacopeia Convention (Twinbrook Parkway, Rockville, Maryland, MD, USA) were used.

2.2. Preparations of Polyelectrolyte Complexes (PECs)

Unloaded CHI-based PECs (named PEC) were prepared by ionotropic gelation method. Briefly, CHI was added to 10 mL of aqueous acetic acid solution (2% v/v); after complete solubilization, the pH of the resulting solution was adjusted to 4.7 with NaOH (1N) and filtration trough 0.2 µm syringe filter. The TPP solution was obtained by solubilizing TPP in 5 mL of distilled water followed by filtration trough 0.2 µm syringe filter. Afterwards, PECs were obtained by adding the anionic solution into the CHI solution and leaving them under magnetic stirring (700 rpm, at room temperature) for 30 min, to allow the cross-linking reaction. The resulted PEC suspension was purified by centrifugation at 10,000 rpm for 20 min (Hettich Zentrifugen, Tuttlingen, Germany) and kept overnight at 4 °C. Various CHI and TPP concentrations, times of interaction between them, as well as surfactant addiction to the formulation were investigated. Drug-loaded PECs were obtained by simply adding Doxo (0.4 mg/mL) to the CHI solution and Zol (0.8 mg/mL) to the TPP solution, prior to proceeding with the PEC preparation, thus leading to Zol-loaded PECs (PEC-Zol), Doxo-loaded PECs (PEC-Doxo), and Zol and Doxo co-loaded PECs (PEC-Doxo-Zol).

2.3. Size, Polydispersity Index (PI) and ζ Potential

The average diameters, polydispersity index (PI) and ζ potential of the obtained formulations were measured via dynamic light scattering (N5, Beckman Coulter, Brea, California, CA, USA and Nano-Z, Malvern Instruments, Malvern, UK). For the analysis, each PEC formulation was properly diluted with ultrapure water and measured at room temperature. Results were calculated as the average of five runs of three independent samples. To evaluate the PEC dimensional stability, size and potential measurements were monitored for at least 30 days, in water at 4 °C (i.e., storage conditions).

2.4. Doxo and Zol Encapsulation Efficiency and Yield of the PECs

The preparation yield of the PECs was calculated from previously freeze-dried formulations (0.01 atm, 24 h; Modulyo, Edwards, Waltham, Massachusetts, UK). In particular, it was gravimetrically obtained from the entire mass of recovered freeze-dried PECs. For the encapsulation efficiency (EE), the supernatant obtained after purification of the loaded PECs containing free drug(s) was submitted to quantitative analyses. In particular, the percentage of Doxo entrapped into PECs was evaluated by spectrophotometric assay (UV-1800, Shimadzu Laboratory World, Kyoto, Japan) at $\lambda = 480$ nm. The linearity of the response was verified over the concentration range 62.5–0.06 µg/mL ($r^2 > 0.99$). On the other hand, Zol quantification was performed by ultra-high-performance liquid chromatography (UHPLC, Shimadzu Nexera Liquid Chromatograph LC-30AD, Kyoto, Japan), with a Gemini C18, 110 Å column (250 mm × 4.6 mm, 5 µm) at $\lambda = 220$ nm, using a mobile phase composed of 20:80 (v/v) acetonitrile:tributyl-ammonium-phosphate buffer (pH = 7). The flow rate was 1 mL/min and the run time was set at 15 min. The drug EE was calculated using the following Equation (1):

$$EE = (\text{Total amount of drugs in formulations-free drugs})/(\text{Total amount of drugs in formulations}) \times 100 \quad (1)$$

The values of the EE (%) were collected from three different batches.

2.5. Cell Culture

The cancer cell lines used were wild-type human osteosarcoma cells (SAOS), wild-type human bone osteosarcoma epithelial cells (U-2 OS) and their Doxo-resistant variant (SAOS DX and U-2 OS DX, respectively). All cell lines were obtained from American Type Culture Collection (ATCC; Rockville, MD, USA) and were grown in Dulbecco's Modified Eagle's Medium (DMEM). Cell media was supplemented with 10% heat-inactivated fetal bovine serum, 20 mM HEPES, 100 U/mL penicillin, 100 mg/mL streptomycin, 1% L-glutamine, and 1% sodium pyruvate. Cells were cultured at a constant temperature of 37 °C in a humidified atmosphere of 5% carbon dioxide (CO_2).

2.6. Cell Proliferation Assay

After trypsinization, all the cell lines were plated in 100 μL of medium in 96-well plates at a density of 2×10^3 cells/well. One day later, cells were treated with free Doxo, free Zol, PEC, PEC-Doxo, PEC-Zol, and PEC-Doxo-Zol at concentrations ranging from 20 μM to 0.156 μM for Doxo and from 200 μM to 0.312 μM for Zol. Cell proliferation was evaluated by MTT assay. Briefly, cells were seeded in serum-containing media in 96-well plates at a density of 2×10^3 cells/well. After 24 h of incubation at 37 °C, the medium was removed and replaced with fresh medium containing all developed formulations at different concentrations. Cells were incubated under these conditions for 72 h. Then, cell viability was assessed by MTT assay. The MTT solution (5 mg/mL in phosphate-buffered saline) was added (20 μL/well), and the plates were incubated for a further four hours at 37 °C. The MTT-formazan crystals were dissolved in 1N isopropanol/hydrochloric acid 10% solution. The absorbance values of the solution in each well were measured at 570 nm using a Bio-Rad 550 microplate reader (Bio-Rad Laboratories, Milan, Italy). The percentage of cell viability was calculated as described in Equation (2):

$$\text{Cell viability} = (\text{abs sample} - \text{abs blank control})/(\text{abs negative control} - \text{abs blank control}) \times 100 \quad (2)$$

where abs sample is the absorbance of the treated wells, abs blank control is the absorbance of only medium without cells and abs negative control is the absorbance of the untreated cells. Then, the concentrations inhibiting 50% of cell growth (IC_{50}) were obtained and these values were used for subsequent experiments. MTT assay was carried out by triplicate determination on at least three separate experiments. All data are expressed as mean ± SD.

2.7. Evaluation of Synergism

The evaluation of synergism was performed using dedicated software CalcuSyn, version 1.2.1 (Biosoft, Ferguson, MO, USA), which measured the interaction between the drugs by calculating the indexes of combination (CIs). CI values <1, 1, and >1 indicate synergism, additive, and antagonism, respectively. Drug combination studies were based on concentration–effect curves generated as a plot of the fraction of unaffected (surviving) cells versus drug concentration after 72 h of treatment. Assessment of synergy was performed quantifying the drug interaction by the CalcuSyn computer program (Biosoft, Ferguson, MO, USA).

3. Results and Discussion

3.1. PECs Preparation and Characterization

CHI-based PECs were obtained through ionotropic gelation technique thanks to the ability of the amine functional groups of CHI to be protonated in acidic environment, thus providing

-NH3$^+$ groups able to interact with negatively charged groups of TPP [31]. Generally, oppositely charged macromolecules aggregate due to their high charge density fluctuation in solutions [22]. Therefore, PEC formation and stability are affected by several factors [32]. Among these, CHI and TPP concentrations used during the preparation process play an important role. The different polymer concentrations used, the size, and PI of the prepared PEC formulations are shown in Table 1. In all the formulations, the volume ratios between CHI and TPP phases were fixed at 2:1.

Table 1. Size and polydispersity index (PI) of different polyelectrolyte complex (PEC) formulations. All results are expressed as mean ± SD of at least three independent experiments. CHI: chitosan TPP: tripolyphosphate.

Formulation	(CHI) mg/mL	(TPP) mg/mL	D (nm)	PI
PEC(CHI 0.4-TPP 0.5)	0.4	0.5	236.9 ± 31.2	1.14 ± 0.5
PEC(CHI 0.3-TPP 0.5)	0.3	0.5	231.9 ± 9.50	0.23 ± 0.1
PEC(CHI 0.5-TPP 0.4)	0.5	0.4	272.1 ± 86.7	0.42 ± 0.1
PEC(CHI 0.5-TPP 0.3)	0.5	0.3	314.2 ± 14.5	1.03 ± 0.6
PEC(CHI 0.5-TPP 0.5)	0.5	0.5	132.7 ± 11.2	0.43 ± 0.1
PEC(CHI 0.4-TPP 0.4)	0.4	0.4	185.1 ± 0.81	0.27 ± 0.1
PEC(CHI 0.3-TPP 0.3)	0.3	0.3	132.3 ± 6.80	0.42 ± 0.1
PEC(CHI 0.3-TPP 0.5)	0.3	0.4	287.8 ± 15.4	0.15 ± 0.1

Results showed that PECs with the smallest size (in the range from ~130 to ~180 nm) were obtained using the same concentrations of both CHI and TPP. By increasing the TPP/CHI ratio, the PEC size significantly increased. This could be probably ascribed to the excess of TPP in the solution; negative charges of TPP might interact with free amino groups of pre-formed PECs, leading to PEC aggregation. A similar size increase was observed by increasing CHI concentration. This effect was probably due to a higher viscosity of the resulting solution, which slowed down the cross-linking reaction between the polymer chains, with the consequent formation of aggregates. Concentrations greater than 0.5 mg/mL of both components led to the formation of visible macro-aggregates (data not shown). The time of interaction between CHI and the cross-linking agent was found to influence PEC size and PI. More specifically, the optimal CHI and TPP concentrations, which led to the smallest PEC size, were used to prepare PECs with controlled-precipitation flow rate (Q). The results of dimensions, PI, and ζ potential analyses of PEC formulations, prepared by using CHI and TPP concentrations and different Q, are summarized in Table 2. In all formulations, the inner diameter of the syringe used for the precipitation of TPP onto the CHI solution was set at 11.99 mm.

Table 2. Size, PI, and ζ potential values of different PEC formulations. All results are expressed as mean ± SD of at least three independent experiments.

Formulation	(CHI) mg/mL	(TPP) mg/mL	Q (μL/min)	d (nm)	PI	ζ Potential (mV)
PEC(CHI 0.5-TPP 0.5)-A	0.5	0.5	500	223.3 ± 3.8	0.67 ± 0.3	18.1 ± 1.5
PEC(CHI 0.5-TPP 0.5)-B	0.5	0.5	133.3	187.0 ± 9.1	0.45 ± 0.2	21.3 ± 1.1
PEC(CHI 0.4-TPP 0.4)-A	0.4	0.4	500	147.7 ± 2.9	0.49 ± 0.1	19.1 ± 1.9
PEC(CHI 0.4-TPP 0.4)-B	0.4	0.4	133.3	129.4 ± 2.7	0.42 ± 2.7	19.1 ± 0.8
PEC(CHI 0.3-TPP 0.3)-A	0.3	0.3	500	127.5 ± 2.2	0.51 ± 0.3	17.8 ± 2.9
PEC(CHI 0.3-TPP 0.3)-B	0.3	0.3	133.3	104.4 ± 1.4	0.41 ± 0.3	21.4 ± 1.9

As it can be observed, PECs obtained using a lower flow rate showed a smaller diameter. This size trend could be attributed to the time needed for the cross-linking reaction; thus, at lower flow rate, the possibility to achieve a homogeneous distribution of the polymer chains should be greater. This should promote their electrostatic interactions and the formation of PECs with a very small diameter (around ~100 nm). A positive charge, evaluated by ζ potential analysis, was found in all the formulations due to the presence of CHI primary free amino groups. On the basis of these results, the formulation named PEC(CHI 0.3-TPP 0.3)-B, obtained by using a concentration of 0.3 mg/mL of both CHI and TPP and a flow rate of 133.3 µL/min, presented optimal features in terms of mean diameter, although with a high PI (~0.4) indicating a poor homogeneity of the PEC dispersion (see Table 2). For this reason, the authors added the multi-block surfactant copolymer Poloxamer F127, at different concentrations, to the CHI acetic acid solution prior to PEC formation [33]. Table 3 shows the F127 concentrations used to prepare different PEC formulations; in all cases, the concentrations of both CHI and TPP used were 0.3 mg/mL. As expected, the addition of F127 resulted in significant PI reduction, depending on the Poloxamer concentration. In particular, in the case of the PEC(CHI 0.3-TPP 0.3)-B formulation, the addition of F127 at 10% (w/w) allowed more monodisperse PECs (PI < 0.25) to be produced, without significant change in size and ζ potential values (see Table 3).

Table 3. Size, PI, and ζ potential values of different PECs. All results are expressed as mean ± SD of at least three independent experiments.

Formulation	(CHI) mg/mL	(TPP) mg/mL	F127 (% w/w)	d (nm)	PI	ζ Potential (mV)
PEC(CHI 0.3-TPP 0.3)-B20	0.3	0.3	20	114.1 ± 5.1	0.48 ± 0.1	17.2 ± 2.5
PEC(CHI 0.3-TPP 0.3)-B16	0.3	0.3	16	114.8 ± 6.9	0.32 ± 0.2	16.9 ± 2.1
PEC(CHI 0.3-TPP 0.3)-B10	0.3	0.3	10	110.8 ± 3.5	0.23 ± 0.2	21.2 ± 3.3

3.2. Preparation and Characterization of PECs Encapsulating Doxo and Zol

Doxo and Zol were loaded into PEC formulations, to obtain a co-delivery of these drugs for a combined therapy. Doxo and Zol EE and preparation yield of different formulations are summarized in Table 4; in all cases, CHI (0.3 mg/mL) and TPP (0.3 mg/mL) were used.

Table 4. Doxorubicin (Doxo) and zoledronic acid (Zol) encapsulation efficiency (EE) (%) and yield (%) of different formulations prepared. All results are expressed as mean ± SD of at least three independent experiments.

Formulation	(Zol)-Loaded (mg/mL)	(Doxo)-Loaded (mg/mL)	EE Zol (%)	EE Doxo (%)	Yield (%)
PEC	-	-	-	-	80.8 ± 0.1
PEC-Zol	0.8	-	92.3 ± 5.3	-	77.8 ± 1.3
PEC-Doxo	-	0.4	-	25.8 ± 0.5	79.4 ± 0.1
PEC-Doxo-Zol	0.8	0.4	83.1 ± 11	29.2 ± 6.6	81.6 ± 0.1

As shown in Table 4, the prepared formulations were characterized by a high yield, greater than 75% in all cases. Zol and Doxo EE were found to be similar in PECs loaded with one or both drugs. In particular, more than 20% of the initial loaded Doxo was found in the PECs. Surprisingly, Zol showed a very high EE (>80%) into formulation, also in association with Doxo. This result was probably due to its electrostatic interaction with positive charges of CHI, thus resulting in a more stable encapsulation. On the other hand, Doxo encapsulation should be related to its interaction with TPP. The mean size as well as the PI of PECs loaded with one or both drugs, were slightly increased (see Table 5).

Table 5. Size, PI, and ζ potential values of different loaded PEC formulations.

Formulation	d (nm)	PI	ζ Potential (mV)
PEC-Zol	131.1 ± 0.1	0.32 ± 0.1	20.2 ± 1.3
PEC-Doxo	120.5 ± 4.7	0.42 ± 0.4	22.9 ± 1.6
PEC-Doxo-Zol	111.5 ± 0.1	0.39 ± 0.4	23.1 ± 2.3

3.3. Stability Studies

In order to evaluate the stability of prepared formulations in storage conditions, the mean diameters, PI, and ζ potential were analyzed as a function of time, in water at 4 °C. As shown in Figure 1, all formulations underwent a slightly increase in size after 10 days; they then had a narrow size distribution for up to 30 days. Moreover, for all analyzed formulations, ζ potential values remained stable for up to 30 days (data not shown).

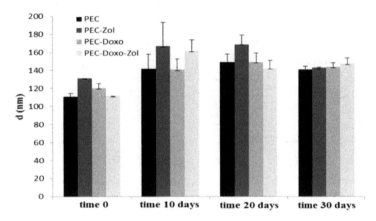

Figure 1. Size and PI of different PEC formulations as a function of time, in water at 4 °C.

3.4. Cell Proliferation Assay

The effects of free Doxo, free Zol, PEC, PEC-Doxo, PEC-Zol, and PEC-Doxo-Zol were evaluated on the proliferation of wild-type SAOS, wild-type U-2 OS, SAOS DX, and U-2 OS DX cancer cell lines by MTT assay. All the tested formulations induced a dose-dependent growth inhibition in all the cell lines analyzed after 72 h, whereas treatment with unloaded PECs did not produce significant cytotoxic effects (see Figure 2).

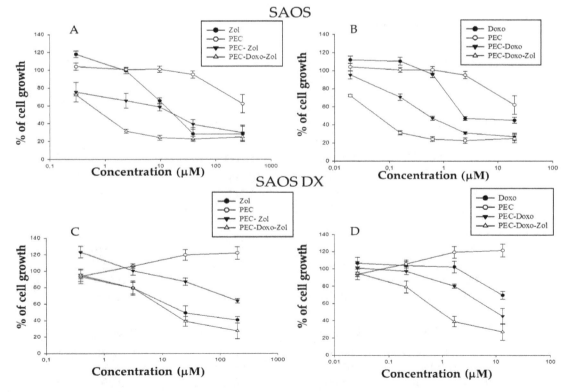

Figure 2. *Cont.*

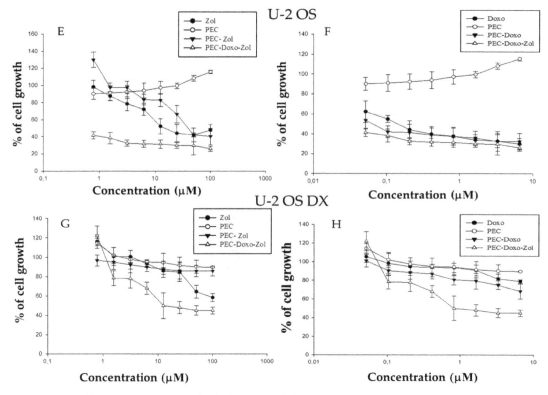

Figure 2. Dose–effect relationship of all developed formulations on wild-type and Doxo-resistant wild-type human osteosarcoma cells (SAOS) and wild-type human bone osteosarcoma epithelial cells (U-2 OS) proliferation. Results are expressed as % of cell growth vs. concentration (µM) of Zol (**A, C, E,** and **G**) or Doxo (**B, D, F,** and **H**). In the case of cells treated with unloaded PECs, the PEC concentration was adjusted as equivalent to the concentration of drug-loaded PECs.

The results of IC_{50} after 72 h of treatment are shown in Table 6.

Table 6. IC_{50} (M) of all developed formulations on wild-type and Doxo-resistant SAOS and U-2 OS, after 72 h of treatment.

SAOS	IC_{50Zol}	SAOS	IC_{50Doxo}
Zol	17	Doxo	2
PEC-Zol	16	PEC-Doxo	0.5
PEC-Doxo-Zol	0.8	PEC-Doxo-Zol	0.05
PEC	-	PEC	-
SAOS DX	IC_{50Zol}	**SAOS DX**	IC_{50Doxo}
Zol	23.4	Doxo	>20
PEC-Zol	>200	PEC-Doxo	10.4
PEC-Doxo-Zol	13.8	PEC-Doxo-Zol	0.9
PEC	-	PEC	-
U-2 OS	IC_{50Zol}	**U-2 OS**	IC_{50Doxo}
Zol	15.60	Doxo	0.14
PEC-Zol	40.40	PEC-Doxo	0.06
PEC-Doxo-Zol	<0.78	PEC-Doxo-Zol	<0.05
PEC	-	PEC	-
U-2 OS DX	IC_{50Zol}	**U-2 OS DX**	IC_{50Doxo}
Zol	>100	Doxo	>6.60
PEC-Zol	>100	PEC-Doxo	>6.60
PEC-Doxo-Zol	13.60	PEC-Doxo-Zol	0.80
PEC	-	PEC	-

The IC_{50} values of free Doxo were equal to 2 μM and superior to 20 μM for wild-type and SAOS DX cells, whereas they were equal to 0.14 μM and superior to 6.60 μM for wild-type and U-2 OS DX cells (see Table 6). The PEC-Doxo induced a 50% growth inhibition at a concentration of 0.5 μM and 10.4 μM for wild-type and SAOS DX, respectively, whereas the concentration was 0.06 μM and superior to 6.60 μM for wild-type and U-2 OS DX, respectively (see Table 6). These data demonstrated that the PECs, even without the co-encapsulation of Zol, were able to strongly increase the cytotoxicity of Doxo in all the tested formulations, except in U-2 OS DX cells. It is noteworthy that Doxo encapsulation in other nanocarriers (e.g., stealth liposomes) results in a reduced Doxo cytotoxicity [34–36]. As previously reported by other authors for different Doxo-encapsulating nanovectors, the cell uptake of Doxo encapsulated into PECs should occur by endocytosis, whereas free Doxo enters cancer cells primarily through passive diffusion across the plasma membrane [37]. Taking into account that unloaded PECs are not cytotoxic at the experimental conditions used here, the enhanced cell toxicity observed with PEC-Doxo should be reasonably due to the enhanced Doxo intracellular concentration. Previously, other authors have demonstrated the possibility of increasing cell apoptosis by modulating Doxo intracellular trafficking [37]. On the other hand, the PEGylated nanocarriers have been shown to reduce drug uptake into the target cells [38]. The IC_{50} values of free Zol were equal to 17 μM for wild-type SAOS and 23.4 μM for SAOS DX, whereas they were equal to 15.60 μM for wild-type U-2 OS and superior to 100 μM for U-2 OS DX cells. The encapsulation of Zol in PECs did not potentiate its antitumor activity; in fact, the IC_{50} values for PEC-Zol were 16 μM and >200 μM for wild-type and SAOS DX, respectively, whereas they were 40.40 μM and superior to 100 μM for wild-type and U-2 OS DX, respectively. These results are in contrast with the authors' previous finding in which different lipid-based nanocarriers encapsulating Zol were useful to increase Zol uptake in different cancer cell lines [20,21]. When incubating wild-type SAOS and U-2 OS with PEC-Zol in this study, a similar or enhanced cytotoxicity was found, when compared to free Zol. This could be ascribed to the strong interaction between CHI and Zol that slows down the delivery of the bisphosphonate into the cytoplasm. Further studies are needed to understand the disappearance of Zol toxicity when incubating cells with Zol-PEC. However, it is noteworthy that PEC-Doxo-Zol inhibited 50% of cell growth at a concentration of 0.05 μM and 0.9 μM for Doxo and 0.8 μM and 13.8 μM for Zol for wild-type and SAOS DX, respectively. On the other hand, it inhibited 50% of cell growth at a concentration inferior to 0.05 μM and 0.80 μM for Doxo and inferior to 0.78 μM and equal to 13.60 μM for wild-type and U-2 OS DX, respectively, by significantly enhancing the effects of both the drugs.

3.5. Evaluation of Synergism

The synergism between Doxo and Zol in PECs was calculated by using the dedicated software CalcuSyn. CI values are shown in Table 7.

Table 7. CIs values between Doxo and Zol on wild-type and Doxo-resistant SAOS and U-2 OS cells.

Cell Lines	CI_{50}	Interpretation
SAOS	0.3	Strong Synergism
SAOS DX	0.4	Strong Synergism
U-2 OS	0.7	Synergism
U-2 OS DX	0.3	Strong Synergism

As summarized in Table 7, a synergic effect was found in wild-type U-2 OS cells, whereas a strong synergism was found in wild-type SAOS, SAOS DX, and U-2 OS DX cells when co-encapsulating Doxo with Zol. Interestingly, the data on SAOX DX and U-2 OS DX strongly confirm the authors' previous finding on the association of Doxo and Zol to revert resistance to Doxo. In particular, Zol is a multi-target chemo-immuno-sensitizing agent, acting on both tumor cell and tumor microenvironment. In fact, nanoparticles (NPs) encapsulating Zol reversed the resistance towards P-gp substrates by decreasing the synthesis of cholesterol, which is critical for the activity of P-gp and the activity of

Ras/ERK1/2/HIF-1α-axis, which mediates the transcription of P-gp [19]. In this study, a synergic effect was also found in wild-type cells, thus suggesting that other mechanisms, different from the inhibition of the P-gp, could be produced when associating these two drugs.

4. Conclusions

In this study, CHI-based PECs co-loaded with Doxo and Zol were successfully prepared with a simple and easily up-scalable method. The results showed that polymer concentration, times of interaction between polymer/cross-linking agent, and surfactant addiction to the formulation are crucial for PEC formation and for their technological features. Finally, this study demonstrated two crucial advantages of PEC-encapsulating Doxo. First, PECs significantly enhance Doxo cytotoxicity, probably due to an enhanced internalization into the cells. Second, the authors' hypothesis was confirmed because PECs co-administrating Zol and Doxo resulted in a significant restoration of cell sensitivity to Doxo, thus providing a promising approach to overcoming MDR.

Author Contributions: S.G. and S.Z. arranged and performed the experiments, prepared the original draft; V.C., A.M.C., and M.A. curated the data; C.L. and M.P. provided cells and took part in the design of the in vitro experiments; L.M. prepared the original draft and reviewed the paper; M.C. provided funding and coordinated the study on cell culture; G.D.R. provided funding and coordinated the formulation study.

Abbreviations

PECs	polyelectrolyte complexes
Doxo	doxorubicin
Zol	zoledronic acid
MDR	multidrug resistance
ABC	ATP-binding cassette family
P-gp	P-glycoprotein
CHI	chitosan
TPP	sodium tripolyphosphate
SAOS	wild-type human osteosarcoma cells
SAOS DX	Doxo-resistant human osteosarcoma cells
U-2 OS	wild-type human bone osteosarcoma epithelial cells
U2-OS DX	Doxo-resistant human bone osteosarcoma epithelial cells
GPC	gel permeation chromatography
PEO	polyethylene oxide
PPO	polypropylene oxide
PI	polydispersity index
EE	encapsulation efficiency
UHPLC	ultra-high-performance liquid chromatography
IC_{50}	concentration inhibiting 50% of cell growth
CIs	indexes of combination
Q	precipitation flow rate

References

1. Krishna, R.; Mayer, L.D. Multidrug resistance (MDR) in cancer: Mechanisms, reversal using modulators of MDR and the role of MDR modulators in influencing the pharmacokinetics of anticancer drugs. *Eur. J. Pharm. Sci.* **2000**, *11*, 265–283. [CrossRef]
2. Liscovitch, M.; Lavie, Y. Cancer multidrug resistance: A review of recent drug discovery research. *IDrugs* **2002**, *5*, 349–355. [PubMed]
3. Stavrovskaya, A.A. Cellular mechanisms of multidrug resistance of tumor cells. *Biochemistry (Moscow)* **2000**, *65*, 95–106. [PubMed]

4. Szakács, G.; Paterson, J.K.; Ludwig, J.A.; Booth-Genthe, C.; Gottesman, M.M. Targeting multidrug resistance in cancer. *Nat. Rev. Drug Discovery* **2006**, *5*, 219–234. [CrossRef] [PubMed]

5. Calcagno, A.M.; Ambudkar, S.V. The molecular mechanisms of drug resistance in single-step and multi-step drug-selected cancer cells. *Methods Mol. Biol.* **2010**, *596*, 77–93. [CrossRef] [PubMed]

6. Thomas, H.; Coley, H.M. Overcoming multidrug resistance in cancer: An update on the clinical strategy of inhibiting p-glycoprotein. *Cancer Control* **2003**, *10*, 159–165. [CrossRef] [PubMed]

7. Choi, C.H. ABC transporters as multidrug resistance mechanisms and the development of chemosensitizers for their reversal. *Cancer Cell Int.* **2005**, *5*, 30. [CrossRef] [PubMed]

8. Gottesman, M.M.; Pastan, I. Biochemistry of multidrug resistance mediated by the multidrug transporter. *Annu. Rev. Biochem.* **1993**, *62*, 385–427. [CrossRef] [PubMed]

9. Gottesman, M.M.; Fojo, T.; Bates, S.E. Multidrug resistance in cancer: Role of ATP-dependent transporters. *Nat. Rev. Cancer* **2002**, *2*, 48–58. [CrossRef] [PubMed]

10. Dean, M.; Rzhetsky, A.; Allikmets, R. The human ATP-binding cassette (ABC) transporter superfamily. *Genome Res.* **2001**, *11*, 1156–1166. [CrossRef] [PubMed]

11. Sharom, F.J. The P-Glycoprotein Efflux Pump: How Does it Transport Drugs? *J. Membr. Biol.* **1997**, *160*, 161–175. [CrossRef] [PubMed]

12. Sharom, F.J. The P-glycoprotein multidrug transporter. *Essays Biochem.* **2011**, *50*, 161–178. [CrossRef] [PubMed]

13. Gimpl, G.; Burger, K.; Fahrenholz, F. Cholesterol as modulator of receptor function. *Biochemistry* **1997**, *36*, 10959–10974. [CrossRef] [PubMed]

14. Kapse-Mistry, S.; Govender, T.; Srivastava, R.; Yergeri, M. Nanodrug delivery in reversing multidrug resistance in cancer cells. *Front. Pharmacol.* **2014**, *5*, 159. [CrossRef] [PubMed]

15. Ozben, T. Mechanism and strategies to overcame multiple drug resistance in cancer. *FEBS Lett.* **2006**, *580*, 2903–2909. [CrossRef] [PubMed]

16. Troost, J.; Lindenmaie, J.; Haefeli, W.E.; Weiss, J. Modulation of cellular cholesterol alters P-glycoprotein activity in multidrug-resistant cells. *Mol. Pharmacol.* **2004**, *66*, 1332–1339. [CrossRef] [PubMed]

17. Caraglia, M.; Marra, M.; Naviglio, S.; Botti, G.; Addeo, R.; Abbruzzese, A. Zoledronic acid: An unending tale for an antiresorptive agent. *Expert Opin. Pharmacother.* **2010**, *11*, 141–154. [CrossRef] [PubMed]

18. Kopecka, J.; Porto, S.; Lusa, S.; Gazzano, E.; Salzano, G.; Giordano, A.; Desiderio, V.; Ghigo, D.; Caraglia, M.; De Rosa, G.; et al. Self-assembling nanoparticles encapsulating zoledronic acid revert multidrug resistance in cancer cells. *Oncotarget* **2015**, *6*, 31461–31478. [CrossRef] [PubMed]

19. Kopecka, J.; Porto, S.; Lusa, S.; Gazzano, E.; Salzano, G.; Pinzòn-Daza, M.L.; Giordano, A.; Desiderio, V.; Ghigo, D.; De Rosa, G.; et al. Zoledronic acid-encapsulating self-assembling nanoparticles and doxorubicin: A combinatorial approach to overcome simultaneously chemoresistance and immunoresistance in breast tumors. *Oncotarget* **2016**, *7*, 20753–20772. [CrossRef] [PubMed]

20. Marra, M.; Salzano, G.; Leonetti, C.; Tassone, P.; Scarsella, M.; Zappavigna, S.; Calimeri, T.; Franco, R.; Liguori, G.; Cigliana, G.; et al. Nanotechnologies to use bisphosphonates as potent anticancer agents: The effects of zoledronic acid encapsulated into liposomes. *Nanomed.: Nano. Biol. Med.* **2011**, *7*, 955–964. [CrossRef] [PubMed]

21. Salzano, G.; Marra, M.; Porru, M.; Zappavigna, S.; Abbruzzese, A.; La Rotonda, M.I.; Leonetti, C.; Caraglia, M.; De Rosa, G. Self-assembly nanoparticles for the delivery of bisphosphonates into tumors. *Int. J. Pharm. (Amsterdam, Neth.)* **2011**, *403*, 292–297. [CrossRef] [PubMed]

22. Lankalapalli, S.; Kolapalli, V.R.M. Polyelectrolyte complexes: A review of their applicability in drug delivery technology. *Indian J. Pharm. Sci.* **2009**, *71*, 481–487. [CrossRef] [PubMed]

23. Patwekar, S.L.; Potulwar, A.P.; Pedewad, S.R.; Gaikwad, M.S.; Khan, S.A.; Suryawanshi, A.B. Review on polyelectrolyte complex as novel approach for drug delivery system. *IJPPR* **2016**, *5*, 97–109.

24. Mayol, L.; De Stefano, D.; Campani, V.; De Falco, F.; Ferrari, E.; Cencetti, C.; Matricardi, P.; Maiuri, L.; Carnuccio, R.; Gallo, A.; et al. Design and characterization of a chitosan physical gel promoting wound healing in mice. *J. Mater. Sci.: Mater. Med.* **2004**, *25*, 1483–1493. [CrossRef] [PubMed]

25. Fan, W.; Yan, W.; Xu, Z.; Ni, H. Formation mechanism of monodisperse, low molecular weight chitosan nanoparticles by ionic gelation technique. *Colloids Surf. B* **2012**, *90*, 21–27. [CrossRef] [PubMed]

26. Gan, Q.; Wang, T.; Cochrane, C.; McCarron, P. Modulation of surface charge, particle size and morphological properties of chitosan-TPP nanoparticles intended for gene delivery. *Colloids Surf. B* **2005**, *44*, 65–73. [CrossRef] [PubMed]

27. Jonassen, H.; Kjøniksen, A.L.; Hiorth, M. Stability of chitosan nanoparticles cross-linked with tripolyphosphate. *Biomacromolecules* **2012**, *13*, 3747–3756. [CrossRef] [PubMed]

28. Nasti, A.; Zaki, N.M.; Leonardis, P.D.; Ungphaiboon, S.; Sansongsak, P.; Rimoli, M.G.; Tirelli, N. Chitosan/TPP and chitosan/TPP-hyaluronic acid nanoparticles: Systematic optimisation of the preparative process and preliminary biological evaluation. *Pharm. Res.* **2009**, *26*, 1918–1930. [CrossRef] [PubMed]

29. Ramasamy, T.; Tran, T.H.; Cho, H.J.; Kim, J.H.; Kim, Y.I.; Jeon, J.Y.; Choi, H.G.; Yong, C.S.; Kim, J.O. Chitosan-Based Polyelectrolyte Complexes as Potential Nanoparticulate Carriers: Physicochemical and Biological Characterization. *Pharm. Res.* **2014**, *31*, 1302–1314. [CrossRef] [PubMed]

30. Serra, M.; Scotlandi, K.; Manara, M.C.; Maurici, D.; Lollini, P.L.; De Giovanni, C.; Toffoli, G.; Baldini, N. Establishment and characterization of multidrug-resistant human osteosarcoma cell lines. *Anticancer Res.* **1993**, *13*, 323–329. [PubMed]

31. Janes, K.A.; Fresneau, M.P.; Marazuela, A.; Fabra, A.; Alonso, M.J. Chitosan nanoparticles as delivery systems for doxorubicin. *J. Controlled Release* **2001**, *73*, 255–261. [CrossRef]

32. Masarudin, M.J.; Cutts, S.M.; Evison, B.J.; Phillips, D.R.; Pigram, P.J. Factors determining the stability, size distribution, and cellular accumulation of small, monodisperse chitosan nanoparticles as candidate vectors for anticancer drug delivery: Application to the passive encapsulation of [14C]-doxorubicin. *Nanotechnol. Sci. Appl.* **2015**, *8*, 67–80. [CrossRef] [PubMed]

33. Hosseinzadeh, H.; Atyabi, F.; Dinarvand, R.; Ostad, S.N. Chitosan–Pluronic nanoparticles as oral delivery of anticancer gemcitabine: Preparation and in vitro study. *Int. J. Nanomed.* **2012**, *7*, 1851–1863. [CrossRef]

34. Alberts, D.S.; Garcia, D.J. Safety aspects of pegylated liposomal doxorubicin in patients with cancer. *Drugs* **1997**, *4*, 30–35. [CrossRef]

35. Gabizon, A.; Martin, F. Polyethylene glycol-coated (pegylated) liposomal doxorubicin. Rationale for use in solid tumours. *Drugs* **1997**, *4*, 15–21. [CrossRef]

36. Working, P.K.; Newman, M.S.; Sullivan, T.; Yarrington, J. Reduction of the cardiotoxicity of doxorubicin in rabbits and dogs by encapsulation in long-circulating, pegylated liposomes. *J. Pharmacol. Exp. Ther.* **1999**, *289*, 1128–1133. [PubMed]

37. Zeng, X.; Morgenstern, R.; Nyström, A.M. Nanoparticle-directed sub-cellular localization of doxorubicin and the sensitization breast cancer cells by circumventing GST-Mediated drug resistance. *Biomaterials* **2014**, *35*, 1227–1239. [CrossRef] [PubMed]

38. Verhoef, J.J.F.; Anchordoquy, T.J. Questioning the Use of PEGylation for Drug Delivery. *Drug Delivery Transl. Res.* **2013**, *3*, 499–503. [CrossRef]

MIL-100(Al) Gels as an Excellent Platform Loaded with Doxorubicin Hydrochloride for pH-Triggered Drug Release and Anticancer Effect

Yuge Feng [1], Chengliang Wang [2], Fei Ke [3], Jianye Zang [2] and Junfa Zhu [1,*]

[1] National Synchrotron Radiation Laboratory and Department of Chemical Physics,
    University of Science and Technology of China, Hefei 230029, China; ygfeng@mail.ustc.edu.cn
[2] Hefei National Laboratory for Physical Sciences at Microscale, CAS Center for Excellence in
    Biomacromolecules, Collaborative Innovation Center of Chemistry for Life Sciences,
    and School of Life Sciences, University of Science and Technology of China, Hefei 230026, China;
    wangcl@ustc.edu.cn (C.W.); zangjy@ustc.edu.cn (J.Z.)
[3] Department of Applied Chemistry and State Key Laboratory of Tea Plant Biology and Utilization,
    Anhui Agricultural University, Hefei 230036, China; kefei@ahau.edu.cn
*   Correspondence: jfzhu@ustc.edu.cn;

Abstract: Slow and controlled release systems for drugs have attracted increasing interest recently. A highly efficient metal-organic gel (MOGs) drug delivery carrier, i.e., MIL-100(Al) gel, has been fabricated by a facile, low cost, and environmentally friendly one-pot process. The unique structure of MIL-100(Al) gels has led to a high loading efficiency (620 mg/g) towards doxorubicin hydrochloride (DOX) as a kind of anticancer drug. DOX-loaded MOGs exhibited high stability under physiological conditions and sustained release capacity of DOX for up to three days (under acidic environments). They further showed sustained drug release behavior and excellent antitumor effects in in vitro experiments on HeLa cells, in contrast with the extremely low biotoxicity of MOGs. Our work provides a promising way for anticancer therapy by utilizing this MOGs-based drug delivery system as an efficient and safe vehicle.

Keywords: metal-organic gels; doxorubicin loading and release; pH-responsiveness; anticancer effect

---

1. Introduction

Most anticancer chemotherapeutics are controlled at high doses to make up for their premature deterioration and non-specific absorption, which typically results in the development of dose-limited toxicity [1–4]. As alternatives, slow and controlled release systems for drugs have recently attracted increasing interest [5,6]. On the one hand, the continuous slow and sustained release of small amounts of drug, instead of several large doses, can weaken patient compliance [7]. On the other hand, delivering the drug by controlled release can reduce the side effects, thus improving therapeutic efficiency [8].

Metal-organic framework (MOFs) is a class of crystalline porous hybrids built from metal ions and organic linkers. Its large surface area, tunable pore size, adjustable composition and structure, and versatile functionality character, make it an ideal carrier for slow and controlled release drug delivery [9–15]. For instance, Horcajada et al. reported that MIL-100(Fe) nanoparticles could load anticancer drugs (doxorubicin, DOX) up to 9%, and a sustained release in phosphate-buffered saline (PBS) within 14 days was observed [16]. Sun et al. reported Cu-metal organic frameworks (MOFs) with mixed ligands, MOFs-2 (40% 1,3,5-benzene tricarboxylate, 60% isophthalic acid) and MOFs-3 (70% 1,3,5-benzene tricarboxylate, 30% isophthalic acid), and their application as the transport vehicles for the delivery of DOX. The MOFs-2 showed the best performance in transport DOX as the consequence of highest loading capacity (95 mg/g). In weak acid solution (pH 5.8), MOFs-2 released 20% DOX in 80 h [17]. Vasconcelos et al. encapsulated the anticancer drug DOX in nano ZIF-8 with a loading capacity of 49 mg/g, which exhibited a progressive release behavior [18]. However, every previous study has its own shortcomings including complicated synthesis routes, intrinsic biotoxicity, low loading capacity, short release time, and poor stability at a physiological pH of 7.4. The shortcomings limit their potential applications in clinical treatment, which requires high qualities of all the performance-indicators above-mentioned.

Metal-organic gels (MOGs), as the emerging carriers, are constructed by the self-assembly of metal ions and suitable ligands through various noncovalent interactions [19,20]. Compared with MOFs, MOGs possess lower density, higher surface area, larger porosity, and can be synthesized in gentle conditions such as cheap and clean solutions, low temperature and short reaction time [21–27]. Inspired by these outstanding features, herein, we designed a kind of MOG, i.e., MIL-100(Al) $(Al_3O(OH)(H_2O)_2(BTC)_2 \cdot nH_2O)$ gels synthesized by a facile, low cost, and environmentally friendly one-pot process as the carrier for anticancer drug doxorubicin (DOX). It is encouraging that MIL-100(Al) gels exhibit high performance in all typical indicators. First, they involve a concise synthetic step, large loading capacity for DOX, and low biotoxicity. Second, DOX-loaded MOGs show a slow and sustainable releasing ability and high anticancer efficiency, thus providing a promising approach for clinical anticancer treatment.

2. Materials and Methods

2.1. Materials and Methods

1,3,5-Benzenetricarboxylic acid (H₃BTC) was purchased from Sigma-Aldrich (St. Louis, MO, USA). Aluminum nitrate nonahydrate $(Al(NO_3)_3 \cdot 9H_2O)$ was obtained from Sinopharm (Shanghai, China) Chemical Reagent Co., Ltd., (Shanghai, China). Doxorubicin (DOX) was purchased from Aladdin Biotech Company (Shanghai, China). Other chemicals obtained from commercial suppliers were of analytical reagent. All chemicals were used without further purification.

The powder X-ray diffraction (PXRD) patterns was collected by using the theta rotating anode X-ray diffractometer with Cu target (40 KV, 200 mA) from 2° to 70°. The Fourier transform infrared spectroscopy (FTIR) spectrum was determined using a Magna-IR 750 spectrometer (Nicolet, Madison, WI, USA) in the range of 500–4000 cm⁻¹ with a resolution of 4 cm⁻¹. The morphologies of the sample were studied using a SIRION200 Schottky field emission scanning electron microscope (FEI, Hillsboro, OR, USA) and JEM-2100F transmission electron microscope (JEOL, Tokyo, Japan) at 200 kV, respectively. Nitrogen adsorption–desorption isotherms were carried out with a Micromeritics TriStar II 3020 adsorption analyzer (Micromeritics, Atlanta, GAM USA) at 77 K. UV-Vis absorption spectra were carried out with a Shimadzu UV-1800 spectrophotometer (Shimadzu, Kyoto, Japan).

2.2. Synthesis of MIL-100(Al) Gels

In a typical synthesis procedure, aluminum nitrate nonahydrate $(Al(NO_3)_3 \cdot 9H_2O, 7.6 \text{ mmol})$ and 1,3,5-Benzentricarboxylic acid (H₃BTC, 5 mmol) were added to 36 mL ethanol [28]. After stirring for 15 min at room temperature to dissolve the solid, the transparent mixture was transferred to a sealed container and heated to 120 °C for one hour. The wet gels were dried in an oven at 80 °C. Finally, the obtained particles were washed by a Soxhlet extractor using ethanol as medium.

2.3. Incorporation of DOX

DOX-anticancer drug (10 mg) was first dissolved in 4 mL deionized water and then the MIL-100(Al) gels (10 mg) were added. The suspension was stirred for 24 h in the dark at room temperature. The obtained materials were then centrifuged, washed with deionized water several times, and dried under vacuum condition for further release tests. The supernatant was collected and measured by a UV-Vis spectrophotometer at a wavelength of 480 nm for the calculation of drug loading content and drug loading efficiency. The drug loading capacity was calculated as follows: drug loading capacity = (weight of DOX in MIL-100(Al) gels/weight of nanoparticles). The drug loading efficiency was calculated by: Drug loading efficiency (wt %) = (weight of DOX in MIL-100(Al) gels/weight of feeding DOX) × 100. The delivery concentration of DOX was derived according to the standard curve which was obtained from measuring the UV-Vis adsorption spectra of DOX with different known concentrations in PBS buffer solution (shown in Figure S1) and then by plotting the absorbance as a function of DOX concentration (shown in Figure S2).

2.4. Drug Release

The drug release experiment was performed by soaking the sample in PBS buffer solutions (pH = 7.4 and pH = 5.5) at 37 °C. Ten mg of DOX-loaded MIL-100(Al) gels (DOX-loaded MOGs) were suspended into 10 mL PBS solution. The mixture solution was stirred at the temperature of 37 °C in a water bath. At predetermined time intervals, 3 mL of PBS solution was removed and assayed. The volume of each withdrawn sample was replaced by the same volume of fresh PBS solution. The amount of released DOX was calculated according to the absorption analyzed by the UV-Vis spectrophotometer at 480 nm and standard absorbance vis DOX concentration curve. The calibration experiment was performed using different known concentrations of DOX in PBS buffer solution (shown in Figure S1). The derived standard absorbance vis DOX concentration curve is shown in Figure S2.

2.5. Cell Cytotoxicity of DOX-Loaded MOGs

HeLa cells were used for cell viability assay. A 96-well plate was used for cell seeding with a total number of about 2×10^3 per well. The cells were first incubated overnight, and then the MIL-100(Al) gels and DOX-loaded MOGs were added in every well with a final concentration ranging from 0.1 μg/mL to 100 μg/mL (0.1 μg/mL, 0.5 μg/mL, 1 μg/mL, 2.5 μg/mL, 5 μg/mL, 10 μg/mL, 25 μg/mL, 50 μg/mL, and 100 μg/mL). Autoclave water was added and treated as the negative control. The cells were incubated with MOGs or DOX-loaded MOGs for 12, 24, 36, 48, and 72 h, respectively. Later, all the medium in the wells were drawn and discharged, and additional MTT solution dissolved in the medium was used to treat the cells for another 4 h. Finally, dimethyl sulfoxide (DMSO) was loaded to replace the medium and dissolve the crystals for further absorbance detection. The absorbance of each well was obtained at the wavelength of 590 nm. Compared to the negative control, the cell viability was calculated. Each sample was repeated five times and the results presented as average values with error bars representing the standard deviation.

2.6. Flow Cytometry

HeLa cells (2×10^5) were seeded on a six-well plate and incubated overnight. The next day, cells were incubated with MIL-100(Al) gels (12.5 μg/mL), DOX-loaded MOGs (12.5 μg/mL), and autoclave water overnight, respectively. The cells were washed twice with 1X PBS followed by treatment with 1X trypsin for 5 min before quenching the cells with culture medium. Thereafter, the cells were washed twice with 1X PBS by centrifugation (1000 rpm, 5 min), and 1X ANNEXIN binding buffer (100 μL) was added to the cell together with PI-PE and ANNEXIN V-FITC conjugate. The cells were incubated in the dark for 20 min. Then, they were immediately analyzed with a flow cytometer.

2.7. Fluorescence Microscopy Images

The fluorescence microscopy studies were performed on HeLa cells in a confocal dish with a total number of 4×10^5 per dish. MIL-100(Al) gels (200 μL) and DOX-loaded MOGs (200 μL) were added into each dish respectively, to give a final concentration of 12.5 μg/mL and the cells were incubated for 12 h. Thereafter, the medium was removed and the cells were washed three times with 1X PBS. The treated cells were re-suspended in 1X PBS. Then, the ANNEXIN V–FITC conjugate was added (25 μL), and the cells incubated for 15 min in the dark. Thereafter, the ANNEXIN containing PBS was removed and the cells were washed three times with 1X PBS before fixing them with paraformaldehyde solution (4% in 1X PBS, 1 mL). After 20 min, the formaldehyde solution was removed and the cells washed twice with 1X PBS. In the end, the cells were incubated with Hoechst solution (5 µg/ mL, 1 mL) in 1X PBS in the dark for 15 min, and washed with twice with 1X PBS to image.

3. Results and Discussion

3.1. Morphology and Structure Characterization of MIL-100(Al) Gels

Transmission electron microscope (TEM) images (Figure 1a,b) showed the irregular structure of the as-synthesized MIL-100(Al) gels. Powder x-ray diffraction (XRD) was applied to identify their microstructure. The result was similar with that of a previous report [29]. As depicted in Figure S3, the pattern for the gel sample revealed a low crystallinity as several broad peaks were observed. However, it also showed that the gel was closely related to the MIL-100(Al) crystal [30]. In each position where a peak appeared for the MIL-100(Al) crystal, there appeared a corresponding broad peak for the gel sample, implying that the gel and the MOF crystal had similar structures. The nitrogen adsorption-desorption isotherm, which was used to evaluate the porous properties of MIL-100(Al) gels, was between those of type-I and type-IV, suggesting the coexistence of micropores and mesopores in the MIL-100(Al) gels sample (Figure S4). The Brunauer–Emmett–Teller (BET) surface area and pore volume of the MIL-100(Al) gels were calculated to be 920 m^2/g and 0.535 cm^3/g, respectively. They were slightly lower than those of MIL-100(Al) (1214 m^2/g and 0.77 cm^3/g). The similar large surface area and high porosity of MIL-100(Al) gels may arise from the intrinsic nature of the MIL-100(Al) [31]. Thus, the large surface area and high porosity make this material a possible candidate for highly efficient drug loading.

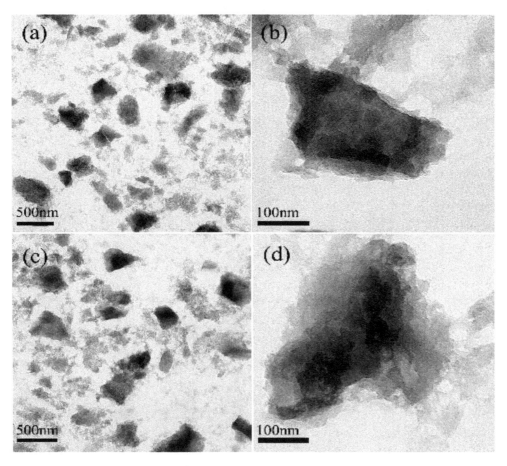

Figure 1. TEM images of (**a,b**) MIL-100(Al) gels. (**c,d**) DOX-loaded MIL-100(Al) gels.

3.2. Drug Loading and Release Behaviors

The TEM images of DOX-loaded MOGs (Figure 1c,d) exhibited almost no change in morphology when compared with MIL-100(Al) gels. Figure 2a is the XRD patterns of MIL-100(Al) gels and DOX-loaded MIL-100(Al) gels (DOX-loaded MOGs). Both of them showed similar features before and after the drug adsorption, indicating that the porous structure of MIL-100(Al) gels was retained after the loading of DOX. Figure 2b shows the FTIR spectra of MIL-100(Al) gels, DOX, and DOX-loaded MOGs. The peak at 3400 cm^{-1} was attributed to the O–H stretching of MIL-100(Al) gels. In the FTIR spectrum of DOX, peaks at 1020 cm^{-1} and 3400 cm^{-1} were caused by –NH$_2$ torsional vibration and O–H stretching vibrations of DOX, respectively. In the case of the DOX-loaded MOGs, peaks of O–H stretching vibrations overlap were broadened and a new adsorption band at 1020 cm^{-1} owing to the torsional vibration of –NH$_2$ from DOX was generated. This FTIR result indicated that MIL-100(Al) gels conjugated with DOX molecules successfully.

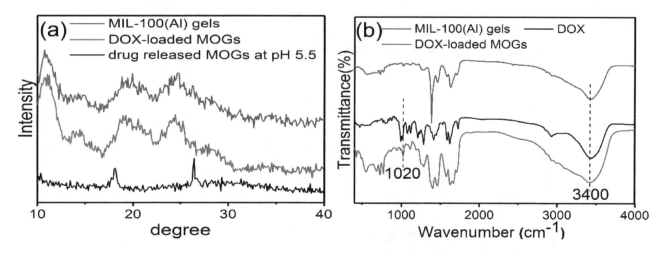

Figure 2. (a) Powder XRD patterns of MIL-100(Al) gels, DOX-loaded MOGs, and drug-released MOGs at pH 5.5; (b) FTIR spectra of MIL-100(Al) gels, DOX, and DOX-loaded MOGs.

It turns out that the loading capacity was reached up to 620 mg of DOX per gram of the sample. This large DOX loading capacity and high loading efficiency (62%) may be attributed to the ultrahigh porosity and enormous internal surface of MIL-100(Al) gels. The driving force of loading of DOX in MOGs may arise from the porous absorption and intermolecular forces. The latter most likely originated from the hydrogen bonds formed between the –NH$_2$, –OH groups in DOX and the surface active –OH, –COOH groups in MOGs [6,32].

The controlled drug release kinetics of DOX from DOX-loaded MOGs were investigated using UV-Vis adsorption spectra in PBS buffer solutions at 37 °C. Figure 3 is the DOX release profiles at two different pH values (pH = 7.4 and 5.5). It can be seen that the release of DOX from DOX-loaded MOGs in pH = 7.4 only reached 10% within 100 h. In contrast, the DOX release rate was significantly increased in pH = 5.5 and this release reached nearly 100% within 100 h. This revealed that under acidic conditions, the drug can be released more easily. Under the weak acidic condition (pH = 5.5), the drug delivery rate gradually decreased with time. Basically, the rate can be clearly divided into three regions: (i) an early rapid release within the first 10 h; (ii) a slow release region in the time range between 10 and 60 h; and (iii) a saturation region after 70 h [33]. The first rapid release was induced by the simple diffusion and dissolution of DOX molecules adsorbed onto the surface of MOGs. The second region revealed a gentle and steady release over a long time due to the desorption, diffusion, and dissolution processes of DOX molecules from channels in the gels to the solution. The last saturated drug release process could be attributed to host-guest interactions between the DOX molecules and the gels. The results revealed that the obtained MIL-100(Al) gels exhibited a high drug loading and long sustained release time under an acidic environment. To further understand the DOX release process from the DOX-loaded MOGs, TEM images were taken from DOX-loaded MOGs after 10 h, 50 h, and 100 h in the release process at pH 5.5 (inset in Figure 3). They revealed the gradual collapse of the MIL-100(Al) gel structure during the procedure. The result was consistent with the XRD pattern of drug-released MOGs at pH 5.5 (Figure 2a), which showed the dissolution of MIL-100(Al) gels in an acidic environment. The reason is that MIL-100(Al) gels self-assemble through multiple non-covalent bonds under preparation conditions such as H-bonds, π–π stacking, electrostatic interactions, and other supramolecular weak interactions [20]. These non-covalent bonds are easily destroyed under acidic conditions, leading to the dissolution of MOGs. The excellent pH-responsive release property may be attributed to the collapse of the MIL-100(Al) gel structure and the reduction of the interaction between DOX and MOGs in acidic conditions (pH 5.5) [34]. In addition, DOX molecules tend to be more hydrophilic at lower pH values [35]. The other possible reason is that the protons can easily penetrate the pores in acidic buffer solution to protonate the amino group of DOX, resulting in the acceleration of drug release [36].

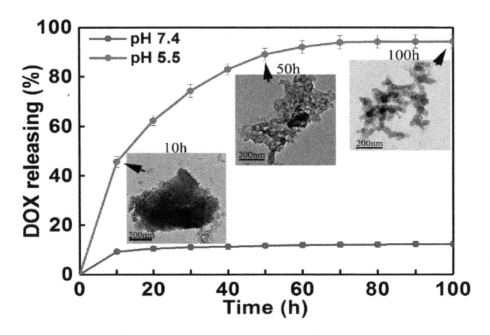

Figure 3. Drug release profiles for DOX-loaded MOGs in PBS buffer solution at pH = 5.5 and pH = 7.4 within 100 h. (Inset are TEM images of DOX-loaded MOGs after 10 h, 50 h, and 100 h in release process at pH 5.5.) Bars denote the standard deviation ($\pm$SD, n = 5).

3.3. Cell Cytotoxicity of DOX-Loaded MOGs

After evaluating the drug loading and release ability of MOGs, in vitro cell viabilities of DOX-loaded MOGs and pure MIL-100(Al) gels on HeLa cells were investigated using the MTT (3-(4,5-Dimethylthiazol-2-yl)-2,5-diphenyltetrazolium bromide) assay. To study the biotoxicity of pure MIL-100(Al) gels and the therapeutic efficiency of DOX-loaded MOGs, HeLa cells were cultured with the DOX-loaded MOGs and pure MIL-100(Al) gels at concentrations ranging from 0.1 μg/mL to 100 μg/mL (0.1, 0.5, 1, 2.5, 5, 10, 25, 50 ,and 100 μg/mL) for 24 h. The results are exhibited in Figure 4. As can be seen, after 24 h incubation with HeLa cells, the pure MIL-100(Al) gels showed no obvious toxicity towards the HeLa cells even at the concentration of MIL-100(Al) gels as high as 100 μg/mL. In contrast, the DOX-loaded MOGs showed high cytotoxicity on HeLa cells. As the concentration of DOX-loaded MOGs increased, the cell viability rapidly decreased. When the concentration of DOX-loaded MOGs reached 25 μg/mL, only ~20% of HeLa cells survived. Therefore, the DOX could be efficiently released from the DOX-loaded MOGs to kill most of the tumor cells, demonstrating that the as-synthesized MIL-100(Al) gels hold great promise for application in the field of drug delivery system for cancer treatment.

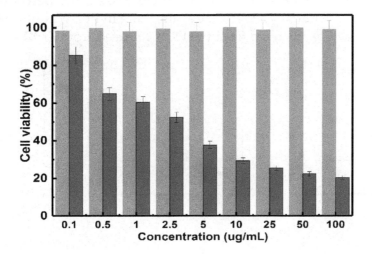

Figure 4. The effect of MIL-100(Al) gels and DOX-loaded MOGs with various concentrations on the cell viability of HeLa cells in 24 h (the orange and blue bars represent the viability of HeLa cancer cells incubated with MIL-100(Al) gels and DOX-loaded MOGs, respectively).

The in vitro drug release behavior of DOX-loaded MOGs on HeLa cells was also investigated. DOX-loaded MOGs and MOGs + free DOX with different concertation were studied. The results are shown in Figure 5a–f. Accordingly, the viability of cells incubated with DOX-loaded MOGs gradually decreased in the time range of 72 h. This was in contrast with the sudden reduction behavior of the viability of cells incubated with MOGs + free DOX, in all the control experiment groups.

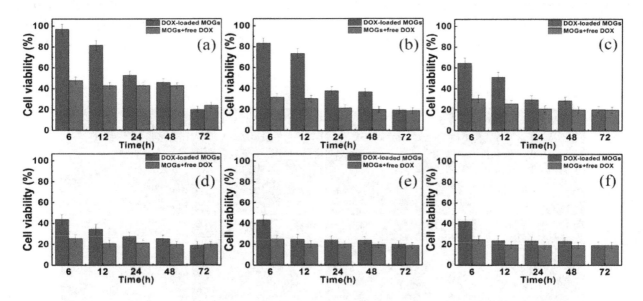

Figure 5. Cell viability of HeLa cells incubated with DOX-loaded MOGs and MOGs + free DOX for different time periods at concentrations of (**a**) 2.5 µg/mL, (**b**) 5 µg/mL, (**c**) 10 µg/mL, (**d**) 25 µg/mL, (**e**) 50 µg/mL, and (**f**) 100 µg/mL.

3.4. Flow Cytometry

In order to further investigate the apoptosis of the cells, we performed the flow cytometry analysis on HeLa cells with 12.5 µg/mL MIL-100(Al) gels and DOX-loaded MOGs. As shown in Figure 6, almost no necrotic and late apoptotic cells were observed in the control experiment (only containing pure autoclave water) (1.49%) and MIL-100(Al) gels (1.88%), revealing the low toxicity of this MOGs-based material. However, when the DOX-loaded MOGs were added, the percentage of apoptotic cells immediately became prominent (89.9%). These results were in line with the MTT assay and further confirmed that apoptotic cell death arose from the DOX released from DOX-loaded MOGs.

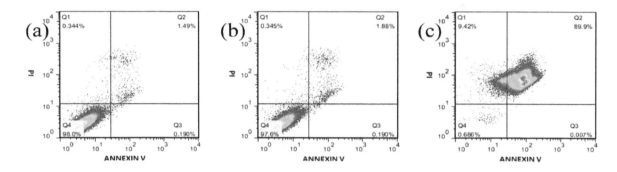

Figure 6. Flow cytometry experiments of HeLa cells when incubated with (**a**) Pure autoclave water as control, (**b**) MIL-100(Al) gels, and (**c**) DOX-loaded MOGs, respectively.

3.5. Fluorescence Microscopy Images

To further confirm the therapeutic efficiency of DOX-loaded MOGs, we performed confocal fluorescence microscopy for HeLa cells incubated with 12.5 µg/mL pure MIL-100(Al) gels and DOX-loaded MOGs for 24 h, followed by staining the nucleus with DAPI and the apoptotic cells with Annexin V-FITC. The results are revealed in Figure 7. Herein, the green fluorescence was attributed to the apoptotic HeLa cells, while the blue and red fluorescence represented the living cell imaging and DOX released, respectively. For the HeLa cells incubated with pure MIL-100(Al) gels, only very small amounts of apoptotic HeLa cells were present (Figure 7c,d). In contrast, for the HeLa cells incubated with DOX-loaded MOGs, a large number of the HeLa cells were apoptotic (Figure 7g,h). This result again demonstrates the high efficiency of the DOX-loaded MOGs in cancer therapeutic treatment.

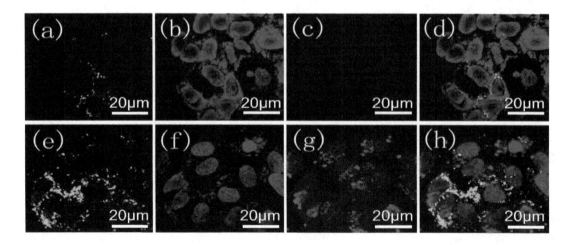

Figure 7. Confocal microscopy images of HeLa cells incubated with 12.5 µg/mL (**a–d**) MIL-100(Al) gels and (**e–h**) DOX-loaded MOGs, respectively. Blue fluorescence represents the living cell imaging. Red fluorescence represents the released DOX from DOX-loaded MOGs within the cancer cells. Green fluorescence represents the apoptosis of cells. (**d,h**) are the merged images of (**a–c**) and (**e–g**), respectively.

4. Conclusions

On the basis of the methods reported in the previous work [5,6,19,20], we reported on a metal-organic gel (MOG)-based drug delivery system for anticancer therapy, i.e., MIL-100(Al) gels, which were synthesized by a facile, low cost, and environmentally friendly one-pot method. The anticancer drug doxorubicin hydrochloride (DOX) was successfully encapsulated in the MIL-100(Al) gels with high loadings (620 mg/g). Through the control experiments, the fabricated DOX-loaded MOGs were comparable with some previous pH-responsive drug delivery systems [16–18]. Specifically, the drug was not released at physiological condition (PBS, pH 7.4), but was released in a controlled manner at acidic conditions (pH 5.5) with approximately 100%, after being delivered over three days. We also conducted in vitro experiments of DOX-loaded MIL-100(Al) gels (DOX-loaded MOGs) toward HeLa cells where it turned out that the DOX-loaded MOGs had excellent efficiency in killing the HeLa cells. The synthetic MIL-100(Al) gels here featured a concise synthetic step, large loading capacity for DOX, and low biotoxicity. Furthermore, the DOX-loaded MOGs showed slow and sustainable releasing ability and high anticancer efficiency. MIL-100(Al) gels exhibited high qualities of all the performance-indicators as above-mentioned, making DOX-loaded MOGs a promising anticancer approach for clinical application.

Author Contributions: Y.F. and J.Z. (Junfa Zhu) conceived and designed the experiments; Y.F. and C.W. performed the experiments; Y.F., C.W. and F.K. analyzed the data; J.Z. (Junfa Zhu) and J.Z. (Jianye Zang) contributed reagents/materials/analysis tools; Y.F. wrote the paper.

Acknowledgments: This work was supported by the National Key R&D Program of China (2017YFA0403402), the Natural Science Foundation of China (Grants U1732272 and 21773222), the Key Program of Research and Development of Hefei Science Center of CAS (2017HSC-KPRD001), and the Collaborative Innovation Center of Suzhou Nano Science and Technology. Thanks to Jilong Wang and Fan Zheng for the assistance of in vivo cell experiments.

References

1. Jain, R.K.; Stylianopoulos, T. Delivering nanomedicine to solid tumors. *Nat. Rev. Clin. Oncol.* **2010**, *7*, 653–664. [CrossRef] [PubMed]
2. Davis, M.E.; Chen, Z.; Shin, D.M. Nanoparticle therapeutics: An emerging treatment modality for cancer. *Nat. Rev. Drug Discov.* **2008**, *7*, 771–781. [CrossRef] [PubMed]
3. Maeda, H.; Nakamura, H.; Fang, J. The EPR effect for macromolecular drug delivery to solid tumors: Improvement of tumor uptake, lowering of systemic toxicity, and distinct tumor imaging in vivo. *Adv. Drug Deliv. Rev.* **2013**, *65*, 71–79. [CrossRef] [PubMed]
4. Chen, Y.; Ai, K.; Liu, J.; Sun, G.Y.; Yin, Q.; Lu, L.H. Multifunctional envelope-type mesoporous silica nanoparticles for pH-responsive drug delivery and magnetic resonance imaging. *Biomaterials* **2015**, *60*, 111–120. [CrossRef] [PubMed]
5. Chowdhuri, A.R.; Singh, T.; Ghosh, S.K.; Sahu, S.K. Carbon dots embedded magnetic nanoparticles @chitosan @metal organic framework as a nanoprobe for pH sensitive targeted anticancer drug delivery. *ACS Appl. Mater. Interfaces* **2016**, *8*, 16573–16583. [CrossRef] [PubMed]
6. Su, Y.Y.; Teng, Z.; Yao, H.; Wang, S.J.; Tian, Y.; Zhang, Y.L.; Liu, W.F.; Tian, W.; Zheng, L.J.; Lu, N.; et al. A multifunctional PB@mSiO$_2$−PEG/DOX nanoplatform for combined photothermal−chemotherapy of tumor. *ACS Appl. Mater. Interfaces* **2016**, *8*, 17038–17046. [CrossRef] [PubMed]
7. Jalvandi, J.; White, M.; Gao, Y.; Truong, Y.B.; Padhye, R.; Kyratzis, I.L. Polyvinyl alcohol composite nanofibres containing conjugated levofloxacin-chitosan for controlled drug release. *Mater. Sci. Eng. C* **2017**, *73*, 440–446. [CrossRef] [PubMed]
8. Wang, D.D.; Zhou, J.J.; Chen, R.H.; Shi, R.H.; Zhao, G.Z.; Xia, G.L.; Li, R.; Liu, Z.B.; Tian, J.; Wang, H.J.; et al. Controllable synthesis of dual-MOFs nanostructures for pH-responsive artemisinin delivery, magnetic

resonance and optical dual-model imaging-guided chemo/photothermal combinational cancer therapy. *Biomaterials* **2016**, *100*, 27–40. [CrossRef] [PubMed]

9.   Zhao, D.; Timmons, D.J.; Yuan, D.; Zhou, H.C. Tuning the Topology and Functionality of Metal–Organic Frameworks by Ligand Design. *Acc. Chem. Res.* **2011**, *44*, 123–133. [CrossRef] [PubMed]

10. Corma, A.; Garcia, H.; Llabres, F.X.; Xamena, I. Engineering Metal Organic Frameworks for Heterogeneous Catalysis. *Chem. Rev.* **2010**, *110*, 4606–4655. [CrossRef] [PubMed]

11. Keskin, S.; Kizilel, S. Biomedical Applications of Metal Organic Frameworks. *Chem. Res.* **2011**, *50*, 1799–1812. [CrossRef]

12. Yang, X.L.; Chen, X.H.; Hou, G.H.; Guan, R.F.; Shao, R.; Xie, M.H. A multiresponsive metal–organic framework: Direct chemiluminescence, photoluminescence, and dual tunable sensing applications. *Adv. Funct. Mater.* **2016**, *26*, 393–398. [CrossRef]

13. Kaur, R.; Kim, K.H.; Paul, A.K.; Deep, A. Recent advances in the photovoltaic applications of coordination polymers and metal organic frameworks. *J. Mater. Chem. A* **2016**, *4*, 3991–4002. [CrossRef]

14. Li, H.; Guo, K.; Wu, C.; Shu, L.; Guo, S.; Hou, J.; Zhao, N.; Wei, L.; Man, X.; Zhang, L. Controlled and Targeted Drug Delivery by a UV-responsive Liposome for Overcoming Chemo-resistance in Non-Hodgkin Lymphoma. *Chem. Biol. Drug Des.* **2015**, *86*, 783–794. [CrossRef] [PubMed]

15. He, Q.; Gao, Y.; Zhang, L.; Zhang, Z.; Gao, F.; Ji, X.; Li, Y.; Shi, J. A pH-responsive mesoporous silica nanoparticles-based multi-drug delivery system for overcoming multi-drug resistance. *Biomaterials* **2011**, *32*, 7711–7720. [CrossRef] [PubMed]

16. Nunzio, M.R.; Agostoni, V.; Cohen, B.; Gref, R.; Douhal, A. A "Ship in a Bottle" Strategy to Load a Hydrophilic Anticancer Drug in Porous Metal Organic Framework Nanoparticles: Efficient Encapsulation, Matrix Stabilizationand Photodelivery. *J. Med. Chem.* **2014**, *57*, 411–420. [CrossRef] [PubMed]

17. Sun, K.K.; Li, L.; Yu, X.L.; Liu, L.; Meng, Q.T.; Wang, F.; Zhang, R. Functionalization of mixed ligand metal-organic frame-works as the transport vehicles for drugs. *J. Colloid Interface Sci.* **2017**, *486*, 128–135. [CrossRef] [PubMed]

18. Vasconcelos, I.B.; Silva, T.G.; Militao, G.C.; Soares, T.A.; Rodrigues, N.M.; Rodrigues, M.O.; Freire, N.B.; Junior, S.A. Cytotoxicity and slow release of the anti-cancer drug doxorubicin from ZIF-8. *RSC Adv.* **2012**, *2*, 9437–9442. [CrossRef]

19. Sengupta, S.; Mondal, R. Metal-Organic-Particle-Supported Metallogel Formation Using a Nonconventional Chelating Pyridine-Pyrazole-Based Bis-Amide Ligand. *Chem. Eur. J.* **2013**, *19*, 5537–5541. [PubMed]

20. Zhang, J.; Su, C.Y. Metal-organic gels: From discrete to coordination polymers. *Coord. Chem. Rev.* **2013**, *257*, 1373–1408. [CrossRef]

21. Xiao, B.; Zhang, Q.; Huang, C.; Li, Y. Luminescent Zn(II)–terpyridine metal organic gel for visual recognition of anions. *RSC Adv.* **2015**, *5*, 2857–2860. [CrossRef]

22. Aiyappa, H.B.; Saha, S.; Wadge, P.; Banerjee, R.S. Fe(III) phytatemetallogel as a prototype anhydrous, intermediate temperature proton conductor. *Chem. Sci.* **2015**, *6*, 603–607. [CrossRef] [PubMed]

23. Huang, M.; Mi, K.; Zhang, J.H.; Liu, H.L.; Yu, T.T.; Yuan, A.; Kong, Q.; Xiong, S. MOF-derived bi-metal embedded N-doped carbon polyhedral nanocages with enhanced lithium storage. *J. Mater. Chem. A* **2017**, *5*, 266–274. [CrossRef]

24. Zhao, X.; Yuan, L.; Zhang, Z.Q.; Wang, Y.S.; Yu, Q.; Li, J. Synthetic Methodology for the Fabrication of Porous Porphyrin Materials with Metal-Organic-Polymer Aerogels. *Inorg. Chem.* **2016**, *55*, 5287–5296. [CrossRef] [PubMed]

25. Li, L.; Xiang, S.L.; Cao, S.Q.; Zhang, J.Y.; Ouyang, G.F.; Chen, L.P.; Su, C.Y. A synthetic route to ultralight hierarchically micro/mesoporousAl(III)-carboxylate metal-organic aerogels. *Nat. Commun.* **2013**, *4*, 1774–1782.

26. Mahmood, A.; Xia, W.; Mahmood, N.; Wang, Q.F.; Zou, R.Q. Hierarchical heteroaggregation of binary metal-organic gels with tunable porosity and mixed valence metal sites for removal of dyes in water. *Sci. Rep.* **2015**, *5*, 10556. [CrossRef] [PubMed]

27. Sutar, P.; Maji, T.K. Coordination polymer gels: Soft metal–organic supramolecular materials and versatile applications. *Chem. Commun.* **2016**, *52*, 8055–8074. [CrossRef] [PubMed]

28. Liu, Y.R.; He, L.; Zhang, J.; Wang, X.; Su, C.Y. Evolution of spherical assemblies to fibrous networked Pd(II) metallo gels from a pyridine-based tripodal ligand and their catalytic property. *Chem. Mater.* **2009**, *21*, 557–563. [CrossRef]

29. Xia, W.; Zhang, X.; Xu, L.; Wang, Y.; Lin, J.; Zou, R. Facile and economical synthesis of metal–organicframework MIL-100(Al) gels for high efficiency removalof microcystin-LR. *RSC Adv.* **2013**, *3*, 11007–11013. [CrossRef]

30. Volkringer, C.; Popov, D.; Loiseau, T.; Ferey, G.; Burghammer, M.; Riekel, C.; Haouas, M.; Taulelle, F. Synthesis, Single-Crystal X-ray Microdiffraction, and NMR Characterizations of the Giant Pore Metal-Organic Framework Aluminum Trimesate MIL-100. *Chem. Mater.* **2009**, *21*, 5695–5697. [CrossRef]

31. Gjmez, G.P.; Cabello, C.P.; Opanasenko, M.; Horacek, M.; Cejka, J. Superior Activity of Isomorphously Substituted MOFs with MIL-100 (M = Al, Cr, Fe, In, Sc, V) Structure in the Prins Reaction: Impact of Metal Type. *ChemPlusChem* **2017**, *82*, 152–159.

32. Tan, S.Y.; Ang, C.Y.; Mahmood, A.; Qu, Q.; Li, P.; Zou, R.; Zhao, Y.L. Doxorubicin-Loaded Metal-Organic Gels for pH and Glutathione Dual-Responsive Release. *ChemNanoMat* **2016**, *2*, 504–508. [CrossRef]

33. Kayal, S.; Ramanujan, R.V. Doxorubicin loaded PVA coated iron oxide nanoparticles for targeted drug delivery. *Mater. Sci. Eng. C* **2010**, *30*, 484–490. [CrossRef]

34. Yang, X.; Grailer, J.J.; Rowland, I.J.; Javadi, A.; Hurley, S.A.; Matson, V.Z. Multifunctional Stable and pH-Responsive Polymer Vesicles Formed by Heterofunctional Triblock Copolymer for Targeted Anticancer Drug Delivery and Ultrasensitive MR Imaging. *ACS Nano* **2010**, *4*, 6805–6817. [CrossRef] [PubMed]

35. Liu, J.; Zong, E.; Fu, H.; Zheng, S.; Xu, Z.; Zhu, D. Adsorption of aromatic compounds on porous covalent triazine-based framework. *J. Colloid Interface Sci.* **2012**, *372*, 99–107. [CrossRef] [PubMed]

36. Hu, X.; Hao, X.; Wu, Y.; Zhang, J.; Zhang, X.; Wang, P.C.; Zou, G.; Liang, X.J. Multifunctional Hybrid Silica Nanoparticles for Controlled Doxorubicin Loading and Release with Thermal and pH Dual Response. *J. Mater. Chem. B* **2013**, *1*, 1109–1118. [CrossRef] [PubMed]

Development of Multifunctional Liposomes Containing Magnetic/Plasmonic MnFe₂O₄/Au Core/Shell Nanoparticles

Ana Rita O. Rodrigues [1], Joana O. G. Matos [1]⬤, Armando M. Nova Dias [1], Bernardo G. Almeida [1], Ana Pires [2], André M. Pereira [2], João P. Araújo [2], Maria-João R. P. Queiroz [3], Elisabete M. S. Castanheira [1]⬤ and Paulo J. G. Coutinho [1],*⬤

1   Centro de Física da Universidade do Minho (CFUM), Campus de Gualtar, 4710-057 Braga, Portugal; ritarodrigues@fisica.uminho.pt (A.R.O.R.); pg26303@alunos.uminho.pt (J.O.G.M.); pg36912@alunos.uminho.pt (A.M.N.D.); bernardo@fisica.uminho.pt (B.G.A.); ecoutinho@fisica.uminho.pt (E.M.S.C.)

2   IFIMUP/IN—Instituto de Nanociência e Nanotecnologia, Universidade do Porto, R. Campo Alegre, 4169-007 Porto, Portugal; ana.pires@fc.up.pt (A.P.); ampereira@fc.up.pt (A.M.P.); jearaujo@fc.up.pt (J.P.A.)

3   Centro de Química da Universidade do Minho (CQUM), Campus de Gualtar, 4710-057 Braga, Portugal; mjrpq@quimica.uminho.pt

*   Correspondence: pcoutinho@fisica.uminho.pt;

Abstract: Multifunctional liposomes containing manganese ferrite/gold core/shell nanoparticles were developed. These magnetic/plasmonic nanoparticles were covered by a lipid bilayer or entrapped in liposomes, which form solid or aqueous magnetoliposomes as nanocarriers for simultaneous chemotherapy and phototherapy. The core/shell nanoparticles were characterized by UV/Visible absorption, X-Ray Diffraction (XRD), Transmission Electron Microscopy (TEM), and Superconducting Quantum Interference Device (SQUID). The magnetoliposomes were characterized by Dynamic Light Scattering (DLS) and TEM. Fluorescence-based techniques (FRET, steady-state emission, and anisotropy) investigated the incorporation of a potential anti-tumor drug (a thienopyridine derivative) in these nanosystems. The core/shell nanoparticles exhibit sizes of 25 ± 2 nm (from TEM), a plasmonic absorption band ($\lambda_{max} = 550$ nm), and keep magnetic character. XRD measurements allowed for the estimation of 13.3 nm diameter for manganese ferrite core and 11.7 nm due to the gold shell. Aqueous magnetoliposomes, with hydrodynamic diameters of 152 ± 18 nm, interact with model membranes by fusion and are able to transport the anti-tumor compound in the lipid membrane, with a high encapsulation efficiency (EE (%) = 98.4 ± 0.8). Solid magnetoliposomes exhibit hydrodynamic diameters around 140 nm and also carry successfully the anticancer drug (with EE (%) = 91.2 ± 5.2), while also being promising as agents for phototherapy. The developed multifunctional liposomes can be promising as therapeutic agents for combined chemo/phototherapy.

Keywords: magnetic/plasmonic nanoparticles; multifunctional liposomes; manganese ferrite; gold shell; anti-tumor drugs; cancer therapy

1. Introduction

In recent years, a revolution in cancer therapy has taken place due to the development of multi-tasked nanostructures or materials for applications in oncology [1,2]. In chemotherapy, the ideal nano-encapsulation system should have biophysical properties that favor the passive accumulation in tumors upon intravenous administration, as well as controlled triggered release of the encapsulated active molecules. In this context, magnetic nano-encapsulation systems are promising since they can enable the magnetic drug targeting by static gradient magnetic fields and magnetic hyperthermia, which produce local heat as a trigger for drug release and a synergistic cytotoxic effect in cancer cells [3–7]. Additionally, systems based on superparamagnetic nanoparticles can generate high-resolution images by T2-weighted magnetic resonance imaging (MRI) for tumor diagnosis [7–9].

Noble metal (Ag, Au) nanoparticles strongly absorb light in the visible region due to coherent oscillations of the metal conduction band electrons in strong resonance with visible frequencies of light. This phenomenon is known as surface plasmon resonance (SPR) [10–13] and is highly dependent on nanoparticles size, shape, surface, and dielectric properties of the surrounding medium [14–16]. Light absorbed by nanoparticles is readily dissipated as heat. Due to their large absorption cross sections, plasmonic nanoparticles can generate a significant amount of heat and increase temperatures in their vicinities [17]. If a sufficient number of nanoparticles are present, the temperature fields overlap and create a substantial global temperature rise [18]. From the point of view of cancer therapeutics, noble metal nanoparticles become very useful as agents for plasmonic photothermal therapy (PTT) on account of their enhanced absorption cross sections, which are four to five orders of magnitude larger than those offered by conventional photo-absorbing dyes [16]. This strong absorption ensures effective laser therapy at relatively lower energies, which render the therapy method minimally invasive. Additionally, metal nanostructures have a higher photo-stability and do not suffer from photo-bleaching [16,19]. Recently, plasmonic nanoparticles have also been used as photoacoustic imaging (PAI) agents to increase tissue penetration, as well as sensitivity and spatial resolution [20].

In nanomedicine, systems with combined magnetic and plasmonic properties are of particular interest for theranostics since they combine simultaneously multiple imaging modalities for diagnosis with complementary synergistic strategies for therapy [21–23]. Gold nanoparticles have been largely used in biomedical applications for their low toxicity, great biocompatibility, easy conjugation with active biomolecules, and their remarkable optical properties, which enable their use as diagnostic and therapeutic agents [19,24]. However, recent works have shown that the conjugation of gold nanoparticles with magnetic ones may decrease the overall magnetization of the nanostructure [25]. Thus, coating magnetic nanoparticles with gold should be carefully considered in order to ensure proper magnetic capabilities for their application. Among all magnetic nanoparticles, those of manganese ferrite have recently received great attention for their high magnetic susceptibility, which suggests that they may be promising as hyperthermia and magnetic drug targeting agents [26,27].

In this study, magnetic/plasmonic nanoparticles possessing a manganese ferrite core and a gold shell were prepared. In order to develop applications in cancer therapy, the prepared nanoparticles were entrapped in liposomes (aqueous magnetoliposomes, AMLs) or covered with a lipid bilayer (solid magnetoliposomes, SMLs). These new nanosystems were tested in this scenario as nanocarriers for a potential anticancer drug, especially active against melanoma, breast adenocarcinoma, and non-small cell lung cancer [28]. In addition, the local heating capability of the developed systems was monitored through the fluorescence quenching of rhodamine B incorporated in the lipid layer when excited with a light source. Considering their potentialities, the new nanosystems developed in this study can be promising for future applications in cancer therapy.

2. Materials and Methods

All the solutions were prepared using spectroscopic grade solvents and ultrapure water of Milli-Q grade (MilliporeSigma, St. Louis, MO, USA).

2.1. Preparation of Manganese Ferrite/Gold Core/Shell Nanoparticles

Manganese ferrite nanoparticles (NPs) were synthesized in 5 mL aqueous solution, by the co-precipitation method, as previously described [26]. First, an aqueous solution containing 612 μL of

50% NaOH solution was heated to 90 °C. Then, a mixture containing 500 µL of 0.5 M MnSO$_4$·H$_2$O solution and 500 µL of 1 M FeCl$_3$·6H$_2$O solution was added, drop by drop, to the previously warmed basic solution under magnetic stirring. After two hours at 90 °C, manganese ferrite nanoparticles were formed. For purification, the obtained sample was washed several times with ethanol, by centrifugation (14,000 g) and magnetic decantation.

For growth of the gold shell, a method adapted from a previously described procedure was used [19]. In addition, 5 mL of an aqueous dispersion of the synthesized MnFe$_2$O$_4$ nanoparticles (with concentration of 4 mg/mL) were added to 25 mL of glycerol and heated up to 200 °C, under vigorous stirring. Then, 2 mL of 0.02 M solution of gold(III) chloride hydrate (HAuCl$_4$), from Sigma-Aldrich (St. Louis, MO, USA), were added dropwise. After 15 minutes under continuous stirring at 200 °C, the gold shell was formed around the MnFe$_2$O$_4$ core NPs. To remove glycerol residues, the synthesized NPs were washed by centrifugation (14,000 g) with ethanol.

2.2. Preparation of Magnetoliposomes

For magnetoliposomes preparation, the lipids L-α-phosphatidylcholine from egg yolk (Egg-PC), and 1,2-dioleoyl-sn-glycero-3-phospho-rac-(1-glycerol) sodium salt (DOPG), from Sigma-Aldrich (St. Louis, MO, USA), were used in a final concentration of 1 mM. The ethanol injection method was employed to obtain aqueous magnetoliposomes (AMLs) [29]. Accordingly, a 20 mM lipid solution in ethanol was injected, under vigorous vortexing, to an aqueous dispersion of manganese ferrite/gold nanoparticles (with 4 mg/mL concentration). After encapsulation, the ferrofluid was washed with water and purified by magnetic decantation to remove all the non-encapsulated NPs.

For the preparation of solid magnetoliposomes (SMLs), a method previously described was used [30]. First, 10 µL of a solution of the synthesized MnFe$_2$O$_4$/Au core/shell nanoparticles (0.02 mg/mL) were ultra-sonicated for one minute at 189 W, and 3 mL of chloroform were added to the solution. Then, immediately after vigorous agitation, 150 µL of a 20 mM methanolic solution of the lipid DOPG (1,2-dioleoyl-sn-glycero-3-phospho-rac-(1-glycerol) sodium salt) were injected under vortexing to form the first lipid layer of the SMLs. To remove the lipid that was not attached to the nanoparticles surface, the particles were washed twice by magnetic decantation with ultrapure water. The lipid bilayer was completed by a new injection of 150 µL of 20 mM lipid methanolic solution, under vortexing, in 3 mL of aqueous dispersion of the particles with the first lipid layer. The SMLs obtained were then washed and purified with ultrapure water by magnetic decantation.

The anti-tumor compound methyl 3-amino-6-(benzo[d]thiazol-2-ylamino)thieno[3,2-b]pyridine-2-carboxylate was incorporated into aqueous magnetoliposomes by the co-injection method (simultaneous injection of compound and lipid) in a final compound concentration of 2 µM. In solid magnetoliposomes, the compound was incorporated by injection of an ethanolic solution (0.2 mM) immediately before the formation of the second lipid layer.

2.3. Preparation of Giant Unilamellar Vesicles (GUVs)

GUVs of soybean lecithin (L-α-phosphatidylcholine from soybean), from Sigma-Aldrich (St. Louis, MO, USA), were obtained by the thin film hydration method [31,32]. For that, a lipid film of 100 µL of soybean lecithin solution (1 mM) was obtained by solvent evaporation under an argon stream, and 40 µL of water were added, followed by incubation at 45 °C for 30 min. Then, 3 mL of glucose aqueous solution (0.1 M) were added and the resulting solution was again incubated at 37 °C for 2 h. After incubation, the GUVs suspension was centrifuged at 14,000 g for 30 minutes at 20 °C, to remove multi-lamellar vesicles and lipid aggregates.

2.4. Spectroscopic Measurements

2.4.1. General Methods

Absorption spectra were performed in a Shimadzu UV-3600 Plus UV-vis-NIR (Shimadzu Corporation, Kyoto, Japan) spectrophotometer. Fluorescence measurements were recorded using a Horiba Fluorolog 3 spectrofluorimeter (HORIBA Jobin Yvon IBH Ltd., Glasgow, UK), equipped with double mono-chromators in both excitation and emission, Glan-Thompson polarizers, and a temperature controlled cuvette holder. Fluorescence spectra were corrected for the instrumental response of the system.

2.4.2. FRET Measurements

Förster Resonance Energy Transfer (FRET) assays were employed to confirm the formation of the lipid bilayer in the solid magnetoliposomes (SMLs). For that purpose, the nitrobenzoxazole labeled lipid NBD-C$_6$-HPC (1-palmitoyl-2-{6-[(7-nitro-2-1,3-benzoxadiazol-4-yl)amino]hexanoyl}-sn-glycero-3-phosphocholine) (from Avanti Polar Lipids, Alabaster, AL, USA) was included in the first lipid layer, while the rhodamine B labeled lipid Rhodamine B-DHPE (1,2-dipalmitoyl-sn-glycero-3-phospho-ethanolamine-N-lissamine rhodamine B sulfonyl (ammonium salt)) (from Avanti Polar Lipids, Alabaster, AL, USA) was included in the second lipid layer.

FRET efficiency, Φ_{RET}, defined as the proportion of donor molecules that have transferred their excess energy to the acceptor molecules, was calculated through donor emission quenching, by taking the ratio of the donor integrated fluorescence intensities in the presence of acceptor (F_{DA}) and in the absence of acceptor (F_D) (Equation (1)) [33].

$$\Phi_{RET} = 1 - \frac{F_{DA}}{F_D} \tag{1}$$

The distance between the donor and acceptor molecules was determined through the FRET efficiency (Equation (2)).

$$r = R_0 \left[\frac{1 - \Phi_{RET}}{\Phi_{RET}} \right]^{1/6} \tag{2}$$

where R_0 is the Förster radius (critical distance), that can be obtained by the spectral overlap, $J(\lambda)$, between the donor emission and the acceptor absorption, according to Equations (3) and (4) (with R_0 in Å, λ in nm, $\varepsilon_A(\lambda)$ in M^{-1} cm^{-1}) [33].

$$R_0 = 0.2108 \left[k^2 \Phi_D^0 n^{-4} J(\lambda) \right]^{1/6} \tag{3}$$

$$J(\lambda) = \int_0^\infty I_D(\lambda) \, \varepsilon_A(\lambda) \, \lambda^4 d\lambda \tag{4}$$

where $k^2 = \frac{2}{3}$ is the orientational factor assuming random orientation of the dyes, n is the refraction index of the medium, $I_D(\lambda)$ is the fluorescence spectrum of the donor normalized so that $\int_0^\infty I_D(\lambda) d\lambda = 1$, and $\varepsilon_A(\lambda)$ is the molar absorption coefficient of the acceptor. Φ_D^0, the fluorescence quantum yield of the donor in the absence of energy transfer, was determined by the standard method (Equation (5)) [34,35].

$$\Phi_D^0 = \frac{A_r F_D n_D^2}{A_D F_r n_r^2} \Phi_r \tag{5}$$

where A is the absorbance at the excitation wavelength, F is the integrated emission area, and n is the refraction index of the solvents used. Subscripts refer to the reference (r) or donor (D). The absorbance at the excitation wavelength was always lower than 0.1 to avoid the inner filter effects. The NBD-C$_6$-HPC molecule intercalated in lipid membranes was used as a reference, $\Phi_r = 0.32$ at 25 °C, as reported by Invitrogen [36].

The hydrophobic dye Nile Red (energy acceptor) was also incorporated in magnetoliposomes labelled with NBD-C_6-HPC (NBD as energy donor) for monitoring the interaction of magnetoliposomes with GUVs by FRET.

2.4.3. Fluorescence Anisotropy Measurements

The steady-state fluorescence anisotropy, r, is calculated by the equation below.

$$r = \frac{I_{VV} - GI_{VH}}{I_{VV} + 2GI_{VH}} \tag{6}$$

where I_{VV} and I_{VH} are the intensities of the emission spectra obtained with vertical and horizontal polarization, respectively (for vertically polarized excitation light), and $G = I_{HV} / I_{HH}$ is the instrument correction factor, where I_{HV} and I_{HH} are the emission intensities obtained with vertical and horizontal polarization (for horizontally polarized excitation light).

2.4.4. Drug Encapsulation Efficiency

The encapsulation efficiency, EE (%), of the potential anti-tumor drug in magnetoliposomes, was determined through fluorescence emission measurements. Therefore, drug loaded magnetoliposomes were subjected to centrifugation at 11,000 rpm for 60 min using Amicon® Ultra centrifugal filter units 100 kDa (Merck Millipore, Darmstadt, Germany). Then, the filtrate (containing the non-encapsulated drug) was pipetted out, the water was evaporated, and the same amount of ethanol was added. After vigorous agitation, its fluorescence was measured, which allowed it to determine the drug concentration using a calibration curve (fluorescence intensity *vs.* concentration) previously obtained in the same solvent. Three independent measurements were performed for each system and standard deviations (SD) were calculated. The encapsulation efficiency was determined using Equation (7).

$$EE(\%) = \frac{(total\ amount - amount\ of\ non\ encapsulated\ compound)}{total\ amount} \times 100 \tag{7}$$

2.5. Structural Characterization

2.5.1. Transmission Electron Microscopy (TEM)

TEM images of nanoparticles and solid magnetoliposomes were acquired using a Transmission Electron Microscope Leica LEO 906E (Leica Microsystems, Wetzlar, Germany) operating at 120 kV, at UME (Electron Microscopy Unit), University of Trás-os-Montes and Alto Douro (Vila Real, Portugal). For SMLs, a negative staining was employed, using a 2% aqueous solution of ammonium molybdate tetrahydrate. In addition, 20 μL of the sample and 20 μL of the staining solution were mixed and a drop of the mixture was placed onto a Formvar grid (Agar Scientific Ltd., Essex, UK), held by tweezers. After 20 s, almost all the solution was removed with filter paper and left to dry. TEM images were processed using *ImageJ* software (National Institutes of Health (NIH), Bethesda, MD, USA) with the addition of a value to all pixels so that a white background resulted, which was followed by inversion and enhanced local contrast. Subsequently, the ParticleSizer plugin [37] was used and was followed by particle analysis. The area of each particle allowed an estimation of the particle diameter. The resulting histogram was fitted to a bimodal Gaussian distribution.

2.5.2. X-Ray Diffraction (XRD)

X-Ray Diffraction (XRD) analyses were performed using a conventional Philips PW 1710 (Royal Philips, Amsterdam, The Netherlands) diffractometer, operating with CuK_α radiation, in a Bragg-Brentano configuration.

2.5.3. Dynamic Light Scattering (DLS)

The mean diameter and size distribution (polydispersity index) of aqueous and solid magnetoliposomes (1 mM lipid concentration) were measured using Dynamic Light Scattering (DLS) equipment NANO ZS Malvern Zetasizer (Malvern Panalytical Ltd., Malvern, UK) at 25 °C, using an He-Ne laser of $\lambda = 632.8$ nm and a detector angle of 173°. The measurements were also carried out for the magnetoliposomes in a solution of human serum albumin (35 mg/mL) in PBS buffer (pH = 7.4). Five independent measurements were performed for each sample.

2.6. Magnetic Measurements

Magnetic measurements of the dry core/shell nanoparticles were performed at room temperature in a Superconducting Quantum Interference Device (SQUID) magnetometer Quantum Design MPMS5XL (Quantum Design Inc., San Diego, CA, USA) using applied magnetic fields up to 5.5 T.

2.7. Measurement of the Photothermal Effect

Solid magnetoliposomes incorporating the labelled lipid Rhodamine B-DHPE were irradiated and Rhodamine B emission was monitored by a function of time, using the detection system of a SPEX Fluorolog 2 spectrofluorimeter (HORIBA Jobin Yvon IBH Ltd., Glasgow, UK). The irradiation setup consisted in a Xenon arc lamp (200 W) and an optical fiber, using a Thorlabs FEL0600 (Thorlabs Inc., Newton, NJ, USA) long pass filter with cut-on wavelength at 600 nm, to ensure the excitation of only the gold nanoparticles (not exciting Rhodamine B dye).

3. Results and Discussion

3.1. Nanoparticles Characterization

3.1.1. Absorption Spectra

Figure 1 displays the UV-Visible absorption spectrum of the synthesized manganese ferrite/gold core/shell nanoparticles. The absorption spectra of net gold nanoparticles and net manganese ferrite nanoparticles are also shown for comparison.

The spectrum of manganese ferrite NPs is typical of an indirect semiconductor, as reported earlier [26], while the spectrum of gold nanoparticles obtained by the standard Turkevish method [38] reveals a characteristic local surface plasmon resonance (LSPR) band, with a maximum around 530 nm. In comparison, the absorption spectrum of manganese ferrite/gold core/shell NPs exhibits a broader and red shifted plasmon band (maximum at 550 nm). The absorption spectrum of gold nanoshells depends on their thickness, as well as on the refraction index of both core and surrounding media [39]. Theoretical studies have shown that, for an air filled core of 10 nm size and a gold shell of 5 nm in water medium, the resonance peak is expected to occur at 538 nm, while, for a 10-nm shell, it should appear at 552 nm [40]. The increase of the core refraction index results in a red shift of the plasmon resonance peak [39]. For a 3-nm gold shell thickness on a 10-nm magnetite core, a resonance peak at 560 nm was found [41].

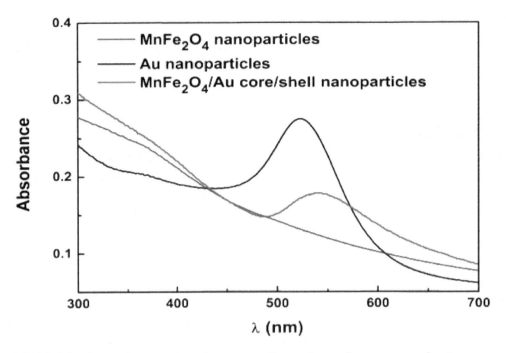

Figure 1. UV-Visible absorption spectra of aqueous dispersions of manganese ferrite nanoparticles, gold nanoparticles, and $MnFe_2O_4$/Au core/shell nanoparticles.

3.1.2. X-Ray Diffraction (XRD) Measurements

XRD analysis confirmed the synthesis of a pure crystalline phase of manganese ferrite/gold nanoparticles, since all their characteristic peaks (CIF 2300618 for manganese ferrite and CIF 9013035 for gold), marked by their indices, were observed (Figure 2b). The percentage amounts obtained for $MnFe_2O_4$ and Au were 59.1% and 40.9%, respectively. Mean sizes of 13.3 nm for manganese ferrite and 11.7 nm for gold, were estimated through a Rietveld analysis using Fullprof software [42]. Table 1 summarizes the main results of the Rietveld analysis. For the net manganese ferrite powdered sample, it resulted in a poor R_F factor of 9.0. It was possible to improve it by optimizing the overall isothermal factor, B_{over}, but an unreasonable value of -2.79 was obtained. A similar improvement was possible by accounting for the effect of sample microstructure (Figure 2a), according to Equation (8) [43], which gives the micro-absorption correction term, P.

$$P = P_0 + C \frac{\tau}{\sin \theta} \left(1 - \frac{\tau}{\sin \theta}\right) \tag{8}$$

where P_0 is the bulk contribution to the micro-absorption effect and τ is the normalized surface roughness parameter [43].

Table 1. Selected Rietveld analysis parameters.

Sample	$O_{x,y,z}$ (*)	i (*)	Micro Absorption Correction	Overall Temperature Factor, B_{over}	Lattice Constant (nm)	Size (nm)	R_f	χ^2
$MnFe_2O_4$	0.251	0.928	No	0 (+)	0.84693	13.8	9.03	1.33
$MnFe_2O_4$	0.251	0.898	No	-2.79	0.84684	13.2	4.45	1.18
$MnFe_2O_4$	0.257	0.60	Yes (#)	0 (+)	0.84685	13.3	3.18	1.18
$MnFe_2O_4$/Au	0.257 (+)	0.60 (+)	Yes (##)	0 (+)	0.84685 (+)	13.3	4.70	1.56
	—	—		0 (+)	0.406945	11.7	0.68	

(#) $P_0 = 0.629$, C = 1.31, $\tau = 0.055$. (##) $P_0 = 0.607$, C = 1.15, $\tau = 0.084$. (+) fixed values. (*) Values in CIF file 2360018 are $O_{x,y,z} = 0.25053$ and $i = 0.33$.

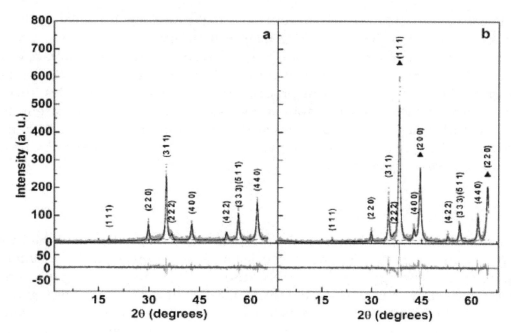

Figure 2. XRD diffractogram of manganese ferrite (**a**) and manganese ferrite/gold core/shell nanoparticles (**b**). Gold diffraction peaks are marked by a filled triangle.

Considering $\mu \bar{l} = 0.01$ (μ is the linear absorption coefficient and $\bar{l}$ is the mean chord length of the powder particle) and the values in Table 1 for Equation (8) parameters, a degree of inversion of $i = 0.60$ is obtained for manganese ferrite. This value is close to the one reported by Chen et al. ($i = 0.67$) [44], using a similar preparation method for $MnFe_2O_4$. The Rietveld analysis of gold phase was not optimal, as the intensity of peak (111) is lower and that of peak (200) is higher than the experimental ones. In addition, the analysis of $MnFe_2O_4$ phase decreased its quality, as the R_F factor increased from 3.18 to 4.70 and the peak (311) got much lower than the experimental one. This could be due to the expected shell morphology of gold in the prepared $MnFe_2O_4/Au$ nanocomposites in which a layer of gold grows on the $MnFe_2O_4$ surface. This morphology, through lattice mismatch induced stress, is predictable to change the intensity of the diffraction peaks [45]. An atomistic modelling of the core/shell nanoparticle is anticipated to yield a better description of the XRD diffractogram [46] and this will be addressed in a future study. The obtained weight fraction of gold was 40.9%, but this is calculated using proportionality factors between diffraction intensity and mass, ATZs [42], that do not take into account the dependence of diffraction intensity on particle size. Since the lattice constant of Au is less than half that of $MnFe_2O_4$, the reduction of diffraction intensity with particle size is much more pronounced for Au than for $MnFe_2O_4$. This means that the value given by Fullprof software is expected to be much lower than the real one. Considering the obtained size of manganese ferrite of 13.3 nm and using the phase densities that resulted from the XRD analysis (5.04 g cm^{-3} for $MnFe_2O_4$ and 19.4 g cm^{-3} for Au), the mass percentage of gold would be 98.7% if the obtained size of gold phase (11.7 nm) corresponds to the shell thickness. This percentage would change to 95.6% if the obtained size value of 11.7 nm corresponds to the double of the shell thickness. This would be true if the effect of the two gold layers in given X-ray crosses contributes equally to the broadening of the diffraction peak. Thus, from XRD data analysis, the thickness of the gold shell is expected to be 5.85 nm. This value is compatible with the observed position of the surface plasmon resonance peak, as discussed in the previous section. Additionally, in magnetite/gold core/shell nanoparticles, reported in Reference [41], the diffraction peak widths were identical for the 10 nm magnetite core and for the 2 nm gold shell (where its dimensions were obtained from HR-TEM measurements). Therefore, the actual value of the gold shell thickness in $MnFe_2O_4/Au$ NPs could be even lower.

A nanostructure consisting of a 5.85 nm gold shell surrounding a cluster of $MnFe_2O_4$ nanoparticles cannot be ruled out. In that case, the calculated mass percentage of gold changes to 91% for a compact over-coating layer of 12 spheres. Nevertheless, in the case of gold shell growth, the magnetic nanoparticles are dispersed in glycerol at a high temperature, before the addition of HAuCl$_4$ solution. This means the magnetic nanoparticles can effectively be dispersed with their surface well stabilized and passivated by the abundant OH groups of glycerol. Furthermore, the formation of the gold shell occurs through oxidation of glycerol. This process originates in other molecules, such as glyceric acid or tartronic acid, which can act as gold surface stabilizers. This is the case in terms of the citric acid in the Turkevish gold nanoparticles synthesis procedure [38]. Therefore, the prepared MnFe$_2$O$_4$/Au core/shell nanoparticles are expected to be surface passivated by hydroxyacids and, as such, well dispersible in aqueous media.

3.1.3. Transmission Electron Microscopy (TEM)

TEM images (Figure 3a) of the MnFe$_2$O$_4$/Au prepared nanoparticles and the corresponding image after processing by *ImageJ* (Figure 3b) revealed a generally spherical shape with the presence of some aggregation. These aggregates probably arise from the sample preparation on TEM grids (slow evaporation of a drop of an aqueous dispersion of nanoparticles). The size histogram that results from the area of the highlighted particles was fitted to a bimodal Gaussian distribution in order to better separate the presence of aggregates from the individual nanoparticles (Figure 3c). A bimodal size distribution of 25 ± 2 nm and 32 ± 6 nm was obtained. The former population is in accordance with the size estimated from XRD measurements, which is 25 nm when the gold shell thickness is 5.85 nm.

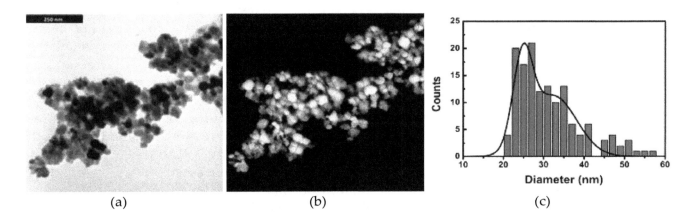

(a)   (b)   (c)

Figure 3. (**a**) TEM image of the synthesized MnFe$_2$O$_4$/Au core/shell nanoparticles. (**b**) TEM image processed by *ImageJ* (same scale of image **a**). (**c**) Particles size histogram and fitting to a bimodal Gaussian distribution (total number of 141 particles).

Below is a critical diameter of 42.9 nm. MnFe$_2$O$_4$ nanoparticles possess a superparamagnetic behavior [47,48], losing at least 90% of the magnetization when an applied magnetic field is removed, which is important for biomedical applications. The size of the nanoparticles obtained in this study is within this limit, and, therefore, these NPs are suitable for applications in biomedicine.

3.2. Magnetic Properties

The magnetic properties of MnFe$_2$O$_4$/Au core/shell nanoparticles (Figure 4) were characterized by measuring their magnetic hysteresis loop, which shows the relationship between the induced magnetic moment and the applied magnetic field (*H*). The core/shell nanoparticles present a superparamagnetic behavior since the ratio between remnant magnetization (M_r) and saturation magnetization (M_s) is below 0.1 [49] (Table 2).

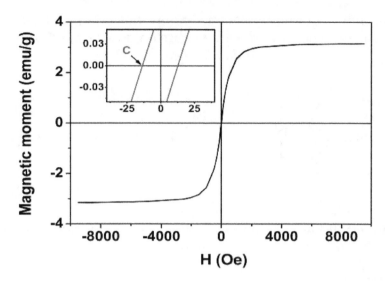

Figure 4. Magnetization hysteresis loop of $MnFe_2O_4$/Au core/shell nanoparticles measured at room temperature. Inset: Enlargement of the loop in the low field region.

Table 2. Coercive field (H_c), saturation magnetization (M_s), remnant magnetization (M_r), and ratio M_r/M_s for $MnFe_2O_4$/Au core/shell nanoparticles at room temperature.

	H_c (Oe)	M_s (emu/g)	M_r (emu/g)	M_r/M_s
$MnFe_2O_4$/Au NPs	13.57	3.15	0.08	0.03

The low saturation magnetization values are due to the presence of a diamagnetic gold layer. The gold shell thickness of $MnFe_2O_4$/Au core/shell nanoparticles was estimated using the magnetic hysteresis cycle. The particles were considered to have a well ordered $MnFe_2O_4$ core covered by a non-magnetic gold shell (with a thickness δ), acting as a "dead layer". Thus, the obtained saturation magnetization, M_s, is proportional to the core volume that possesses a spontaneous magnetization, which is related to the thickness of the dead layer and to the particle diameter, through Equation (9) [49].

$$M_s = M_{s0}\left(1 - \frac{6\delta}{D}\right) \tag{9}$$

where D is the particle diameter and M_{s0} is the saturation magnetization of $MnFe_2O_4$.

Chen et al. [44] observed that the saturation magnetization of manganese ferrite depends on particle size, which is estimated to be a value of 58 emu/g for $MnFe_2O_4$ nanoparticles of 13.3 nm (also prepared by coprecipitation). Using this value, a gold layer thickness of δ = 4.0 nm is obtained for particles with a diameter of 25 nm (from TEM) and M_s = 3.15 emu/g. This is roughly in accordance with XRD results.

3.3. Magnetoliposomes as Drug Nanocarriers

The obtained magnetic/plasmonic nanoparticles were either entrapped in liposomes (aqueous magnetoliposomes, AMLs) or covered by a lipid bilayer that forms the so-called solid magnetoliposomes (SMLs). The potential of both types of magnetoliposomes as drug carriers was investigated. A potential anti-tumor compound, which is a fluorescent thienopyridine derivative (Figure 5), was incorporated into AMLs and SMLs and its fluorescence emission was studied. This compound can be promising as an anticancer agent in oncological therapy, as it exhibited very low growth inhibitory concentrations (GI_{50}), between 3.5 µM (for A375-C5 melanoma cell line) and 6.4 µM (for non-small cell lung cancer, NCI-H460 cell line), when tested in vitro in several human tumor cell lines [28]. Moreover, the same compound has shown a very low affinity for the multi-drug resistance protein (MDR1), which is a protein that promotes drug resistance in cells [50]. This compound exhibits fluorescence in several polar and non-polar media, but not in aqueous solution [50]. Therefore, fluorescence-based methodologies (fluorescence emission, FRET, and fluorescence anisotropy) are advantageous techniques to monitor behavior and location of this compound in magnetoliposomes.

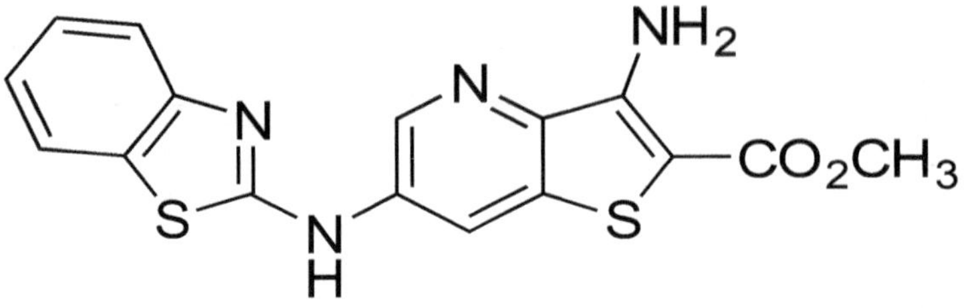

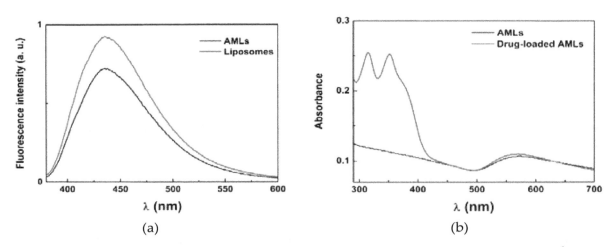

Figure 5. Structure of the potential anti-tumor thienopyridine derivative.

3.3.1. Aqueous Magnetoliposomes

The emission of the thienopyridine derivative in AMLs and liposomes (the latter without nanoparticles and with the same concentration of compound) is shown in Figure 6a. Since this potential drug is not fluorescent in aqueous media [50], the emission observed is indicative of the encapsulation of the compound in magnetoliposomes. A quenching of the compound fluorescence is observed in AMLs relative to the liposomes, which confirms its incorporation in the magnetic nanocarriers since this effect is attributed to the presence of the nanoparticles that absorb in a wide wavelength range [26]. Figure 6b displays the absorption spectra of AMLs containing the core/shell nanoparticles, with and without the anti-tumor drug, which confirms the successful loading of the drug into the magnetoliposomes and shows the overlap of the absorption spectra of nanoparticles with the compound fluorescence emission. This indicates that the nanoparticles can quench, by energy transfer, the compound fluorescence, as already observed [26]. Additionally, the gold shell can also introduce a quenching effect through electron transfer processes.

Figure 6. (a) Fluorescence spectra (λ_{exc} = 360 nm) of the anti-tumor compound (2×10^{-6} M) in liposomes and AMLs of Egg-PC containing $MnFe_2O_4$/Au core/shell nanoparticles; (b) Absorption spectra of AMLs containing the core/shell nanoparticles with and without the anti-tumor drug.

Moreover, the fluorescence anisotropy measurements (Table 3) confirmed that the anti-tumor compound is located mainly in the lipid bilayer. The anisotropy values were analogous to those previously determined in liposomes of the same lipids [50]. The behavior observed is similar to the one previously reported for magnetoliposomes containing manganese ferrite nanoparticles (without the gold shell) [26], which indicates that gold does not influence compound location in magnetoliposomes.

Table 3. Steady-state fluorescence anisotropy (r) values, at 25 °C, for the anti-tumor compound in magnetoliposomes in comparison with the values in neat liposomes.

	Lipid	r
Liposomes [50]	Egg-PC	0.176
	DOPG	0.181
AMLs	Egg-PC	0.173
	DOPG	0.168
SMLs	DOPG	0.175

The size of DOPG AMLs containing the magnetic/plasmonic nanoparticles were determined by Dynamic Light Scattering (DLS), which exhibit hydrodynamic diameters of 152 ± 18 nm and with a low polydispersity index (PDI = 0.19 ± 0.04). This size is larger than the one reported for Egg-PC aqueous magnetoliposomes containing manganese ferrite nanoparticles [26], but very similar to the one of DOPG solid magnetoliposomes based on $MnFe_2O_4$ [26]. In the presence of human serum albumin (HSA), 35 mg/mL (typical concentration in serum) in PBS buffer, the size of AMLs slightly increases and possesses hydrodynamic diameters of 157 ± 29 nm with a slightly higher polydispersity (PDI = 0.23 ± 0.09). For enhanced permeability and a retention (EPR) effect of loaded drugs, the diameter of (magneto)liposomes must be small. A successful extravasation into tumors has been shown to occur for nanocarriers with sizes below 200 nm [51]. Moreover, an encapsulation efficiency of $EE\ (\%)$ = 98.4 ± 0.8 was obtained for the anti-tumor thienopyridine derivative in these aqueous magnetoliposomes, which anticipate that these systems contain $MnFe_2O_4$/Au NPs as very promising nanocarriers for anti-cancer drugs.

The interaction of AMLs containing $MnFe_2O_4$/Au nanoparticles with Giant Unilamellar Vesicles (GUVs), used as models of biological membranes, was also investigated. The aim of this study was to evaluate the ability of magnetoliposomes to release drugs by fusing with cell membranes, considering future applications in cancer therapy/theranostics. Taking into account the fluorescence quenching caused by the presence of the core/shell nanoparticles, the emission of the anti-tumor compound incorporated in aqueous magnetoliposomes was measured before and after interaction with GUVs (Figure 7a). After interaction with GUVs, the observed unquenching effect indicates the occurrence of membrane fusion between AMLs and the model membranes, with an increase in the distance between the drug and the nanoparticles (decreasing the interaction that leads to emission quenching).

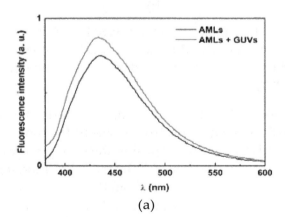

(a)

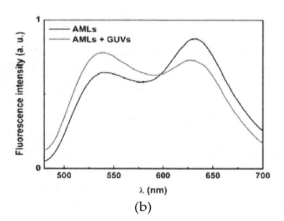

(b)

Figure 7. (a) Fluorescence spectra (λ_{exc} = 360 nm) of the thienopyridine derivative (2 × 10^{-6} M) in AMLs of Egg-PC containing $MnFe_2O_4$/Au nanoparticles, before and after interaction with GUVs. (b) Fluorescence spectra (λ_{exc} = 400 nm) of AMLs containing both NBD-C_6-HPC (2 × 10^{-6} M) and Nile Red (2 × 10^{-6} M), before and after interaction with GUVs.

To further confirm that this unquenching is, in fact, due to fusion between AMLs and GUVs, the interaction between these two systems was also monitored by FRET (Förster Resonance Energy Transfer). For that purpose, AMLs containing both the labeled lipid NBD-C_6-HPC and the lipid probe Nile Red [52–54] were prepared. In this case, the NBD moiety acted as the energy donor and the dye Nile Red acted as the energy acceptor [55]. Exciting only the donor NBD, a strong band due to Nile Red emission was observed (with maximum around 630 nm), which resulted from energy transfer to Nile Red (Figure 7b). After interaction with GUVs, the donor fluorescence (λ_{max} = 535 nm) increased and the acceptor emission band decreased, which showed the diminution of FRET process efficiency and, consequently, proved the membrane fusion between AMLs and GUVs.

3.3.2. Solid Magnetoliposomes

The preparation of solid magnetoliposomes, where a cluster of nanoparticles is successively covered by two lipid layers, was performed using a methodology previously developed [30]. This method has proven to be successful for solid magnetoliposomes containing magnetic nanoparticles of manganese ferrite [26], nickel ferrite [30], and magnetite [56]. To confirm that the same procedure can be applied to nanoparticles with a gold shell, the formation of the lipid bilayer around $MnFe_2O_4$/Au nanoparticles was confirmed by FRET.

The labeled lipid NBD-C_6-HPC (NBD as energy donor) was included in the first lipid layer of the SMLs and the lipid Rhodamine B-DHPE (rhodamine as the acceptor) was included in the second lipid layer. The emission of SMLs containing only the NBD-labelled lipid and SMLs containing both donor and acceptor labeled lipids were measured (Figure 8a), exciting only the donor NBD.

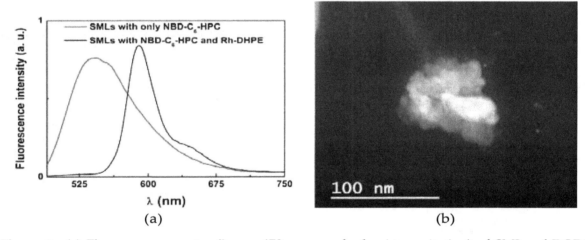

(a)   (b)

Figure 8. (**a**) Fluorescence spectra (λ_{exc} = 470 nm, no rhodamine excitation) of SMLs of DOPG containing $MnFe_2O_4$/Au core/shell nanoparticles labeled with only NBD-C_6-HPC and labeled with both NBD-C_6-HPC and rhodamine B-DHPE; (**b**) TEM image (dark field mode) of SMLs containing core/shell nanoparticles (obtained with a negative staining).

The fluorescence spectrum of SMLs with only the donor shows, as expected, a characteristic NBD emission band (λ_{max} = 535 nm). On the other hand, the fluorescence spectrum of the SMLs containing both donor and acceptor rates reveals a decrease in the NDB emission opposing the strong rise in the rhodamine B emission band, which shows the energy transfer of the excited NBD moiety to rhodamine B. A distance between donor and acceptor of r_{DA} = 3.1 nm was determined, from the calculated FRET efficiency of 0.65 (Equations (2)–(5)). Considering that donor and acceptor are each in one of the lipid layers, the distance between them proves the bilayer formation in SMLs, considering the typical cell membrane thickness (7–9 nm) [57]. TEM images of solid magnetoliposomes (Figure 8b) containing the core/shell nanoparticles point to nanosystems with diameters around 100 nm. DLS measurements revealed that these solid liposomes exhibit hydrodynamic diameters of 138 ± 19 nm and a low value for the polydispersity index (PDI = 0.20 ± 0.07). In the presence of HSA (PBS buffer, pH = 7.4), the size determined by DLS rises to 160 ± 32 nm (PDI = 0.24 ± 0.08), but is still below 200 nm.

The incorporation of the anti-tumor thienopyridine derivative in SMLs and the fusion with model membranes (GUVs) were confirmed in a similar way to the AMLs. As such, the emission of compounds loaded in SMLs was measured, as well as the emission after interaction of the SMLs with GUVs (Figure 9a). It was observed that a quenching effect of the compound fluorescence emission by the presence of magnetic/plasmonic nanoparticles (relative to the observed in liposomes) indicates incorporation of the thienopyridine derivative in the SMLs membrane. This quenching is more pronounced than for AMLs due to the lower distance between the NPs cluster and the drug. Figure 9b shows the absorption spectra of drug loaded and unloaded SMLs. Like in the case of AMLs, SMLs can also absorb (through the core/shell nanoparticles) in the compound emission region.

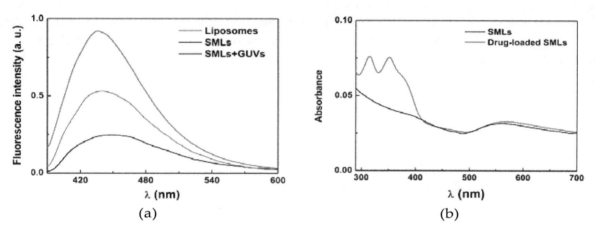

(a)   (b)

Figure 9. (a) Fluorescence spectra (λ_{exc} = 360 nm) of the thienopyridine derivative (2×10^{-6} M), in SMLs of DOPG containing MnFe$_2$O$_4$/Au core/shell nanoparticles, before and after interaction with GUVs. (b) Absorption spectra of SMLs containing the core/shell nanoparticles, with and without the anti-tumor drug.

The fluorescence anisotropy value of the anti-tumor drug in these SMLs is also similar to the one in liposomes and AMLs of the same lipid (Table 3). This indicates that the main location of the compound is in the lipid membrane, as reported for liposomes [50]. The drug encapsulation efficiency in SMLs is slightly lower than the one for AMLs, *EE (%)* = 91.2 ± 5.2, but still quite high.

The unquenching effect detected upon interaction with GUVs proves membrane fusion of SMLs with the model membranes. Again, these results are similar to the ones in magnetoliposomes containing net MnFe$_2$O$_4$ nanoparticles [26] and, hence, the SMLs containing magnetic/plasmonic nanoparticles are promising nanocarriers for this anti-tumor drug.

3.4. Magnetoliposomes as Agents for Phototherapy

For the study of photo thermal ability, solid magnetoliposomes containing MnFe$_2$O$_4$/Au core/shell nanoparticles and including the labeled lipid Rhodamine B-DHPE were synthesized and Rhodamine B emission was measured under irradiation (λ > 600 nm) along time (Figure 10). The local heating produced by gold propagates by heat diffusion, resulting in quenching of the rhodamine emission, due to the increase of efficiency of the non-radiative decay pathways. This effect is observed in Figure 10, where a monotonic decrease in Rhodamine fluorescence intensity is detected along the irradiation time, which leads to a local temperature increase. The solution temperature raised only 2 °C during irradiation time, but this increase also occurred in the absence of irradiation. This indicates that the excitation light from the spectrofluorometer, which is always incident in the sample during measurement, has higher intensity than the irradiation light (at λ > 600 nm), so that the effect of the latter is negligible. When only the excitation light hits the sample, the rhodamine emission intensity is approximately constant (Figure 10). On the contrary, upon irradiation at λ > 600 nm, an emission quenching occurs, that can only originate from a local temperature increase. The corresponding heat must, therefore, originate from the photo-thermal effect of the gold nanoshell upon light irradiation with λ > 600 nm. Huang et al. [58] studied local heating produced by laser irradiation of gold nanoparticles in the interior of a cell, both experimentally and theoretically. It was found that, for a 50 mW laser power focused into a 0.1 mm spot, the temperature at the vicinity of gold nanoparticles would increase from 25 °C to approximately 38 °C, after 4 min of irradiation and for an absorption at the plasmon resonance wavelength of 0.1. Using a light power meter (Thorlabs PM100USB with a S140C sensor), the light intensity through the λ > 600 nm filter was ~5 mW. Assuming 50% loss upon the used coupling to an optical fiber with a 1-mm diameter, and considering the final irradiation time of 120 min, the equivalent light power in the conditions of the calculations of Huang et al. [58] would be ~18 mW. According to the reported linear relation between the calculated temperature near gold nanoparticles and irradiation time [58], a local temperature increase of ~5 °C is expected. This temperature increase is compatible with the observed rhodamine fluorescence quenching. A much higher local temperature increase using laser irradiation of the developed magnetic/plasmonic lipid covered systems is then expected.

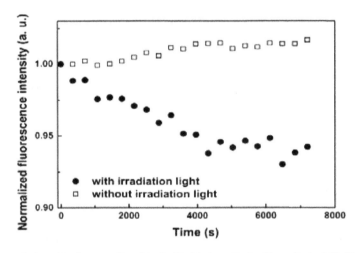

Figure 10. Fluorescence intensity (normalized to initial intensity) of irradiated SMLs with $MnFe_2O_4$/Au core/shell nanoparticles labelled with Rhodamine B-DHPE, as a function of time. For comparison, the behavior without irradiation light is also shown.

Therefore, these results show that solid magnetoliposomes based on manganese ferrite/gold core/shell nanoparticles are promising agents for plasmonic photothermal therapy. The local temperature increase caused by irradiation of the core/shell nanoparticles will also promote an increase in fluidity of the lipid membrane of liposomes, which enhances drug release.

4. Conclusions

In this work, liposomes containing magnetic/plasmonic nanoparticles with manganese ferrite core and a gold shell were prepared. The multifunctional liposomes obtained, with sizes around or below 150 nm, were revealed to be suitable nanocarriers for an anticancer drug (a thienopyridine derivative), exhibiting high encapsulation efficiencies. Drug-loaded aqueous magnetoliposomes (with the nanoparticles entrapped in liposomes) were able to interact with model membranes by fusion. The solid magnetoliposomes (where the core/shell nanoparticles are covered by a lipid bilayer) have shown the ability to be used in photothermia applications. Therefore, the multifunctional liposomes containing $MnFe_2O_4$/Au core/shell nanoparticles were found to be promising agents for combined chemo/phototherapy.

Author Contributions: E.M.S.C. and P.J.G.C. conceived and designed the experiments. A.R.O.R., J.O.G.M., and A.M.N.D. performed the synthesis and structural characterization of magnetic/plasmonic nanoparticles, liposomes, and magnetoliposomes, and the photo physical studies. P.J.G.C. supervised the structural characterization and analysis of the results. A.P., A.M.P., and J.P.A. performed the experimental magnetic measurements. B.G.A. and A.M.P. performed the analysis of the magnetic properties and the corresponding discussion. M.J.R.P.Q. synthesized the anti-tumor compound and contributed to the interpretation of the results. E.M.S.C. supervised the photo physical measurements and the interpretation of the results. A.R.O.R. and E.M.S.C. participated in the draft of the manuscript. P.J.G.C. wrote the final manuscript. All the authors revised and approved the manuscript.

Acknowledgments: The authors acknowledge the Center for Biological Engineering (CEB) of University of Minho for the availability of DLS equipment.

References

1. Piktel, E.; Niemirowicz, K.; Watek, M.; Wollny, T.; Deptula, P.; Bucki, R. Recent insights in nanotechnology-based drugs and formulations designed for effective anti-cancer therapy. *J. Nanobiotechnol.* **2016**, *14*, 1–33. [CrossRef] [PubMed]

2. Su, C.W.; Chiang, C.S.; Li, W.M.; Hu, S.H.; Chen, S.Y. Multifunctional nanocarriers for simultaneous encapsulation of hydrophobic and hydrophilic drugs in cancer treatment. *Nanomedicine* **2014**, *9*, 1499–1515. [CrossRef] [PubMed]

3. Zeng, H.; Sun, S. Synthesis, Properties, and Potential Applications of Multicomponent Magnetic Nanoparticles. *Adv. Funct. Mater.* **2008**, *18*, 391–400. [CrossRef]

4. Silva, S.M.; Tavallaie, R.; Sandiford, L.; Tilley, R.D.; Gooding, J.J. Gold coated magnetic nanoparticles: From preparation to surface modification for analytical and biomedical applications. *Chem. Commun.* **2016**, *52*, 7528–7540. [CrossRef] [PubMed]

5. Stafford, S.; Garcia, R.S.; Gun'ku, Y.K. Multimodal Magnetic-Plasmonic Nanoparticles for Biomedical Applications. *Appl. Sci.* **2018**, *8*, 97. [CrossRef]

6. Espinosa, A.; Di Corato, R.; Kolosnjaj-Tabi, J.; Flaud, P.; Pellegrino, T.; Wilhelm, C. Duality of Iron Oxide Nanoparticles in Cancer Therapy: Amplification of Heating Efficiency by Magnetic Hyperthermia and Photothermal Bimodal Treatment. *ACS Nano* **2016**, *10*, 2436–2446. [CrossRef] [PubMed]

7. Huang, L.; Ao, L.; Hu, D.; Wang, W.; Shend, Z.; Su, W. Magneto-Plasmonic Nanocapsules for Multimodal-Imaging and Magnetically Guided Combination Cancer Therapy. *Chem. Mater.* **2016**, *28*, 5896–5904. [CrossRef]

8. Felton, C.; Karmakar, A.; Gartia, Y.; Ramidi, P.; Biris, A.S.; Gosh, A. Magnetic nanoparticles as contrast agents in biomedical imaging: Recent advances in iron- and manganese-based magnetic nanoparticles. *Drug Metab. Rev.* **2014**, *46*, 142–154. [CrossRef]

9. Ahmas, A.; Bae, H.; Rhee, I. Highly stable silica-coated manganese ferrite nanoparticles as high-efficacy T2 contrast agents for magnetic resonance imaging. *AIP Adv.* **2018**, *8*, 55019–55028. [CrossRef]

10. Kerker, M. *The Scattering of Light and Other Electromagnetic Radiation*, 1st ed.; Academic Press: New York, NY, USA, 1969; pp. 27–96. ISBN 978-0-12-404550-7.

11. Papavassiliou, C.G. Optical properties of small inorganic and organic metal particles. *Prog. Solid State Chem.* **1979**, *12*, 185–271. [CrossRef]

12. Bohren, C.F.; Huffman, D.R. *Absorption and Scattering of Light by Small Particles*, 1st ed.; Wiley-VCH: Weinheim, Germany, 1998; pp. 286–324. ISBN 978-0-47-129340-8.

13. Kreibig, U.; Vollmer, M. *Optical Properties of Metal Clusters*, 1st ed.; Springer: Heidelberg, Germany, 1995; pp. 30–68. ISBN 978-3-642-08191-0.

14. Ozbay, E. Plasmonics: Merging photonics and electronics at nanoscale dimensions. *Science* **2006**, *13*, 189–193. [CrossRef] [PubMed]

15. Noguez, C. Surface Plasmons on Metal Nanoparticles: The Influence of Shape and Physical Environment. *J. Phys. Chem. C* **2007**, *111*, 3806–3819. [CrossRef]

16. Huang, X.; Jain, P.K.; El-Sayed, I.; El-Sayed, M.A. Plasmonic photothermal therapy (PPTT) using gold nanoparticles. *Lasers Med. Sci.* **2008**, *23*, 217–228. [CrossRef] [PubMed]

17. Govorov, A.O.; Richardson, H.H. Generating Heat with Metal Nanoparticles. *Nano Today* **2007**, *2*, 30–38. [CrossRef]

18. Keblinski, P.; Cahill, D.G.; Bodapati, A.; Sullivan, C.R.; Taton, T.A. Limits of Localized Heating by Eletromagnetically Excited Nanoparticles. *J. Appl. Phys.* **2006**, *100*, 54301–54305. [CrossRef]

19. Elsherbini, A.A.M.; Saber, M.; Aggag, M.; El-Shahawy, A.; Shokier, H.A.A. Laser and radiofrequency-induced hyperthermia. *Int. J. Nanomed.* **2011**, *6*, 2155–2165. [CrossRef] [PubMed]

20. Kim, C.; Favazza, C.; Wang, L.V. In Vivo Photoacoustic Tomography of Chemicals: High-Resolution Functional and Molecular Optical Imaging at New Depths. *Chem. Rev.* **2010**, *110*, 2756–2782. [CrossRef]

21. Perez-Lorenzo, M.; Vaz, B.; Salgueirin, V.; Correa-Duarte, M.A. Hollow-Shelled Nanoreactors Endowed with High Catalytic Activity. *Chem. Eur. J.* **2013**, *19*, 12196–12211. [CrossRef]

22. He, Q.; Guo, S.; Qian, Z.; Chen, X. Development of Individualized Anti-Metastasis Strategies by Engineering Nanomedicines. *Chem. Soc. Rev.* **2015**, *44*, 6258–6286. [CrossRef]

23. Li, Z.; Yi, S.; Cheng, L.; Yang, K.; Li, Y.; Liu, Z. Magnetic Targeting Enhanced Theranostic Strategy Based on Multimodal Imaging for Selective Ablation of Cancer. *Adv. Funct. Mater.* **2014**, *24*, 2312–2321. [CrossRef]

24. Larsen, G.K.; Farr, W.; Murph, S.E.H. Multifunctional Fe$_2$O$_3$-Au Nanoparticles with different shapes: Enhanced catalysis, photothermal effects, and magnetic recyclability. *J. Phys. Chem. C* **2016**, *120*, 15162–15172. [CrossRef]

25. Sood, A.; Arora, V.; Shah, J.; Kotnala, R.K.; Jain, T.K. Multifunctional gold coated iron oxide core-shell nanoparticles stabilizedusing thiolated sodium alginate for biomedical applications. *Mater. Sci. Eng. C* **2017**, *80*, 274–281. [CrossRef] [PubMed]

26. Rodrigues, A.R.O.; Ramos, J.M.F.; Gomes, I.T.; Almeida, B.G.; Araújo, J.P.; Queiroz, M.-J.R.P.; Coutinho, P.J.G.; Castanheira, E.M.S. Magnetoliposomes based on manganese ferrite nanoparticles as nanocarriers for anti-tumor drugs. *RSC Adv.* **2016**, *6*, 17302–17313. [CrossRef]

27. Pereira, C.; Pereira, A.M.; Fernandes, C.; Rocha, M.; Mendes, R.; Garcia, M.P.F.; Guedes, A.; Tavares, P.B.; Grenèche, J.-M.; Araújo, J.P.; et al. Superparamagnetic MFe$_2$O$_4$ (M = Fe, Co, Mn) Nanoparticles: Tuning the Particle Size and Magnetic Properties through a Novel One-Step Coprecipitation Route. *Chem. Mater.* **2012**, *24*, 1496–1504. [CrossRef]

28. Queiroz, M.-J.R.P.; Calhelha, R.C.; Vale-Silva, L.; Pinto, E.; Nascimento, M.S.-J. Novel [6-(hetero)arylamino]thieno[3,2-*b*]pyridines: Synthesis and anti-tumoral activities. *Eur. J. Med. Chem.* **2010**, *45*, 5732–5738. [CrossRef] [PubMed]

29. Kremer, J.M.H.; Esker, M.W.J.V.D.; Pathmamanoharan, C.; Wiersema, P.H. Vesicles of variable diameter prepared by a modified injection method. *Biochemistry* **1977**, *16*, 3932–3935. [CrossRef] [PubMed]

30. Rodrigues, A.R.O.; Gomes, I.T.; Almeida, B.G.; Araújo, J.P.; Castanheira, E.M.S.; Coutinho, P.J.G. Magnetoliposomes based on nickel ferrite nanoparticles for biomedical applications. *Phys. Chem. Chem. Phys.* **2015**, *17*, 18011–18021. [CrossRef]

31. Tamba, Y.; Terashima, H.; Yamazaki, M. A membrane filtering method for the purification of giant unilamellar vesicles. *Chem. Phys. Lipids* **2011**, *164*, 351–358. [CrossRef]

32. Tanaka, T.; Tamba, Y.; Masum, S.M.; Yamashita, Y.; Yamazaki, M. La^{3+} and Gd^{3+} induce shape change of giant unilamellar vesicles of phosphatidylcholine. *Biochim. Biophys. Acta* **2002**, *1564*, 173–182. [CrossRef]

33. Valeur, B. *Molecular Fluorescence—Principles and Applications*, 1st ed.; Wiley-VCH: Weinheim, Germany, 2001; pp. 247–261. ISBN 3-527-29919-X.

34. Demas, J.N.; Crosby, G.A. The measurement of photoluminescence quantum yields—Review. *J. Phys. Chem.* **1971**, *75*, 991–1024. [CrossRef]

35. Fery-Forgues, S.; Lavabre, D. Are fluorescence quantum yields so tricky to measure? A demonstration using familiar stationery products. *J. Chem. Educ.* **1999**, *76*, 1260–1264. [CrossRef]

36. Johnson, I.; Spence, M.T.Z. *Molecular Probes Handbook: A Guide to Fluorescent Probes and Labeling Technologies*, 11th ed.; Life Technologies: Carlsbad, CA, USA, 2010; pp. 545–587. ISBN 978-0982927915.

37. Wagner, T.; Eglinger, J. Thorstenwagner/Ij-Particlesizer: v1.0.9 Snapshot Release (Version v1.0.9-SNAPSHOT). Zenodo: Genève, Switzerland, June 2017. [CrossRef]

38. Kimling, J.; Maier, M.; Okenve, B.; Kotaidis, V.; Ballot, H.; Plech, A. Turkevich method for gold nanoparticle synthesis revisited. *J. Phys. Chem. B* **2006**, *110*, 15700–15707. [CrossRef] [PubMed]

39. Wu, D.; Xu, X.; Liu, X. Influence of dielectric core, embedding medium and size on the optical properties of gold nanoshells. *Solid State Commun.* **2008**, *146*, 7–11. [CrossRef]

40. Qian, X.; Bai, J. Theoretical Studies of the Optical Properties of Hollow Spherical Metallic Nanoshells. *J. Comput. Theor. Nanosci.* **2013**, *10*, 2354–2360. [CrossRef]

41. Xu, Z.; Hou, Y.; Sun, S. Magnetic Core/Shell Fe_3O_4/Au and Fe_3O_4/Au/Ag Nanoparticles with Tunable Plasmonic Properties. *J. Am. Chem. Soc.* **2007**, *129*, 8698–8699. [CrossRef] [PubMed]

42. Rodriguez-Carvajal, J. Recent advances in magnetic structure determination by neutron powder diffraction. *Phys. B* **1993**, *192*, 55–69. [CrossRef]

43. Pitschke, W.; Hermann, H.; Mattern, N. The influence of surface roughness on diffracted X-ray intensities in Bragg–Brentano geometry and its effect on the structure determination by means of Rietveld analysis. *Powder Diffr.* **1993**, *8*, 74–83. [CrossRef]

44. Chen, J.P.; Sorensen, C.M.; Klabunde, K.J.; Hadjipanayis, G.C.; Devlin, E.; Kostikas, A. Size-dependent magnetic properties of $MnFe_2O_4$ fine particles synthesized by coprecipitation. *Phys. Rev. B* **1996**, *54*, 9288–9296. [CrossRef]

45. Yeh, J.-W.; Chang, S.-Y.; Hong, Y.-D.; Chen, S.-K.; Lin, S.-J. Anomalous decrease in X-ray diffraction intensities of Cu-Ni-Al-Co-Cr-Fe-Si alloy systems with multi-principal elements. *Mat. Chem. Phys.* **2007**, *103*, 41–46. [CrossRef]

46. Neder, R.B.; Korsunskiy, V.I.; Chory, C.; Müller, G.; Hofmann, A.; Dembski, S.; Graf, C.; Rühl, E. Structural characterization of II-VI semiconductor nanoparticles. *Phys. Status Solidi C* **2007**, *4*, 3221–3233. [CrossRef]

47. Rafique, M.Y.; Li-Qing, P.; Javed, Q.; Iqbal, M.Z.; Hong-Mei, Q.; Farooq, M.H.; Zhen-Gang, G.; Tanveer, M. Growth of monodisperse nanospheres of $MnFe_2O_4$ with enhanced magnetic and optical properties. *Chin. Phys. B* **2013**, *22*, 107101–107107. [CrossRef]

48. Huang, J.-R.; Cheng, C. Cation and magnetic orders in $MnFe_2O_4$ from density functional calculations. *J. Appl. Phys.* **2013**, *113*, 33912–33918. [CrossRef]

49. Smit, J. *Magnetic Properties of Materials*; McGraw Hill: New York, NY, USA, 1971; p. 89. ISBN 978-0070584457.

50. Costa, C.N.C.; Hortelão, A.C.L.; Ramos, J.M.F.; Oliveira, A.D.S.; Calhelha, R.C.; Queiroz, M.-J.R.P.; Coutinho, P.J.G.; Castanheira, E.M.S. A new anti-tumoral heteroarylaminothieno[3,2-*b*]pyridine derivative: Its incorporation into liposomes and interaction with proteins monitored by fluorescence. *Photochem. Photobiol. Sci.* **2014**, *13*, 1730–1740. [CrossRef] [PubMed]

51. Sawant, R.R.; Torchilin, V.P. Challenges in development of targeted liposomal therapeutics. *AAPS J.* **2012**, *14*, 303–315. [CrossRef]

52. Greenspan, P.; Mayer, E.P.; Fowler, S.D. Nile red: A selective fluorescent stain for intracellular lipid droplets. *J. Cell Biol.* **1985**, *100*, 965–973. [CrossRef]

53. Coutinho, P.J.G.; Castanheira, E.M.S.; Rei, M.C.; Real Oliveira, M.E.C.D. Nile Red and DCM fluorescence anisotropy studies in $C_{12}E_7$/DPPC mixed systems. *J. Phys. Chem. B* **2002**, *106*, 12841–12846. [CrossRef]

54. Feitosa, E.; Alves, F.R.; Niemiec, A.; Oliveira, M.E.C.D.R.; Castanheira, E.M.S.; Baptista, A.L.F. Cationic liposomes in mixed didodecyldimethylammonium bromide and dioctadecyldimethylammonium bromide aqueous dispersions studied by differential scanning calorimetry, Nile Red fluorescence, and turbidity. *Langmuir* **2006**, *22*, 3579–3585. [CrossRef]

55. Rodrigues, A.R.O.; Gomes, I.T.; Almeida, B.G.; Araújo, J.P.; Castanheira, E.M.S.; Coutinho, P.J.G. Magnetoliposomes based on nickel/silica core/shell nanoparticles: Synthesis and characterization. *Mater. Chem. Phys.* **2014**, *148*, 978–987. [CrossRef]

56. Rodrigues, A.R.O.; Mendes, P.M.F.; Silva, P.M.L.; Machado, V.A.; Almeida, B.G.; Araújo, J.P.; Queiroz, M.J.R.P.; Castanheira, E.M.S.; Coutinho, P.J.G. Solid and aqueous magnetoliposomes as nanocarriers for a new potential drug active against breast cancer. *Colloids Surf. B Biointerfaces* **2017**, *158*, 460–468. [CrossRef]

57. Curtis, H.; Barnes, N.S. *Biology*, 5th ed.; Worth Publishers: New York, NY, USA, 1989; Part 1; ISBN 978-0879013943.

58. Huang, X.; Jain, P.K.; El-Sayed, I.H.; El-Sayed, M.A. Determination of the minimum temperature required for selective photothermal destruction of cancer cells with the use of immunotargeted gold nanoparticles. *Photochem. Photobiol.* **2006**, *82*, 412–417. [CrossRef]

Systemic Administration of Polyelectrolyte Microcapsules: Where Do They Accumulate and When? In Vivo and Ex Vivo Study

Nikita A. Navolokin [1,2], Sergei V. German [1,3], Alla B. Bucharskaya [2], Olga S. Godage [2], Viktor V. Zuev [2], Galina N. Maslyakova [1,2], Nikolaiy A. Pyataev [4], Pavel S. Zamyshliaev [4], Mikhail N. Zharkov [4], Georgy S. Terentyuk [1,2], Dmitry A. Gorin [1,3] and Gleb B. Sukhorukov [1,5,*]

[1] Remote Controlled Theranostic Systems Lab, Saratov State University, Saratov 410012, Russia; nik-navolokin@yandex.ru (N.A.N.); gsv0709@mail.ru (S.V.G.); gmaslyakova@yandex.ru (G.N.M.); vetklinikanew@mail.ru (G.S.T.); gorinda@mail.ru (D.A.G.)

[2] Scientific Research Institute of Fundamental and Clinical Uronephrology, Saratov Medical State University, Saratov 410000, Russia; allaalla_72@mail.ru (A.B.B.); olgabess@yandex.ru (O.S.G.); zuev.viktor.sgmu@gmail.com (V.V.Z.)

[3] Biophotonics Laboratory, Skoltech Center for Photonics and Quantum Materials, Skolkovo Institute of Science and Technology, Moscow 121205, Russia

[4] Laboratory of Pharmacokinetics and Targeted Drug Delivery, Medicine Institute, National Research Ogarev Mordovia State University, Saransk 430005, Russia; pyataevna@mail.ru (N.A.P.); zamyshlyaev@gmail.com (P.S.Z.); mikhail.zharkov.92@mail.ru (M.N.Z.)

[5] School of Engineering and Materials Science, Queen Mary University of London, London E1 4NS, UK

[*] Correspondence: g.sukhorukov@qmul.ac.uk;

Abstract: Multilayer capsules of 4 microns in size made of biodegradable polymers and iron oxide magnetite nanoparticles have been injected intravenously into rats. The time-dependent microcapsule distribution in organs was investigated in vivo by magnetic resonance imaging (MRI) and ex vivo by histological examination (HE), atomic absorption spectroscopy (AAS) and electron spin resonance (ESR), as these methods provide information at different stages of microcapsule degradation. The following organs were collected: Kidney, liver, lung, and spleen through 15 min, 1 h, 4 h, 24 h, 14 days, and 30 days after intravenous injections (IVIs) of microcapsules in a saline buffer at a dosage of 2.5×10^9 capsule per kg. The IVI of microcapsules resulted in reversible morphological changes in most of the examined inner organs (kidney, heart, liver, and spleen). The capsules lost their integrity due to degradation over 24 h, and some traces of iron oxide nanoparticles were seen at 7 days in spleen and liver structure. The morphological structure of the tissues was completely restored one month after IVI of microcapsules. Comprehensive analysis of the biodistribution and degradation of entire capsules and magnetite nanoparticles as their components gave us grounds to recommend these composite microcapsules as useful and safe tools for drug delivery applications.

Keywords: polymer microcapsules; magnetite nanoparticles; biodistribution; magnetic resonance imaging; electron spin resonance spectroscopy; histological examination; atomic absorption spectroscopy; intravenous injections

1. Introduction

Novel drug delivery systems have been in the focus of research in bio-nanotechnology in the past decades. Substantial progress in biomedicine and applied chemistry resulted in the development of reasonably effective delivery systems aimed to bring bioactive compounds via chemical targeting to a particular site of the body, organs and tissues. The major demand in the area is how to direct the vesicles to the tumor site, which remains challenging due to side effects. Most of the elaborated delivery systems are "passive" in terms of external navigation and control over their delivery. Recent developments in nanobiotechnology have made an essential contribution, as they deal with fabrication of constructs enabling multimodal functioning, carrying bioactive molecules and being visible and addressable externally. Logically, if a delivery system represents a sort of vesicle in order to make it visible and addressable, these vesicles should also incorporate nanoparticles such as magnetite nanoparticles, which can be seen by full-body imaging techniques such as magnetic resonance imaging (MRI).

Among the technologies available so far for drug delivery, in general, there are a limited number of techniques enabling multifunctionality. Multifunctionality in this particular context is the combination of the following: Ability to carry bioactive substances, navigate to a specific site, be biodegradable after deploying the cargo, and susceptible to external activation and visualization. Obviously, the components of these multifunctional delivery systems should be responsive to local media or external stimuli. Use of externally guided nanostructured carriers for drug delivery is a promising method in bio-nanotechnology, which can be used in areas such as diagnostics of tumors [1,2] for enhanced contrast at MRI visualization [3,4], targeted delivery of drugs to specific organs and tissues [5–7] and for magnetic hyperthermia of tumors [8–10]. This research has been undertaken to illustrate the promise of addressed delivery to particular sites in the body with the help of magnetic nanoparticles externally navigated with a magnetic field [11], which might also work as an accomplishing method with biological targeting performed by conjugation of nanoparticles with tumor-specific antibodies, followed by accumulation of nanoparticles in the targets [12].

In light of the development of multifunctional delivery systems more than a decade ago, the principles of layer-by-layer (lbl) assembly were applied to construct micron and submicron sized delivery systems, where various components can be simply tailored via incorporation of responsive and charge species as shell components of the capsules [13].

These capsules, proposed as delivery systems a while ago, were intensively studied mostly for their physical and chemical properties. At present, these capsules can be made of a defined size in a range from about 100 nm to several microns, contain various bioactive molecules including proteins, nucleic acids as well as small molecules, and can be externally addressed via a magnetic field, light or ultrasound [14,15]. These capsules can be taken up by various cells types, including endothelial cells, mesenchymal stem cells, microphages, neuroblastoma and others [16–18]. The mechanism of cell uptake is relevant to endocytosis and, as most reports have demonstrated, there is a minimal or absent effect on cell viability. Various cell types showed high percentages of survival at an excess of capsules per cell ratio. Capsule degradation inside the cells varied from a few to up to 24 h, depending on the cell type and capsule composition. The release of encapsulated materials inside the cells can be gradual or triggered externally if light is used to open the capsules while inside the cells and releases the cargo to cytoplasm [19–23].

Despite the intense study on capsule properties and their interaction with cells, there is a lack of reported data on how the capsules would behave if administered systemically in vivo. So far, there have been few reports on lbl capsules administered in vivo either via subcutaneous injection or nasal gavage [24–27]. There are attempts for MRI imaging of iron oxide modified capsules. However, there are no systematic studies of lbl capsule distribution in organs or at what time point they are accumulated in a particular part of the body once they are introduced systemically.

The aim of this study was to examine capsule distribution in vivo upon systemic delivery via the tail and to explore major organs, such as the liver, lung, heart, spleen, and kidney for capsule presence at different time points in rats. Particular attention was given to evaluating for how long the capsules and debris of capsule degradation were present in these organs and what their degradation times were. A detailed analysis of capsule fate in vivo is very complex and requires various methods for the unambiguous identification of capsules and their components. In order to facilitate capsule identification, capsules were made of biodegradable polymers to ensure their degradation was modified with magnetite nanoparticles sandwiched between the layers. Complex analysis was conducted in vivo using MRI visualization and on ex vivo samples using atomic absorption spectroscopy (AAS), electron spin resonance (ESR) for detection of iron as an element and as superparamagnetic nanoparticles, respectively, and direct histology visualization of selected organs.

2. Materials and Methods

2.1. Magnetic Microcapsule Preparation

Magnetic microcapsules were prepared using the layer-by-layer technique [28]. Poly-L-arginine hydrochloride (Parg, MW ~70 kDa), dextran sulfate sodium salt (Dex, MW ~70 kDa), and sodium chloride (anhydrous) were used without further purification and were purchased from Sigma-Aldrich GmbH, Germany. The water used in all experiments was prepared in a UVOI-1M purification system (Mediana-filter, Moscow, Russia) and had a resistivity higher than 14 MΩ•cm.

The following materials were used for the microcapsule preparation: $CaCO_3$ microparticles (diameter, 4 ± 0.7 μm), poly-L-arginine and dextran sulfate sodium salt diluted in 0.15 M NaCl water solution; magnetite hydrosol (diameter, 13 ± 5 nm and zeta potential, -31 ± 9 mV measured by the DLS method) (Figure S1). In this work, the method described previously by Massart was used for iron oxide nanoparticle synthesis [29]. Synthesis was carried out using the setup described in reference [30].

The nanocomposite polyelectrolyte shells were formed on the surface of calcium carbonate microparticles. Polyelectrolyte shells were prepared by lbl assembly technique via alternate treating microparticles in solutions of oppositely charged polyelectrolytes and nanoparticles. These were poly-L-arginine (Parg), dextran sulfate sodium salt (Dex) and magnetite nanoparticles (MNPs). The consecutive adsorption of Parg and MNPs was repeated three times and finally, the capsules had the following composition: Parg/Dex/(Parg/MNPs)₃/Parg/Dex (Figure 1a). The microcapsule with each freshly deposited layer was washed two times with deionized water before starting the next deposition step. Optical and transmission electron microscopy (TEM) images of magnetic microcapsules are presented in Figure 1b. The concentration of the microcapsules was determined using a hemocytometer and it was of the order of 5×10^8 mL^{-1}.

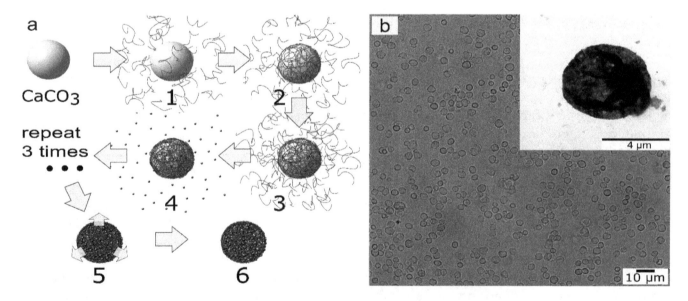

Figure 1. (a) Scheme of microcapsule preparation: 1, 3–adsorption of Parg, 2–adsorption of Dex, 4–adsorption of magnetite nanoparticles (MNP)s, 5–dissolution of core, 6–magnetic polyelectrolite microcapsule. (b) Optical and transmission electron microscopy (TEM) (inset figure) images of biodegradable microcapsules containing magnetite MNPs.

The polyelectrolyte composites containing this type of magnetite nanoparticles exhibit the superparamagnetic behavior which was shown on the planar polyelectrolyte composite coatings. [31].

Variation of the volume fraction of inorganic nanoparticles led us to control the physical properties of microcapsule shells as well as MRI contrast. Contrast enhancement of magnetic microcapsules increases with increasing average distance between magnetite nanoparticles in the shell [32]. In agreement with the analyses of some already published articles, we can conclude that size stability of such type of microcapsule in vitro is very high [33].

2.2. Dynamic Light Scattering, Atomic Force Microscopy, and Transmission Electron Microscopy

The measurements of the zeta-potential and size distribution of nanoparticles were performed using a Zetasizer Nano-ZS instrument (Malvern Instruments Ltd., Malvern, UK).

Atomic force microscopy (AFM) images of microcapsules were obtained with a Ntegra Spectra microscope (NT-MDT, Zelenograd, Moscow, Russia) in tapping mode. For image acquisition, NSG10 probes from NT-MDT with a resonant frequency of about 220 kHz, a force constant of 3.1–37.6 N/m and a tip curvature below 10 nm were used. Samples were prepared by drying a drop of the microcapsule suspension on the cover glass slide surface. All image processing was done with Gwyddion software [34].

Transmission electron microscopy (TEM) images were obtained using a Libra-120 transmission electron microscope (Carl Zeiss, Jena, Germany) operating at 120 kV. The samples were prepared by deposition of a capsule suspension onto a formvar film supported by the copper grid.

2.3. Animal Study. Ex Vivo Organ Preparation

Animal experiments were performed in accordance with the University's Animal Ethics Committee and the relevant international agency [35] in Core Facilities of Saratov State Medical University. In experiments, 42 white outbred male rats weighing 200 ± 20 g were used. Thirty-six rats were intravenously injected with a single dose of a microcapsule suspension dispersed in physiological saline at 2.5×10^9 capsules per kg. Then, the animals were randomly divided into 6 groups of 6 rats in each group; the control group consisted of 6 rats. The duration of the experiment was different in different groups; i.e., the lifetime of the animals after administration of the microcapsules was 15 min, 1 h, 4 h, 24 h, 7 days and 30 days. These time intervals were chosen as they are most frequently used for the biodistribution study [36].

An MRI study was performed and after that, the animals were decapitated. The following organs were collected: Kidney, liver, lung, and spleen at the indicated time points after microcapsule administration. The time dependence of microcapsule and iron distribution inside the rats was investigated by histological examination, AAS and ESR.

2.4. Magnetic Resonance Imaging

Magnetic resonance imaging in vivo was performed using a Philips Achieva 1.5T high field MRI scanner with a phased array coil. Immobilization of animals was carried out for 60 min in the supine position with the fixation of the limbs. Zoletil 50 (Virbac, France) was administered intramuscularly at a dose of 40 μg/kg for anesthesia. T1 and T2-weighted quick "Spin Echo" protocols (Turbo Spin Echo–TSE), and T1-weighted "Fast Field Echo" (is equal to the "Gradient Echo") were used. The presence of contrast agents in the test object which mainly reduces the longitudinal relaxation time T1 (substances containing gadolinium, for example, gadobutrol [37]), in the tissue causes a hyperintense signal on T1-weighted images (lighter staining). Contrast agents which mainly reduce the transverse relaxation time T2 (iron oxides) cause a hypointense signal on T2-weighted images. After in vivo MRI study, the animals were decapitated.

2.5. Histological Examination

The sampling of internal organs (spleen, liver, kidneys, lungs, and heart) for morphological studies and determination of microcapsule accumulation were conducted after removing the animals from the experiment. Samples of internal organs were fixed in a 10% solution of buffered neutral formalin for morphological examination and subjected to standard wiring alcohol. The standard histological techniques with hematoxylin and eosin staining were used.

The capsules were counted in 10 fields of vision in each section of organ, but not less than in 3 sections, with an increase of 774 on Microvizor medical of transmitted light mVizo-103 (LOMO, St. Petersburg, Russia). The standard magnification allows one to obtain more objective data and to compare them, so it will be possible to study the dynamics of microcapsule movement and determine the time points for the accumulation of microcapsules in the organs.

2.6. Atomic Absorption Spectrometry

A Thermo Scientific iCE 3500 instrument (Thermo Scientific, Bartlesville, OK, USA) was used for the quantitative determination of iron in the tumor. The operating principle of the method is based on the transfer of elements defined in the atomic state. Fiery atomizer was used in the work. The element concentration was determined by the intensity of the light absorption with the characteristic wavelength of atomic vapor of the element. The wavelength was 248.3 nm for Fe, the slit width was 0.2 nm, and the lamp current was 75%. A hollow cathode lamp was used as the light source. A standard sample of metal ions (GSO 7330-96, Saint Petersburg, Russia) was used for the calibration of the spectrometer.

2.7. Quantitative Magnetite Content Analysis via Electron Spin Resonance (ESR) Spectroscopy

In order to evaluate microcapsules presence in organs, a quantitative magnetite content analysis of ex vivo samples was performed using the ESR method according to the procedure described by Chertok et al. [38] with modification given below in this section.

The modified procedure of ESR spectroscopy in this study is based on the recording of ferromagnetic resonance spectra reflecting the magnetite content in a specimen. The paramagnetic peaks of the ionized iron become totally smooth and really cannot influence the intensity and other characteristics of the signal. Thus, the endogenous iron does not interfere with determination of ferromagnetic capsules. Furthermore, the constant distribution of magnetite over the capsules and the uniform environment for the incorporated magnetite (the polyelectrolytes surrounding the magnetite) guarantee that the resonance field and the spectrum forms are not different for any specimens containing microcapsules. This makes it possible to calibrate the spectrometer with in vitro specimens of a microcapsules suspension and to measure the microcapsule and magnetite content in ex vivo specimens without further corrections, including the control correction.

Before ESR analysis, pieces of extracted organs weighing 150–200 mg were dried in a vacuum oven and fixed to the quartz rod. After that, they were inserted into a recording unit (block) of the ESR spectrometer (The scheme is shown in Supporting Information (Figure S3)).

ESR spectra were obtained using a CMS 8400 X-band ESR spectrometer (Adani, Belarus) with the following parameters: Resonant frequency, ~9.2 GHz; center field, 3100 G; sweep width, 3400 G; modulation amplitude, 1 G.

In our studies, the ESR method originally proposed in the paper [38] has been modified: ESR spectra were recorded in dry samples at room temperature (21 °C) in contrast to low-temperature (−128 °C) measurements in frozen samples used by Chertok et al. This modification makes the recording easier to use without significant loss of accuracy. The obtained calibration curve for the contain/signal relationship have proved the relation to be linear in the investigated concentration range (from 0.5 to 20 μg of magnetite per sample) for dry capsules. The calibration curve is given in SI (Figure S4).

Spectra were recorded as the first derivative of absorbed microwave power (P) versus the applied magnetic field (B) and are given as (dP/dB). The double integral of the collected spectra ($\int\int$(dP/dB)dBdB) is known to be proportional to the number of resonating electronic spins in a measured sample. Double integral values were obtained from spectra using the EPRCMD 4.0 program (Adani, Minsk, Belarus).

The concentration of magnetite in the samples was obtained with the help of a calibration curve, which was made using samples with the known content of magnetite in form of a dried suspension of magnetite microcapsules of known concentration. The samples were dried in vacuum at ESR-neutral substrate and then investigated by the procedure mentioned above.

Control experiments, conducted with blood and tissue samples without any magnetite in the system, showed no ferromagnetic signal; therefore, the background correction was negligible and was not taken into account (Figure S5). It should be noted that the addition of blood and organ homogenates to the calibration samples does not alter the shape of the spectra (Figure S6) and the resonance field. This fact underpins the possibility of application of the ESR method to the quantitative analysis of magnetite microcapsules in ex vivo samples.

3. Results

3.1. In Vivo MRI Study of Intravenously Injected Capsules

Initial assessment of capsule distribution was done by MRI. Magnetite nanoparticles mainly reduce the transverse relaxation time T2 and cause the darker staining of corresponding marked tissue areas on T2-weighted images (Figure 2). The microcapsules with magnetite NPs in the shell do not enhance contrast in the region of interest ROI compared to magnetite hydrosol in the same concentration, but upon enzyme degradation liberated nanoparticles enhance contrast in magnetic resonance (MR) images (Figure 2, Figure S2).

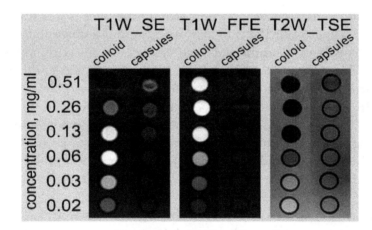

Figure 2. The MRI contrast of the magnetite colloid and magnetic microcapsules at a different concentrations of magnetite in the probe tubes. Different pulse sequences are presented from left to right: T1 weighted "Spin-echo" (T1W_SE), T1 weighted "Fast Field Echo" (T1W_FFE), and T2 weighted "Turbo Spin Echo" (T2W_TSE).

Figure 3 shows the T1 and T2 weighted MR images of rats obtained 24 h after injection of microcapsules containing magnetite nanoparticles. Solid orange lines indicate liver in a rat after microcapsule injection. Dotted orange lines indicate liver in a control rat. Magnetite distributed in liver leads to a decrease in the MR signal intensity in the region of interest (ROI) in the T1 weighted MR images (Figure 3a). This can be explained by the fact that the concentration of magnetite in the ROI was higher than 0.4 mg/mL. At high concentrations of magnetite nanoparticles, the effect of the T2 relaxation process on the measured MR signal intensity was higher than the effect of the T1 relaxation process. This leads to a decrease in the MR signal intensity in the T1 weighted images. The T2 relaxation time affects the MR signal intensity in the T1 weighted images because in clinical MRI the images are weighted by T1 and T2 but not calculated from only T1 or T2 relaxation times. Pure T1 and T2 images are not useful in clinical MRI, because the T1 and T2 values could not be applied for differential diagnosis or characterization of pathology [39].

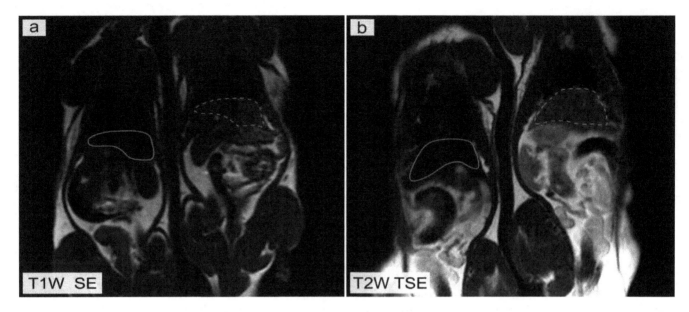

Figure 3. Magnetic resonance (MR) images of rats obtained 24 h after injection of a microcapsule suspension. (**a**) T1 weighted MR image. (**b**) T2 weighted image. The rat on the right is a control rat, without injection of microcapsules.

The average magnetite nanoparticles concentration in the liver is less than 1 mg/mL, taking into account volume of the rat's liver so artifacts in MR images are not observed.

According to MRI investigation, immediately after intravenous administration of microcapsules, the contrast of the region of interest is not observed. This fact is related to the high volume fraction of magnetite NPs in the microcapsules used. Microcapsules with a high volume fraction of magnetite NPs have no effect on the MR signal intensity, but upon enzyme degradation the liberated nanoparticles enhance contrast (Figure 2, Figure S2) [32]. It was established that the dependence of the MR signal on the volume fraction of magnetite was related to the interparticle distance (d) in the microcapsule shell (Figure S2). The further histological study demonstrated that the microcapsules were destroyed in the liver within 24 h and the realized magnetite nanoparticles exhibited contrast properties within 7 days (Figure 3).

Then, the distribution of the microcapsules in the organs was analyzed postmortem at selected time points by the three methods mentioned above: AAS, histology, and ESR. Appropriate qualitative and quantitative assay methods need to be established and be sensitive enough to detect the presence of microcapsules in cells and tissues.

3.2. Comparative Analysis of Histology Data with AAS and ESR

The time dependence of microcapsule and iron distribution inside the internal organs of rats after intravenous injection (IVI) of biodegradable microcapsules was investigated by histological examination, AAS, and ESR.

Liver. At the histologic examination the content of the microcapsules increased most 1 h after IVI, while pronounced changes were noted in the form of circulatory disorders and dystrophy of hepatocytes. Four hours after IVI, the number of whole capsules decreased, but the amount of pigment increased (Figure 4a,b). At the same time, the morphological changes in the tissue were less pronounced, although there were signs of an allergic reaction with eosinophils in the lumen of the vessels. Twenty-four hours after IVI of microcapsules, the dissolution of the capsules in the Kupffer cells was noted and the hepatocytes with the release of its contents into the cytoplasm of a cell, eosinophilia was not already marked. A week later, the content of the pigment was large, and the whole capsules were only between hepatocytes or their fragments. A month later a normalized structure of the liver was observed, and the pigment was absent. According to AAS, the maximum amount of iron in the liver was observed 1 h after IVI of microcapsules. According to ESR analysis, the dynamics of magnetite distribution had a different character. Starting at a relatively small fraction at first time point of 15 min it consistently increased over 24 h and reached a maximum at the end of the first day after administration. After a week, the concentration of magnetite in the liver dropped 7-fold lower than that at the maximum (Figure 5).

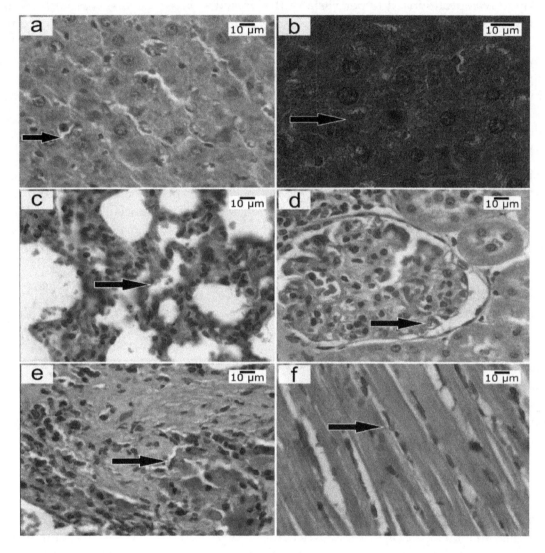

Figure 4. (a) Liver 4 h after intravenous injection (IVI) of the microcapsules—the conglomerates of the microcapsules in sinusoids. Hematoxylin and eosin (H&E), magnification 774×. **(b)** Liver 4 h after IVI of microcapsules, the conglomerates of the microcapsules were painted in blue. Prussian blue staining, magnification 1199.7×. **(c)** Lung 15 min after IVI of the microcapsules, microcapsules in capillaries of lung tissue. H&E, magnification 774×. **(d)** Kidneys 15 min after IVI of the microcapsules—the microcapsules in vascular loops of glomeruli. H&E, magnification 774×. **(e)** Spleen one day after IVI of the microcapsules—the microcapsules and magnetite were observed in spleen tissue. H&E, magnification 774×. **(f)** Heart 1 h after IVI of microcapsules—the individual microcapsules in myocardium. H&E, magnification 774×. The arrow indicates microcapsules or their clusters in the organs.

Lung. At the histological examination, the maximum changes appeared 4 h after IVI of microcapsules in the form of pronounced congestion of large vessels, focal hemorrhages, and peribronchial eosinophilic infiltration. The severity of these changes was reduced after 24 h. A large number of capsules were also noted 15 min after IVI of microcapsules in an average amount of 8.75 ± 1.03 units in the field of view in the lumen of medium caliber vessels, between the bronchi and in the stroma (Figure 4c). One week after IVI of microcapsules, the severity of the allergic reactions increased with the involvement of the bronchi and blood vessels. One month after IVI of the microcapsules, the appearance of a large number of lymphocytes in the lungs was noted, which were in the form of widespread infiltrates located around the main bronchus. Infiltrates occupied the area in several fields of view at the lowest magnification eye field. There was pronounced hyperplasia of the muscular layer of vessels of various sizes, with ring-shaped lymphoid infiltration around blood vessels of all calibers. The area of perivascular infiltration was significantly less than that around the bronchi. According to AAS, the maximum amount of iron in the lungs was observed 4 h after IVI of microcapsule suspension. According to ESR analysis in lungs, the concentration of magnetite was highest in the early stages of ex vivo analysis (between 15 min and 4 h after administration). It was significantly decreased at the time point of 24 h, and the magnetite was not determined in the lungs in the subsequent phases of observation for week and month time (Figure 5). Unfortunately, it was not confirmed by MRI, because normal lung tissue has low proton density; therefore, magnetite-containing microcapsules were not visualized in lungs by MRI in vivo.

It should also be noted that in the lungs, a marked allergic reaction was observed during all time intervals, which was manifested by the appearance of perivascular lymphoid infiltration, and further abrupt thickening of the vessel walls, as well as more pronounced hyperplasia of bronchial lymphoid tissue, which was observed one month after the intravenous administration of the capsules. The absence of marked toxicity in the internal organs after IVI of microcapsules are consistent with our data obtained earlier [32].

Spleen. At the histological examination the maximum changes occurred 4 h after IVI of microcapsules in the form of pronounced congestion, increase in the number of microcapsules (up to 9 in the field of view in the white pulp. In red pulp, up to 4). After one day, the largest accumulation of microcapsules was noted, and there were also indirect signs of their degradation (Figure 4e). An important fact is that the signs of degradation were observed at all time intervals. After one week, single capsules were observed in the white pulp, and the pigment was located diffusely. One month after, the pigment disappeared in the red pulp and it remained in the white pulp. According to AAS, the maximum amount of iron in the spleen was observed after 4 h. According to ESR, the dynamics of magnetite accumulation in the spleen was similar to that in the liver (increasing in the first day with subsequent decreasing), but after 24 h, the concentration of magnetite in the spleen was two times higher than that in the liver (Figure 5).

Kidneys. At the histological examination, the maximum changes were observed 24 h after injection in the form of hemorrhages in the cortex, dilatation of capillary loops of the glomeruli, and marked degradation of the capsules with accumulation of content in the epithelium of convoluted tubules. This does not allow us to make an unambiguous conclusion: The capsules pass through the urinary filter and their contents are reabsorbed from the urine back into the tubules or capsules entered into the epithelium through the capillaries which nourish epithelium. The maximum content of whole capsules was observed in the first time points after IVI—in 15 min and 1 h (Figure 4d). After one week, the whole capsules were not detected, but the appearance of magnetite in the epithelium of convoluted tubules was noted. After one month, a normal structure of the kidney and the absence of pigment were observed. According to AAS, the maximum amount of iron in the kidneys was observed after 15 min. According to ESR analysis in kidneys the absence of magnetite may be explained as follows: The concentration of magnetite in kidneys is lower than the limit of determination even at the time of first measurement (Figure 5).

Heart. At the histological examination the maximum changes were observed within 1 h after administration in the form of marked edema, single diapedetic hemorrhages, swelling and necrosis of cardiomyocytes. The maximum content of the capsules was up to 2–3 in the field of view (Figure 4f). Four hours after IVI of microcapsules, the severity of changes was reduced, and capsules were not detected; moderate swelling and granular degeneration were saved to the week after the introduction and after a month, the normal structure of the myocardium was seen. AAS and ERS investigations were not carried out in the heart tissue.

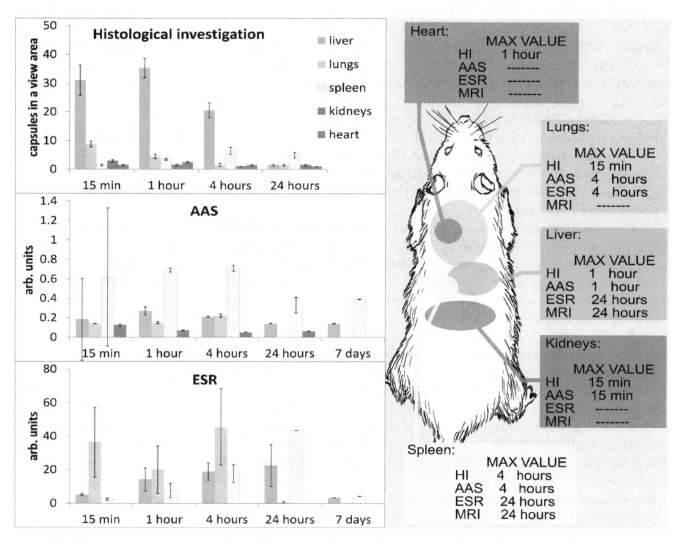

Figure 5. Biodistribution of magnetic microcapsules at intravenous injections. Left side: Microcapsule biodistribution data obtained by histological investigation, atomic absorption spectrometry (AAS) and electron spin resonance (ESR). Right side: maximum accumulation of microcapsules and MR signal for each organ observed.

4. Discussion

Since the nanocomposite microcapsules are multicomponent systems consisting of three components (cationic and anionic polyelectrolytes and inorganic nanoparticles), the components have different biodegradation times and as a result, the polymer shells are degraded more quickly than the magnetite nanoparticles. Therefore, as far as the degradation of the magnetic capsule is concerned, one should consider it as a multistep process. There is an initial state before biodegradation starts, then it is likely the polymer shell degradation occurs, releasing magnetite nanoparticles which later degrade, and iron ions could be free from the nanoparticles. Such a complex process of degradation requires different complementary methods for evaluating the biodistribution of magnetic microcapsules. Morphological methods, such as histology, allow comprehensive determination of the quantitative content of capsules in sections of internal organs, time points the capsules appear there, maximum accumulation and the delocalization of whole capsules between internal organs, and, at the end, to evaluate complete capsule destruction and elimination of their components at certain time points after intravenous administration. ESR allows evaluation of the biodistribution of magnetite nanoparticles once they are intact either in capsules or released from capsules but still intact and exhibit superparamagnetic properties. MRI makes possible the visualization of magnetite nanoparticles before and after polymer shell degradation, since these peculiarities of MRI capsule degradation imaging are discussed in detail [32]. After the beginning of capsule destruction, the morphological method ceases to be adequate for further quantification, since the capsules cannot be identified any longer. Since capsule integrity is lost, one can follow the fate of magnetite nanoparticles released from the destroyed capsules by using the MRI (in vivo) and ESR (ex vivo) methods. Both of these methods can monitor magnetite nanoparticles till their degradation, leaving only iron ions, which cannot be detected any longer by MRI and ESR. Along with that, AAS allows detection of iron element biodistribution at all stages of capsule accumulation and degradation, including monitoring of iron before and after microcapsule and nanoparticle degradation. In addition, the complexity of application of these methods makes it possible to identify more clearly the time periods of biodegradation of capsules with magnetite nanoparticles in certain organs.

Comparative analysis of microcapsule biodistribution showed that a significant correlation was observed between the temporal dynamics of microcapsule content in the liver, spleen, and kidneys, according to the histological and AAS data. At histological examination, the maximum amount of magnetite microcapsules was obtained in the kidneys and lungs at 15 min, in the liver and heart at 1 h, and in the spleen at 24 h after IVI of microcapsules. At AAS the maximum amount of magnetite microcapsules was observed in the kidneys at 15 min, in the liver at 1 h, and in the spleen and lungs at 4 h after IVI of microcapsules.

ESR analysis demonstrated the magnetite distribution dynamics in various tissues. Magnetite was found in the lungs, liver, and spleen and was not detected in the kidney at the selected time point. According to ESR analysis, the maximum of magnetite accumulation developed in the lungs after 4 h, and in the liver and spleen at 24 h after intravenous administration of capsules, Biodegradation of the capsules and the release of their content begin on the first day after administration of the capsules. Additionally, the examined organs showed no presence of magnetite 30 days after IVI of microcapsules. Although the discrepancy of the results obtained by ESR and MRI could be explained by the sensitivity of both methods to magnetite nanoparticle conditions and the integrity of the microcapsule shells. According to the histological investigation, the microcapsules were degraded within 24 h, which resulted in the different behavior of MRI and ESR signals.

The differences in the tissue distributions of magnetite and microcapsules can be explained by the action of several factors. Firstly, our study has demonstrated a significant accumulation of magnetite in the tissues with a highly developed reticuloendothelial system (liver and spleen). These data are consistent with the data from other studies [40,41], in which it was shown that nanoparticles are actively phagocytosed and accumulated in the organs with a large content of tissue macrophages.

Another factor which plays an important role in biodistribution may be the specific features of particle passage through the microcirculatory system. We assume that early-stage accumulation and the subsequent rapid decrease in the particle concentration in lungs is caused by mechanical embolization of some pulmonary capillaries with microcapsules at their first passage. The embolization is possible because the diameter of the capsules is close to the size of the pulmonary capillaries. The properties of microcirculation can also contribute to the accumulation of the microcapsules and magnetite in the liver and spleen. These organs contain open sections of the circulatory system, which makes possible the transition of the microcapsules from the blood flow to the interstitium.

5. Conclusions

In this study, we showed what happens with polyelectrolyte capsules modified with magnetic nanoparticles when they are systemically administered. The intravenous administration of microcapsules brings about changes in tissue morphology in most organs (kidney, heart, liver, spleen), but it is reversible and after a month, the structure of the tissue is completely restored.

Whole capsules were not observed demonstrating their complete degradation, and the pigment indicating iron disappeared. Although the timeline of organ localization for capsules is coherent for other delivery systems, showing at first the accumulation in liver with traces of iron oxide seen in the spleen after 7 days, the overall picture illustrates the applicability of using these capsules for systemic delivery without visible pathological observation.

The reported data gave us more understanding about the distribution of capsules in the animal body in the dynamic time frames over hours and days and provide information about what organ and when one could expect the capsules potentially bearing bioactive cargo. The polyelectrolyte microcapsules, being on the research agenda for decades, can deliver the substance of interest to organs at a certain time after injection. Thus, the long-standing potential for application of these capsules can be further explored on particular delivery to organs. The magnetic nanoparticles have not been used here as their magnetic properties, but their addressing with magnetic field and/or electromagnetic irradiation is subject for further study where the expectations of multifunctional microcapsules to be used as multimodal drug delivery systems could be fulfilled.

Author Contributions: Conception and design of study, D.A.G., G.N.M. and G.B.S.; investigation, N.A.N., S.V.G., A.B.B., O.S.G., V.V.Z., M.N.Z., G.S.T. and P.S.Z.; analysis and interpretation of the experimental data, N.A.N., S.V.G., A.B.B., V.V.Z., G.N.M., N.A.P., P.S.Z. and G.S.T.; writing the manuscript, A.B.B., S.V.G., O.S.G., P.S.Z., M.N.Z. and N.A.P.; writing and revising of the manuscript, N.A.N., G.N.M., D.A.G. and G.B.S.; supervision, G.B.S.

Acknowledgments: In this section you can acknowledge any support given which is not covered by the author contribution or funding sections. This may include administrative and technical support, or donations in kind (e.g., materials used for experiments).

References

1. Stark, D.D.; Weissleder, R.; Elizondo, G.; Hahn, P.F.; Saini, S.; Todd, L.E.; Wittenberg, J.; Ferucci, J.T. Superparamagnetic Iron Oxide: Clinical Application as A Contrast Agent for MR Imaging of the Liver. *Radiology* **1988**, *168*, 297–301. [CrossRef] [PubMed]

2. Krishnan, K.M. Biomedical Nanomagnetics: A Spin Through Possibilities in Imaging, Diagnostics, and Therapy. *IEEE Trans. Magn.* **2010**, *46*, 2523–2558. [CrossRef] [PubMed]

3. Rosen, J.E.; Chan, L.; Shieh, D.B.; Gu, F.X. Iron Oxide Nanoparticles for Targeted Cancer Imaging and Diagnostics. *Nanomed.-Nanotechnol.* **2012**, *8*, 275–290. [CrossRef] [PubMed]

4. Ito, A.; Honda, H.; Kobayasi, T. Medical Application of Functionalized Magnetic Nanoparticles. *J. Biosci. Bioeng.* **2005**, *100*, 1–11. [CrossRef] [PubMed]

5. Suzuki, M.; Honda, H.; Kobayashi, T.; Wakabayashi, T.; Yoshida, J.; Takahashi, M. Development of a Target Directed Magnetic Resonance Contrast Agent Using Monoclonal Antibody-Conjugated Magnetic Particles. *Brain Tumor Pathol.* **1996**, *13*, 127–132.

6. Gaumet, M.; Vargas, A.; Gurny, R.; Delie, F. Nanoparticles for Drug Delivery: The Need for Precision in Reporting Particle Size Parameters. *Eur. J. Pharm. Biopharm.* **2008**, *69*, 1–9. [CrossRef] [PubMed]

7. Kievit, F.M.; Zhang, M. Surface Engineering of Iron Oxide Nanoparticles for Targeted Cancer Therapy. *Acc. Chem. Res.* **2011**, *44*, 853–862. [CrossRef] [PubMed]

8. Johannsen, M.; Gneveckow, U.; Thiesen, B.; Taymoorian, K.; Cho, C.H.; Waldofner, N.; Scholz, R.; Jordan, A.; Loening, S.A.; Wust, P. Thermotherapy of Prostate Cancer Using Magnetic Nanoparticles: Feasibility, Imaging, And Three-Dimensional Temperature Distribution. *Eur. Urol.* **2007**, *52*, 1653–1661. [CrossRef] [PubMed]

9. Ito, A.; Tanaka, K.; Honda, H.; Abe, S.; Yamaguchi, H.; Kobayashi, T. Complete Regression of Mouse Mammary Carcinoma with a Size Greater than 15 mm by Frequent Repeated Hyperthermia Using Magnetite Nanoparticles. *J. Biosci. Bioeng.* **2003**, *96*, 364–369. [CrossRef]

10. Wu, K.; Wang, J.-P. Magnetic Hyperthermia Performance of Magnetite Nanoparticle Assemblies under Different Driving Fields. *AIP Adv.* **2017**, *7*, 056327. [CrossRef]

11. Estelrich, J.; Escribano, E.; Queralt, J.; Busquets, M.A. Iron Oxide Nanoparticles for Magnetically-Guided And Magnetically-Responsive Drug Delivery. *Int. J. Mol. Sci.* **2015**, *16*, 8070–8101. [CrossRef] [PubMed]

12. Wankhede, M.; Bouras, A.; Kaluzova, M.; Hadjipanayis, C.G. Magnetic Nanoparticles: an Emerging Technology for Malignant Brain Tumor Imaging and Therapy. *Expert Rev. Clin. Pharmacol.* **2012**, *5*, 173–186. [CrossRef] [PubMed]

13. Timin, A.; Gao, H.; Voronin, D.; Gorin, D.; Sukhorukov, G. Inorganic/Organic Multilayer Capsule Composition for Improved Functionality and External Triggering. *Adv. Mater. Interfaces* **2017**, *4*, 1600338. [CrossRef]

14. Becker, A.L.; Johnston, A.P.; Caruso, F. Layer-by-layer-assembled Capsules and Films for Therapeutic Delivery. *Small* **2010**, *6*, 1836–1852. [CrossRef] [PubMed]

15. Delcea, M.; Möhwald, H.; Skirtach, A.G. Stimuli-Responsive LbL Capsules and Nanoshells for Drug Delivery. *Adv. Drug Deliv. Rev.* **2011**, *63*, 730–747. [CrossRef] [PubMed]

16. Zebli, B.; Susha, A.S.; Sukhorukov, G.B.; Rogach, A.L.; Parak, W.J. Magnetic Targeting and Cellular Uptake of Polymer Microcapsules Simultaneously Functionalized with Magnetic and Luminescent Nanocrystals. *Langmuir* **2005**, *21*, 4262–4265. [CrossRef] [PubMed]

17. De Geest, B.G.; Vandenbroucke, R.E.; Guenther, A.M.; Sukhorukov, G.B.; Hennink, W.E.; Sanders, N.N.; Demmster, J.; De Smedt, S.C. Intracellularly Degradable Polyelectrolyte Microcapsules. *Adv. Mater.* **2006**, *18*, 1005–1009. [CrossRef]

18. Yu, W.; Zhang, W.; Chen, Y.; Song, X.; Tong, W.; Mao, Z.; Gao, C. Cellular Uptake of Poly(Allylamine Hydrochloride) Microcapsules with Different Deformability and Its Influence on Cell Functions. *J. Colloid Interface Sci.* **2016**, *465*, 149–157. [CrossRef] [PubMed]

19. De Geest, B.G.; Sanders, N.N.; Sukhorukov, G.B.; Demeester, J.; De Smedt, S.C. Release Mechanisms for Polyelectrolyte Capsules. *Chem. Soc. Rev.* **2007**, *36*, 636–649. [CrossRef] [PubMed]

20. Loretta, L.; Rivera-Gil, P.; Abbasi, A.Z.; Ochs, M.; Ganas, C.; Zins, I.; Sönnichsen, C.; Parak, W.J. LbL Multilayer Capsules: Recent Progress and Future Outlook for Their Use in Life Sciences. *Nanoscale* **2010**, *2*, 458–467. [CrossRef]

21. Bédard, M.F.; De Geest, B.G.; Skirtach, A.G.; Möhwald, H.; Sukhorukov, G.B. Polymeric Microcapsules with Light Responsive Properties for Encapsulation and Release. *Adv. Colloid Interface Sci.* **2010**, *158*, 2–14. [CrossRef] [PubMed]

22. Abbaspourrad, A.; Carroll, N.J.; Kim, S.H.; Weitz, D.A. Polymer Microcapsules with Programmable Active Release. *J. Am. Chem. Soc.* **2013**, *135*, 7744–7750. [CrossRef] [PubMed]

23. Ambrosone, A.; Marchesano, V.; Carregal-Romero, S.; Intartaglia, D.; Parak, W.J.; Tortiglione, C. Control of Wnt/β-Catenin Signaling Pathway in Vivo via Light Responsive Capsules. *ACS Nano* **2016**, *10*, 4828–4834. [CrossRef] [PubMed]

24. De Koker, S.; De Geest, B.G.; Cuvelier, C.; Ferdinande, L.; Deckers, W.; Hennink, W.E.; De Smedt, S.C.; Mertens, N. In Vivo Cellular Uptake, Degradation, and Biocompatibility of Polyelectrolyte Microcapsules. *Adv. Funct. Mater.* **2007**, *17*, 3754–3763. [CrossRef]

25. Zheng, C.; Zhang, X.G.; Sun, L.; Zhang, Z.P.; Li, C.X. Biodegradable and Redox-Responsive Chitosan/poly (L-aspartic acid) Submicron Capsules for Transmucosal Delivery of Proteins and Peptides. *J. Mater. Sci. Mater. Med.* **2013**, *24*, 931–939. [CrossRef] [PubMed]

26. Voronin, D.V.; Sindeeva, O.A.; Kurochkin, M.A.; Mayorova, O.; Fedosov, I.V.; Semyachkina-Glushkovskaya, O.; Gorin, D.A.; Tuchin, V.V.; Sukhorukov, G.B. In Vitro and In Vivo Visualization and Trapping of Fluorescent Magnetic Microcapsules in a Bloodstream. *ACS Appl. Mater. Interfaces* **2017**, *9*, 6885–6893. [CrossRef] [PubMed]

27. Yi, Q.; Li, D.; Lin, B.; Pavlov, A.M.; Luo, D.; Gong, Q.; Song, B.; Ai, H.; Sukhorukov, G.B. Magnetic Resonance Imaging for Monitoring of Magnetic Polyelectrolyte Capsule In Vivo Delivery. *Bionanoscience* **2014**, *4*, 59–70. [CrossRef]

28. Donath, E.; Sukhorukov, G.B.; Caruso, F.; Davis, S.A.; Möhwald, H. Novel Hollow Polymer Shells by Colloid-Templated Assembly of Polyelectrolytes. *Angew Chem. Int. Ed. Engl.* **1998**, *37*, 2201–2205. [CrossRef]

29. Massart, R. Preparation of Aqueous Magnetic Liquids in Alkaline and Acidic Media. *IEEE Trans. Magn.* **1981**, *17*, 1247–1248. [CrossRef]

30. German, S.V.; Inozemtseva, O.A.; Markin, A.V.; Metvalli, K.; Khomutov, G.B.; Gorin, D.A. Synthesis of Magnetite Hydrosols in Inert Atmosphere. *Colloid J.* **2013**, *75*, 483–486. [CrossRef]

31. Dincer, I.; Tozkoparan, O.; German, S.V.; Markin, A.V.; Yildirim, O.; Khomutov, G.B.; Gorin, D.A.; Venig, S.B.; Elerman, Y. Effect of the Number of Iron Oxide Nanoparticle Layers on the Magnetic Properties of Nanocomposite LbL Assemblies. *J. Magn. Magn. Mater.* **2012**, *324*, 2958–2963. [CrossRef]

32. German, S.V.; Bratashov, D.N.; Navolokin, N.A.; Kozlova, A.A.; Lomova, M.V.; Novoselova, M.V.; Burilova, E.A.; Zuev, V.V.; Khlebtsov, B.N.; Bucharskaya, A.B.; et al. In vitro and in vivo MRI Visualization of Nanocomposite Biodegradable Microcapsules with Tunable Contrast. *Phys. Chem. Chem. Phys.* **2016**, *18*, 32238–32246. [CrossRef] [PubMed]
33. Zyuzin, M.V.; Díez, P.; Goldsmith, M.; Carregal-Romero, S.; Teodosio, C.; Rejman, J.; Feliu, N.; Escudero, A.; Almendral, M.J.; Linne, U.; et al. Comprehensive and Systematic Analysis of the Immunocompatibility of Polyelectrolyte Capsules. *Bioconjug. Chem.* **2017**, *28*, 556–564. [CrossRef] [PubMed]
34. Nečas, D.; Klapetek, P. Gwyddion: An Open-Source Software for SPM Data Analysis. *Open Phys.* **2012**, *10*, 181–188. [CrossRef]
35. International Guiding Principles for Biomedical Research Involving Animals. December 2012. CIOMS&ICLAS. Available online: https://olaw.nih.gov/sites/default/files/Guiding_Principles_2012.pdf (accessed on 3 October 2014).
36. Yang, L.; Kuang, H.; Zhang, W.; Aguilar, Z.P.; Wei, H.; Xu, H. Comparisons of the Biodistribution and Toxicological Examinations after Repeated Intravenous Administration of Silver and Gold Nanoparticles in Mice. *Sci. Rep.* **2017**, *7*, 3303. [CrossRef] [PubMed]
37. Huppertz, A.; Rohrer, M. Gadobutrol, a Highly Concentrated Mr-Imaging Contrast Agent: Its Physicochemical Characteristics and the Basis for Its Use in Contrast-Enhanced MR Angiography and Perfusion Imaging. *Eur. Radiol.* **2004**, *14*, M12–M18. [PubMed]
38. Chertok, B.; Cole, A.J.; David, A.E.; Yang, V.C. Comparison of Electron Spin Resonance Spectroscopy and Inductively-Coupled Plasma Optical Emission Spectroscopy for Biodistribution Analysis of Iron-Oxide Nanoparticles. *Mol. Pharm.* **2010**, *7*, 375e85. [CrossRef] [PubMed]
39. Rinck, P.A. *Magnetic Resonance in Medicine: The Basic Textbook of the European Magnetic Resonance Forum*, 4th ed.; Wiley-Blackwell: Berlin, Germany, 2001; p. 252.
40. Arami, H.; Khandhar, A.; Liggitt, D.; Krishnan, K.M. In Vivo Delivery, Pharmacokinetics, Biodistribution and Toxicity of Iron Oxide Nanoparticles. *Chem. Soc. Rev.* **2015**, *44*, 8576–8607. [CrossRef] [PubMed]
41. Patil, U.S.; Adireddy, S.; Jaiswal, A.; Mandava, S.; Lee, B.R.; Chrisey, D.B. In Vitro/in Vivo Toxicity Evaluation and Quantification of Iron Oxide Nanoparticles. *Int. J. Mol. Sci.* **2015**, *16*, 24417–24450. [CrossRef] [PubMed]

Intratumoral Delivery of Doxorubicin on Folate-Conjugated Graphene Oxide by In-Situ Forming Thermo-Sensitive Hydrogel for Breast Cancer Therapy

Yi Teng Fong [1,2,†], Chih-Hao Chen [2,†] and Jyh-Ping Chen [1,2,3,4,*]

[1] Department of Chemical and Materials Engineering, Chang Gung University, Taoyuan 33302, Taiwan; evausatw@cgmh.org.tw

[2] Department of Plastic and Reconstructive Surgery and Craniofacial Research Center, Chang Gung Memorial Hospital, Linkou, Kwei-San, Taoyuan 33305, Taiwan; cjh5027@cgmh.org.tw

[3] Research Center for Chinese Herbal Medicine and Research Center for Food and Cosmetic Safety, College of Human Ecology, Chang Gung University of Science and Technology, Kwei-San, Taoyuan 33302, Taiwan

[4] Department of Materials Engineering, Ming Chi University of Technology, Tai-Shan, New Taipei City 24301, Taiwan

* Correspondence: jpchen@mail.cgu.edu.tw;

† These authors contributed equally to this paper.

Abstract: By taking advantage of the pH-sensitive drug release property of graphene oxide (GO) after intracellular uptake, we prepared folic acid (FA)-conjugated GO (GOFA) for targeted delivery of the chemotherapeutic drug doxorubicin (DOX). GOFA-DOX was further encapsulated in an injectable in-situ forming thermo-sensitive hyaluronic acid-chitosan-g-poly(N-isopropylacrylamide) (HACPN) hydrogel for intratumoral delivery of DOX. As the degradation time of HACPN could be extended up to 3 weeks, intratumoral delivery of GOFA-DOX/HACPN could provide controlled and targeted delivery of DOX through slow degradation HACPN and subsequent cellular uptake of released GOFA-DOX by tumor cells through interactions of GOFA with folate receptors on the tumor cell's surface. GOFA nano-carrier and HACPN hydrogel were first characterized for the physico-chemical properties. The drug loading experiments indicated the best preparation condition of GOFA-DOX was by reacting 0.1 mg GOFA with 2 mg DOX. GOFA-DOX showed pH-responsive drug release with ~5 times more DOX released at pH 5.5 than at pH 7.4 while only limited DOX was released from GOFA-DOX/HACPN at pH 7.4. Intracellular uptake of GOFA by endocytosis and release of DOX from GOFA-DOX in vitro could be confirmed from transmission electron microscopic and confocal laser scanning microscopic analysis with MCF-7 breast cancer cells. The targeting effect of FA was revealed when intracellular uptake of GOFA was blocked by excess FA. This resulted in enhanced in vitro cytotoxicity as revealed from the lower half maximal inhibitory concentration (IC50) value of GOFA-DOX (7.3 µg/mL) compared with that of DOX (32.5 µg/mL) and GO-DOX (10 µg/mL). The flow cytometry analysis indicated higher apoptosis rates for cells treated with GOFA-DOX (30%) compared with DOX (8%) and GO-DOX (11%). Animal studies were carried out with subcutaneously implanted MCF-7 cells in BALB/c nude mice and subject to intratumoral administration of drugs. The relative tumor volumes of control (saline) and GOFA-DOX/HACPN groups at day 21 were 2.17 and 1.79 times that at day 0 with no significant difference. In comparison, the relative tumor volumes of treatment groups at the same time were significantly different at 1.02, 0.67 and 0.48 times for DOX, GOFA-DOX and GOFA-DOX/HACPN groups, respectively. The anti-tumor efficacy was also supported by images from an in vivo imaging system (IVIS) using MCF-7 cells transfected with luciferase (MCF-7/Luc). Furthermore, tissue biopsy examination and blood analysis indicated that intratumoral delivery of DOX using GOFA-DOX/HACPN did not elicit acute toxicity. Taken together,

GOFA-DOX/HACPN could be deemed as a safe and efficient intratumoral drug delivery system for breast cancer therapy.

Keywords: thermo-sensitive hydrogel; graphene oxide; folic acid; intratumoral delivery; cancer therapy

---

1. Introduction

In recent years, an effective cancer treatment platform has always been the focus of developing advanced drug delivery systems based on different nano-sized drug carriers [1,2]. Such systems used liposomes and/or polymer nanoparticles as the drug carrier, combining triggered release of an anticancer drug under the characteristic environment of cancer cells and protect the drug until it enters the cell to increase the intracellular drug concentration [3]. Thus, the ideal drug delivery system should be not only to improve the treatment efficacy but also to decrease the systemic toxicity effects. Graphene, a novel two-dimensional (2D) honeycomb material, has been recognized as one of the most promising nanomaterials used as a filler in polymer matrices [4]. With a 2D planar structure composed of sp^2 mixed-layer trajectories, graphene-based nanomaterials have been widely studied for applications in biotechnology [5]. When used as a drug carrier, graphene is usually modified to increase its hydrophilicity and reduce the thickness by converting it into an oxidized form (i.e., graphene oxide, GO) [6,7]. Indeed, GO was shown to be a functional nano-sized carrier for delivery of anticancer drugs based on π–π stacking, such as camptothecin (camptothecin, CPT), camptothecin derivatives (SN38) and adriamycin (doxorubicin, DOX) [8]. The hydrogen bond interactions between GO and the drug can result in a large amount of drug being adsorbed onto GO due to its large specific surface area [9,10]. An added advantage of GO for chemotherapeutic drug delivery is the pH-dependent drug release behavior, where enhanced drug release at a low pH value (pH 5.0 to pH 5.5) will provide efficient intracellular drug release after its endocytosis by the cell for drug release in the endosome [11,12].

Targeted delivery of anticancer drugs for cancer therapy could be more effective than traditional chemotherapy. The targeting therapy could be divided into active targeting and passive targeting [13,14]. For active targeting therapy, the drug carrier is modified with a ligand or a monoclonal antibody on the surface to increase the ability of the carrier to be specifically recognized by diseased cells. Folic acid (FA) is a group of water-soluble vitamin B that exists in green leaves, vegetables and other plants. It is an important element for all cells and involved in DNA synthesis or cell division. Folic acid is transported into healthy cells or cancer cells through their folate receptors on cell surface. As cancer cells require more FA for maintaining cell differentiation and proliferation, there are over-expressed folate receptors on the cell membrane of cancer cells, compared with healthy and/or normal cells [15]. Thus, modifying an anticancer drug nano-carrier, such as GO, with FA could enhance its ability to be recognized and its intracellular uptake efficiency by cancer cells through ligand-mediated targeting drug delivery [16,17]. Previously, we have used FA-conjugated multi-walled carbon nanotubes (a 1D carbon nanomaterial) for targeted delivery of DOX to cancer cells [18].

In-situ forming thermo-sensitive hydrogel undergoes physical sol-to-gel phase transition as temperature increases. It can be easily administered via injection using a conventional syringe needle after in-situ gelation at the physiological temperature [19]. Poly(N-isopropylacrylamide) (PNIPAm) is one of the most studied thermo-sensitive hydrogel showing reversible sol-gel phase transition behavior around its lower critical solution temperature (LCST) at ~32 °C [20,21]. PNIPAm end capped with a carboxylic acid group could be synthesized for subsequent conjugating with carbohydrate polymers, e.g., chitosan and hyaluronic acid, to form injectable thermo-sensitive copolymer, hyaluronic acid-chitosan-g-poly(N-isopropylacrylamide) (HACPN) with a similar LCST to PNIPAm [22].

Compared to traditional intravenous administration of anticancer drugs, intratumoral drug delivery systems have the potential to enable the loading and release of insoluble anticancer drugs through in-situ forming thermo-sensitive hydrogel. This drug delivery system can deliver anticancer drugs locally to the tumor site, leading to low dose requirements and reduce multiple drug administration cycles, which could reduce or eliminate adverse effects of the drug due to local delivery and prevention of systemic drug uptake [23]. Injectable gelling depots with thermo-sensitive hydrogel and pre-shaped implant systems are two types of intratumoral delivery systems for anticancer drugs [24]. The injectable gelling depot based on in-situ phase separation of thermo-sensitive hydrogel has been shown to be less invasive and lead to less pain upon injection as compared to pre-formed implants, making them a desirable system for local administration of anticancer drugs [25]. A typical injectable gelling depot system is formulated by simple mixing of drug and polymer solution below the LCST of the polymer hydrogel. After injection, sol-gel transition occurs to transform the minimally viscous solution into a drug delivery gel depot. The advantage of this method is the avoidance of invasive surgery for implantation, a high water content of the hydrogel to improve the compatibility, biodegradability of the thermo-sensitive polymer for excretion from the body once achieving its intended purpose and flexibility of the design of the drug release rate by changing the formulation [26].

However, thermo-sensitive hydrogels present challenges in anticancer drug delivery applications, i.e., initial burst release [27]. The burst release may lead to systemic toxicity due to the high dosage of drug released. The main reasons for burst release stems from the fact that a solid gel is not formed immediately upon injection into the body. A highly hydrophilic drug trapped in the aqueous phase of the gel may diffuse into the body fluid uncontrollably fast before and after gelation induced by a temperature change. To solve the burst release problem, we postulate that embedding drug-loaded GO in in-situ forming HACPN hydrogel could provide an ideal drug delivery platform for intratumoral delivery of anticancer drugs. A key requirement of in-situ depot-forming systems for local delivery, and more specifically for intratumoral delivery, could be fulfilled easily by HACPN hydrogel with its injectability through standard gauge needles [28]. Therefore, we first prepared FA-conjugated GO as the targeted drug delivery carrier for doxorubicin (DOX) (GOFA-DOX). Then, GOFA-DOX was encapsulated into the thermo-sensitive and biodegradable polymer hydrogel HACPN for local drug delivery. We demonstrated that GOFA, with its high loading capacity for DOX, showed enhanced intracellular uptake by breast cancer cell MCF-7 and pH-responsive drug release. The targeted drug delivery in concomitant with the degradation of HACPN could alleviate burst DOX release and enhance cytotoxicity toward MCF-7 cells in vitro. Furthermore, an efficient and safe breast cancer therapy employing intratumoral delivery of GOFA-DOX/HACPN in xenograft tumor mouse models with MCF-7 implanted subcutaneously in nude mice could be expected (Figure 1).

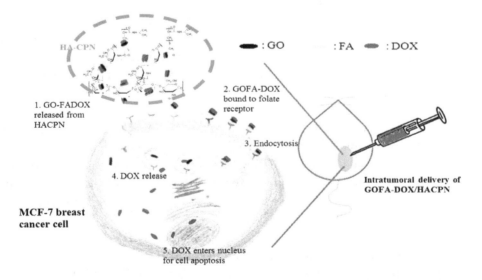

Figure 1. The schematic illustration of the antitumor effect by intratumoral delivery of DOX-loaded GOFA in HACPN hydrogel (GOFA-DOX/HACPN) in a xenograft tumor mouse model with MCF-7 cells implanted subcutaneously in nude mice.

2. Results and Discussion

2.1. Synthesis and Characterization of GO and GOFA

The nano-sized GO was prepared by using commercial GO as raw material through modified Hummer method, followed by prolong (30 min) ultrasonication [29]. This reduced GO size and introduced abundant carboxyl groups for conjugating with FA. The morphology of as-prepared GO was characterized by transmission electron microscope (TEM) and atomic force microscope (AFM). As shown in Figure 2, the size of GO was 150~200 nm while the thickness was about 4.0 ± 0.2 nm, which was in agreement with previous studies [30]. Using 1-ethyl-3-(3-dimethylaminopropyl) carbodiimide (EDC) as a crosslinking agent, we synthesized GOFA by covalently conjugating GO with FA through amide bond formation between the amine groups of FA and carboxyl groups of GO in an aqueous solution. The EDC-mediated conjugation works by activating carboxyl groups for direct reaction with primary amines via amide bond formation. Because no portion of the EDC chemical structure becomes part of the final bond between GO and FA, it is considered a zero-length carboxyl-to-amine crosslinker. GOFA showed a light brownish color stable solution in phosphate buffered solution (PBS) with no aggregation occurred up to 1 day at 0.1 mg/mL, ensuring proper suspension during DOX loading. After FA was conjugated to GO to form GOFA, the size remained the same but the thickness increased to 12.0 ± 0.3 nm from TEM and AFM observation (Figure 2). The roughness also increased from 1.5 ± 0.4 nm to 5.3 ± 0.5 nm. Controlling the size of GOFA within 200 to 500 nm was very important for its efficient intracellular uptake into cells [31].

The modified Hummer method used here oxidized commercial GO with concentrated sulfuric acid and introduced more oxygen molecules, including abundant carboxyl groups, to GO. An aqueous suspension of GO exhibits a zeta potential of -33.0 ± 1.1 mV, indicative of negatively charged surfaces caused by the presence of hydrophilic carboxyl groups. The zeta potential of GO changed to -24.7 ± 0.9 mV after conjugation with FA as the carboxyl groups was consumed after reacting with the primary amine groups of FA. The changes in thickness, roughness and zeta potential indicated successful conjugation of FA with GO nano-sheet.

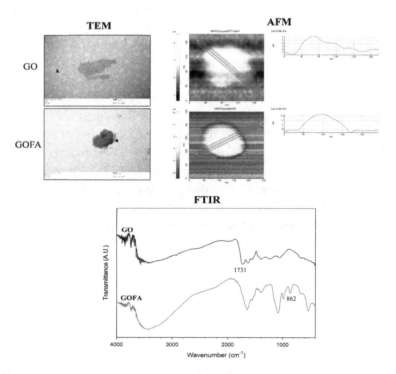

Figure 2. Transmission electron microscopic (TEM), atomic force microscopic (AFM) and Fourier transform infrared (FTIR) spectroscopic analysis of GO and GOFA.

From Fourier transform infrared (FTIR) spectroscopy analysis, major peaks of GO at 3400 cm^{-1} (OH), 1731 cm^{-1} (C=O), 1640 cm^{-1} (C=C), 1246 cm^{-1} (C–OH) and 1060 cm^{-1} (C–O) were identified (Figure 2). After FA conjugation to GO, the absorption peaks at 1731 cm^{-1} disappeared due to consumption of carboxylic acid C=O with concomitant appearance of the additional aromatic C–H bending at 862 cm^{-1} due to FA. Taken together, the FTIR analysis indicated successful incorporation of FA in GOFA. This was also supported by quantitative analysis of the amount of FA conjugated to GO, which is 98.2 μg FA/mg GOFA with 92.8% loading efficacy.

2.2. Synthesis and Characterization of HACPN

Due to the toxicity of PNIPAm, copolymers containing PNIPAm and other biocompatible natural polymers were preferred for biomedical applications. Modification of PNIPAm by grafting with other biocompatible polymers could fortify the mechanical properties of the hydrogel and reduce its cytotoxicity [32]. Thus, the HACPN hydrogel is more practicable as an injectable hydrogel vehicle for drug delivery [33]. The relative compositions of chitosan, hyaluronic acid and PNIPAm in HACPN could be calculated to be 12.6% (w/w), 5.5% (w/w) and 81.9% (w/w), respectively [28]. The HACPN solution was free free-flowing at 25 °C and transformed into gels at 37 °C [32]. Furthermore, the solid hydrogel remained stationary when the sample vial was inverted, verifying the high structural strength of the injectable thermo-sensitive polymer hydrogel at the physiological temperature. The LCST was determined from the sol-gel phase transition by measuring the turbidity of a 10% (w/v) polymer solution. The relative absorbance of the polymer solution increased with temperature and the LCST could be calculated to be 30.5 and 30.3 °C for 5% and 10% (w/v) HACPN solutions, respectively, by defining the LCST being the temperature corresponding to half of the maximum change in the absorbance (Figure 3A). The gelling processes of HACPN was also thermo-reversible as subsequent cooling cycle resulted in gel-sol transition and fully reversible gel melting [28].

The phase transition kinetics analysis was carried out to investigate the gel formation time of HACPN solutions. As shown in Figure 3B, the relative absorbance rose sharply as the temperature was shifted from 25 to 37 °C. The gel formation kinetics of 5% HACPN was slower than that of 10% HACPN albeit both completed gel formation in less than 5 min. The fast gel formation will ensure fast in-situ gel formation to entrap DOX-loaded GOFA and prevent burst release of the drug. It should be noted that the volume of polymer solution used here (2 mL) for in vitro gel forming kinetics measurements was much larger than the volume used for in vivo injection (0.2 mL). Therefore, we expect the gel formation time will be shorter than that shown in Figure 3B (~4 min). With comparable LCST but faster gel formation kinetics, 10% HACPN was chosen for further studies.

The effect of GOFA on the phase transition of HACPN was studied using differential scanning calorimetry (DSC). From DSC analysis (Figure 3C), the temperatures at the onsets of the differential scanning calorimetry (DSC) endotherms were at 28.70 and 29.53 °C for HACPN and GOFA/HACPN, respectively, while the corresponding peak temperatures were 29.95 and 30.07 °C, which could be referred to as the LCST [34]. Moreover, the enthalpy change of the phase transition, which was calculated by integration of peak area, increased from 0.9763 to 1.299 J/g during the heating process of the DSC cycle, indicating the replacement of water molecules around the hydrophilic polar groups by GOFA at a temperature lower than the LCST and the endothermic heat caused by the dehydration of polar groups increased [35].

The drug release behaviors from a hydrogel matrix depended on several factors, such as diffusion through the matrix, osmosis, degradation or weight loss of the matrix and physical parameters of the polymer matrix [36]. Taking advantage of the weight loss of HACPN hydrogel is an attractive characteristic for intratumoral drug delivery since the hydrogel does not need to be removed after local application [37]. From the weight loss at 37 °C in phosphate buffered saline (PBS), HACPN showed quick degradation rate initially with ~65% remaining weight at day 7 (Figure 3D). After this period, the degradation rate slowed down moderately with ~12% remaining weight at day 28. The degradation of HACPN hydrogel in vitro implies that GOFA/DOX could be continuously released in vivo after intratumoral delivery, followed by intracellular uptake of the nano-drug by cancer cells.

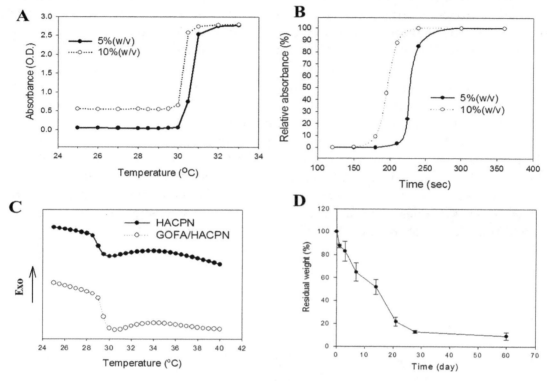

Figure 3. (**A**) Phase transition behavior of thermo-sensitive polymer HACPN at 5% and 10% (w/v) from 25 to 33 °C; (**B**) Kinetics of phase transition of 5% and 10% (w/v) HACPN solutions during heating with instantaneous temperature change from 25 to 37 °C; (**C**) Thermal properties of HACPN and GOFA/HACPN with 0.1% (w/w) GOFA from differential scanning calorimetry; (**D**) The weight loss of 10% (w/v) HACPN in pH 7.4 PBS at 37 °C.

2.3. DOX Loading and Release

Drug loading and release behavior are the most important characteristics to evaluate a drug delivery system. Figure 4A shows the drug loading performance of GOFA. The high surface area and conjugate structure of GO could facilitate strong π–π stacking interactions with DOX and to achieve high DOX loadings [9]. By increasing the amount of DOX used during drug loading, the loading content (the weight of DOX to the weight of GOFA) of DOX increased sharply and reached as high as 25 mg DOX/mg GOFA when 3 mg DOX reacted with 0.1 mg GOFA. On the contrary, the DOX loading efficiency (the weight percentage of initial DOX bound to GOFA) decreased with increasing amount of DOX used and reduced from 95.5% to 37.6% when 3 mg DOX was used. Thus, reacting 2.0 mg DOX with 0.1 mg GOFA (DOX/GOFA = 20) was deemed the best condition for preparing GOFA-DOX considering both drug loading efficiency and loading content with the former being 51.2% and the latter being 14.2 mg/mg. It should be noted the DOX loading content reported here is much higher than the values (32 µg/mg and 1.84 mg/mg) reported previously using FA-conjugate carbon nanotubes [18,38]. For DOX loading to GO, the loading contents reported previously were 2.35 and 0.294 mg/mg [10,39]. These results indicated that GOFA is a highly efficient nano-carrier for loading and delivery of DOX.

The release of drug from GOFA-DOX at 37 °C in PBS at pH 7.4 and 5.5 is presented in Figure 4B. The pH values for evaluating drug release were chosen based on the physiological and the endosomal pH value of cancer cells, respectively. The drug release curves showed that DOX loaded on GOFA was released at a slow and controlled manner at pH 7.4, to the extent of 18.7% in 216 h. The release rate of DOX was significantly enhanced at pH 5.5 and the amount of drug released was 89.4% within the same time period.

That the release rate of DOX at pH 5.5 was significantly higher than that at pH 7.4 may be caused by weakening of hydrogen bonds between DOX and GOFA. Noncovalent attachment of DOX to GOFA involves hydrogen bonds between –COOH of GOFA and –OH of DOX and between –OH of GOFA and –OH of DOX [18]. The degree of hydrogen bond interactions between DOX and GOFA is a function of the pH value. The H^+ in solution would compete with the hydrogen bond-forming group and weaken the hydrogen bond interactions at pH 5.5, leading to greater release of DOX. Alternatively, the high release rate at acidic conditions may be caused by the amine ($-NH_2$) groups of DOX getting protonated to result in partial dissociation of hydrogel-bonding interaction [40]. The high drug loading and the pH-sensitive release of DOX suggest that GOFA is a promising delivery vehicle for the anticancer drug.

The drug release behavior of DOX from GOFA-DOX/HACPN showed the same pH dependence as GOFA but is much slower than GOFA (Figure 4B). Thus, we can anticipate effective modulation of the burst release of DOX by entrapping GOFA-DOX in HACPN at the physiological pH extracellularly, followed by copious DOX release at the endosomal pH in cancer cells to exert enhanced cytotoxicity following the intracellular uptake of GOFA-DOX.

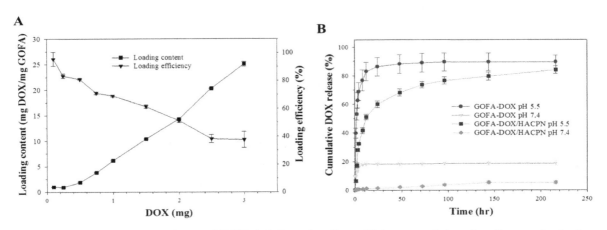

Figure 4. The loading and release of DOX. (**A**) Drug loading efficiency and drug loading content when 0.1 mg GOFA was reacted with different amount of DOX; (**B**) Drug release from GOFA-DOX and GOFA-DOX/HACPN at pH 7.4 and pH 5.5 in PBS (37 °C).

2.4. In Vitro Cell Culture

2.4.1. Cellular Uptake

Eukaryotic cells could form endocytotic vesicles to enclose extracellular substances through invagination of their plasma membrane segments. The specific uptake of GOFA by MCF-7 cells could be strongly suggested by receptor-mediated endocytosis to show efficient and targeted delivery of DOX by GOFA-DOX [9]. Folate receptor is a common tumor marker expressed at high levels on the surfaces of various cancer cells, which can facilitate cellular internalization of GO through receptor-mediated endocytosis after conjugating FA to GO. Confocal microscopy revealed intracellular fluorescence corresponding to quantum dot (QD)-labeled GOFA when MCF-7 cells were exposed to GOFA for 1 h and quenched with trypan blue to eliminate the residual fluorescence bound to cell membrane (Figure 5A). When folate receptors on MCF-7 cell surface were blocked by FA before contacting with GOFA, less receptor-mediated intracellular uptake was expected for GOFA. Indeed, we observed drastically diminished intracellular fluorescence signal of GOFA by blocking with excess FA (Figure 5B). This difference is due to the efficient blockage of folate receptor on MCF-7 cell surface with free FA in solution, which competitively inhibited the affinity of folate receptor toward GOFA. Overall, our result was in agreement with previous studies that revealed folate receptor-dependent cellular uptakes by cancer cells for anticancer drug delivery [41].

Two possible mechanisms of cellular DOX uptake from nanoparticles have been suggested: (1) DOX is released from the nanoparticle outside the cells, or (2) DOX is carried by the nanoparticle and released inside the cells [42]. Folic acid modification could increase the cytotoxicity of DOX encapsulated in nanoparticles toward MCF-7 cells by minimizing extracellular DOX release [43]. Upon incubation of MCF-7 with free DOX at 37 C for 1 h, red fluorescence was found mostly confined within the nucleus of shrunken cells, where DOX is chelated with DNA (Figure 5C). For GOFA-DOX, green fluorescence of GOFA appears in the cytoplasm of shrunken cells (Figure 5D). This provides a direct evidence for endocytosis of GOFA, which accumulated in the cytoplasm after internalization. Red fluorescence was only observed in the cell nucleus, indicating DOX released from GOFA in the cytoplasm could translocate across the nuclear membrane to interact with DNA molecules in the cell nucleus (Figure 5D). That the red signal due to DOX is much stronger for GOFA-DOX than DOX also implied GOFA could facilitate DOX diffusion across the cell membrane through intracellular uptake of GOFA-DOX to enhance the cytotoxicity toward cancer cells. Taken together, the results suggest that DOX-loaded GOFA could be transported across cell membrane via endocytosis and DOX was subsequently released under the acidic intracellular environment.

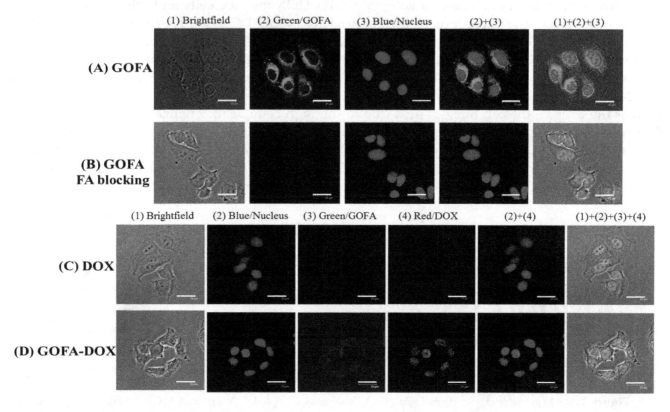

Figure 5. Confocal microscopy images of MCF-7 cells after incubated with GOFA for 1 h (**A**); incubated with 0.1 mg/mL folic acid for 1 h to block cell surface folate receptors and then treated with GOFA for 1 h (**B**); incubated with free DOX for 1 h (**C**); incubated with GOFA-DOX for 1 h (**D**). Bar = 25 μm.

Internalization of GOFA by MCF-7 cells was also observed by transmission electron microscope (TEM) to confirm endocytosis. Intracellular uptake was evident after contacting GOFA with cells, which were found within the endosomes in the cytoplasmic region (Figure 6). The presence of GOFA in close proximity to the nuclear region could be also observed. In vitro confocal and TEM images therefore strongly support efficient entry of GOFA into cancer cells through endocytosis after releasing from HACPN. It could be postulated that GOFA could potentially enhance the apoptotic effects of DOX via its efficient endocytosis by the cancer cells and increase the intracellular anticancer activity of the drug [44].

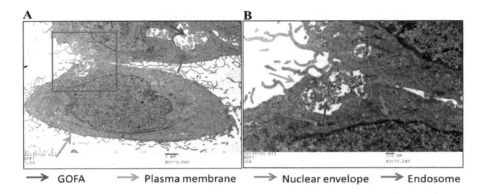

Figure 6. (**A**) Transmission electron microscope (TEM) micrographs of MCF-7 cells treated with GOFA for 1 h. (**B**) is an enlarged view of the square in (**A**). (**A**) Bar = 2 μm, (**B**) Bar = 500 nm.

2.4.2. In Vitro Cytotoxicity and Biocompatibility Studies

After confirming the successful entry of GOFA-DOX into the cells and release the drug, cell viability assay was used to compare the cytotoxicity of GO-DOX, GOFA-DOX and free DOX at different DOX concentrations toward MCF-7 cells (Figure 7A). When treated with an equivalent concentration of DOX, MCF-7 cells showed the lowest viability when treated with GOFA-DOX, followed by GO-DOX and free DOX. The IC50 values were calculated to be 7.3, 10 and 32.5 μg/mL for GOFA-DOX, GO-DOX and free DOX, respectively. This suggests GOFA-DOX can efficiently deliver the drug to the cell nucleus area due to the high cellular internalization of FA-conjugated GO via receptor-binding endocytosis. The biocompatibility of GOFA was confirmed over a broad concentration range using MCF-7 cells (Figure 7B), where the relative cell viability is above 90% up to 100 μg/mL, which covers the concentrations of GOFA studied in Figure 7A, indicating cell cytotoxicity shown by GOFA-DOX was indeed from DOX released but not from the drug carrier itself.

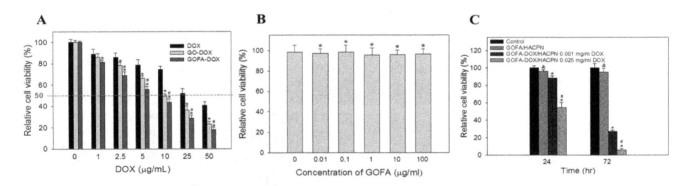

Figure 7. (**A**) Cytotoxicity of free DOX, GO-DOX and GOFA-DOX against MCF-7 cells. The cells were treated for 24 h. The relative cell viability was compared to the control without DOX. * $p < 0.05$ compared with DOX, # $p < 0.05$ compared with GO-DOX; (**B**) Viability of MCF-7 cells after incubated with different concentration of GOFA for 24 h. The relative cell viability was compared to the control without GOFA. * $p > 0.05$ compared with control; (**C**) Cell viability of MCF-7 cells after incubated with GOFA/HACPN and GOFA-DOX/HACPN at different DOX concentrations for 24 and 72 h. The control is cell culture medium. & $p > 0.05$ compared with control, * $p < 0.05$ compared with control, # $p < 0.05$ compared with GOFA-DOX/HACPN 0.001 mg/mL DOX. Data are presented as mean ± standard deviation (SD), $n = 6$.

For the cytotoxicity of GOFA-DOX/HACPN toward MCF-7 cells, when cells were incubated at a low DOX concentration (0.001 mg/mL), cell survival rate was 90% after 24 h (Figure 7C). When MCF-7 cells were cultured for 72 h in the presence of GOFA-DOX/HACPN, cell viability was further decreased to ~30%. At a higher DOX concentration (i.e., 0.025 mg/mL), the same cytotoxicity effect could be observed. That the cytotoxicity of GOFA-DOX/HACPN was both DOX dose and time-dependent, indicating GOFA-DOX could be released from HACPN continuously to exert the cytotoxicity effect toward MCF-7 cells. The biocompatibility of GOFA/HACPN could be also observed from Figure 7C with the relative cell viability not significantly different from the control, indicating GOFA/HACPN does not elicit cytotoxicity toward MCF-7 cells in vitro.

2.4.3. Cell Apoptosis Induced by DOX In Vitro

Doxorubicin is known as an anthracycline antibiotic effective in treating a variety of cancers. It functions primarily at the DNA level by blocking the replication and transcription processes [45,46]. DOX also activates damage-inducible DNA repair and prevent the triggering of programmed cell death by spontaneous and induced DNA damage [47]. To confirm the cytotoxicity of GO-DOX and GOFA-DOX toward MCF-7 cells was induced by apoptosis as of free DOX and compare the apoptosis ratio, Annexin V-FITC/PI staining assays was performed and the apoptotic and necrotic cells were quantified by flow cytometry. The percentages of necrotic (Q1), late apoptotic (Q2), early apoptotic (Q3) and live cells (Q4) are shown in Figure 8. The flow cytometry analysis revealed that early and late apoptosis represented the major death mode of MCF-7 cells, which was caused by free DOX or DOX released form GO (GOFA). The ratio of apoptosis cells treated with GOFA-DOX was 30.3%, compared with that of free DOX (8.6%). Most importantly, it is worth noting that the ratio of apoptosis cells treated with GOFA-DOX was markedly higher than that in cells treated with GO-DOX (11.2%), endorsing the targeting effect of FA. In general, the results of flow cytometry were consistent with the cell viability results by 3-(4,5-dimethyl-2-thiazolyl)-2,5-diphenyl-2H-tetrazolium bromide (MTT) assays (Figure 7A), underlining the importance of using GOFA to facilitate the entrance of DOX-loaded nano-carrier into the cells through endocytosis and subsequently release DOX that enters the nucleus to exert the cell cytotoxicity (Figure 5C,D). Furthermore, the FA-mediated intracellular uptake of GOFA could enhance the endocytosis of the nano-carrier to substantially increase the extent of cytotoxicity of DOX toward MCF-7 though cell apoptosis (Figure 5A,B).

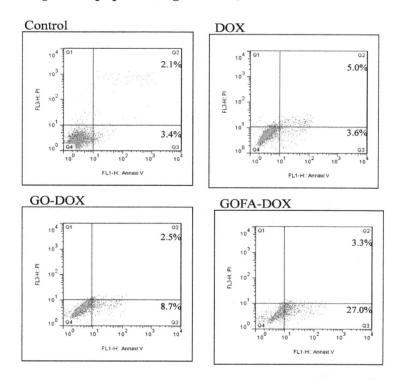

Figure 8. Flow cytometer analysis of the apoptotic and necrotic cells by Annexin V-FITC/PI staining (Q1: necrotic; Q2: late apoptotic; Q3: early apoptotic; Q4: live) after 24 h incubation with free DOX, GO-DOX and GOFA-DOX, respectively. The numbers in Q1 to Q3 indicate the percentage of cells after the treatment.

2.5. Animal Study

2.5.1. Antitumor Effect

With an aim to improve antitumor therapeutic effects and to decrease the side effects of DOX, we have successfully demonstrated that GOFA nano-carrier could conjugate with DOX and be encapsulated in HACPN to enhance its cytotoxicity toward MCF-7 breast cells in vitro. To validate those data in vivo, we administered the DOX-loaded GOFA in HACPN by taking advantage of the in-situ gelling property of the thermo-sensitive hydrogel. All BALB/c nude mice with an aggressive subcutaneous MCF-7 cells tumor were injected intratumorally with formulations containing saline (control), GOFA/HACPN, free DOX, GOFA-DOX or GOFA-DOX/HACPN, followed by measuring the tumor size and mouse body weight. In order to successful determining the anti-tumor effects in vivo, the size of the tumor was controlled within 60–100 mm^3 when the treatment started.

As shown in Figure 9A, the same trends of tumor growth were observed in the control group and the GOFA/HACPN group. The relative tumor volume increased rapidly during the treatment period and reached 2.17 ± 0.02 (control) and 1.79 ± 0.16 (GOFA/HACPN) at day 21 with no significant difference between groups. In contrast, the tumor growth rate was inhibited at different levels in all DOX-treated groups. The DOX, GOFA-DOX and GOFA-DOX/HACPN groups showed 0.82 ± 0.10, 0.67 ± 0.02 and 0.48 ± 0.07 relative tumor sizes at day 21, respectively, with significant difference among groups. Indeed, in vitro cytotoxicity results also endorsed the substantial enhancement of cytotoxicity of GOFA-DOX toward MCF-7 cells over free DOX at the same drug dosage (Figures 7A and 8). Intratumoral injection of DOX showed associated cytotoxic effects only at the early stage of treatment and short-term inhibition of tumor growth. The tumor volume rapidly dropped as early as 3 days after treatment and lasted for 4 days, followed by a rebound phenomenon in tumor volume at the later stage of treatment. For the GOFA-DOX group, with the targeting effect of FA, DOX could be more efficiently delivered to MCF-7 cells and the relative tumor volume could be significantly reduced throughout the test period after day 7 and showed minimal recovery 7 days after treatment. Nonetheless, the most efficient cytotoxic effect and continuous inhibition of tumor growth was observed only in the GOFA-DOX/HACPN group where the tumor size was continuously reduced up to 11 days to resulted in the highest tumor inhibition ratio of 52% (based on tumor volume changes) after 21 days, suggesting the in vivo anti-tumor efficacy using a combinatory GOFA-DOX/HACPN intratumoral drug delivery platform. These results demonstrated that thermo-sensitive HACPN hydrogel loading GOFA-DOX for cancer in-situ treatment could lead to more extensive destruction of tumor tissues and enhance the therapeutic efficiency. The enhanced intracellular uptake of GOFA-DOX contributed to the higher tumor-killing ability when compared with the free DOX dosage form. For comparison with GOFA-DOX, in-situ forming HACPN thermo-sensitive hydrogel can be retained around the tumor tissue and slowly released GOFA-DOX in concomitant with hydrogel degradation, which could raise local DOX concentration in the tumor and enhance the topical bioavailability of DOX for the best antitumor effect toward MCF-7 cells.

To assess the potential for adverse effects associated with treatments, mice were observed for changes in their body weight and appetite, for diarrhea and abnormal behavior over the course of treatments. Neither control nor drug-treated mice showed abnormalities in appetite and behavior throughout the 21 days observation period and there was no significant difference in weight for all treatment groups from the control (Figure 9B).

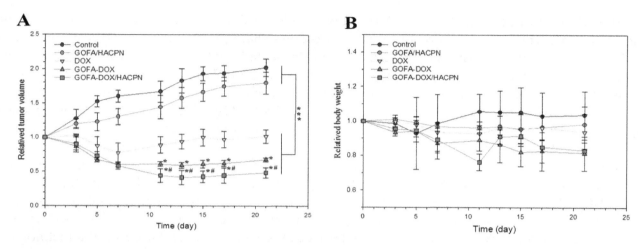

Figure 9.   Antitumor activity induced by DOX in nude mice bearing MCF-7 cancer cells. DOX (30 mg/kg) was administered intratumorally and tumor volume (**A**) and body weight (**B**) changes were recorded. The data are shown as mean $\pm$ standard deviation (SD), $n = 6$. * $p < 0.05$ compared with DOX, [#] $p < 0.05$ compared with GOFA-DOX, *** $p < 0.001$.

2.5.2. Histological and Systemic Toxicity Analysis

At day 21, the tumors were harvested for histological analysis. As shown in Figure 10A, there was no evidence of necrosis in the H&E staining slide for the tumor in the control group. Minimum necrosis was observed in the GOFA/HACPN group whereas some necrosis regions were observed in the free DOX and GOFA-DOX groups. There was significantly more necrosis regions in tumors treated with GOFA-DOX/HACPN when compared with other DOX-treated groups. Indeed, the H&E staining revealed that the cavitation phenomenon in coagulative necrosis was more obvious in the GOFA-DOX/HACPN group (Figure 10A). These results demonstrated that intratumoral delivery of GOFA-DOX/HACPN enhanced the anti-tumor efficacy, suggesting it is an excellent treatment for breast cancer.

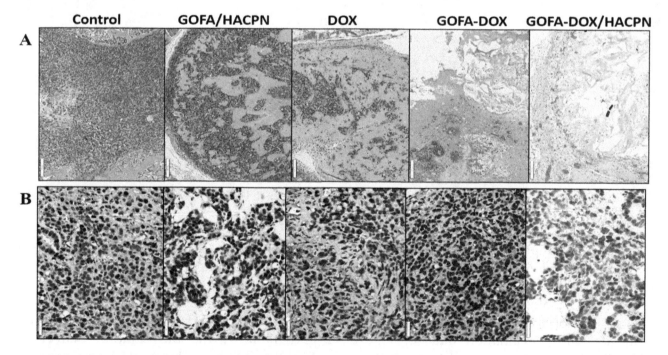

Figure 10. (**A**) H&E (Bar = 100 μm) and (**B**) proliferating cell nuclear antigen (PCNA) immunohistochemical (Bar = 20 μm) staining of retrieved tumor tissues at day 21.

Improved tumor delivery of DOX should also inhibit proliferation of cancer cells. Immunohistochemical examination of tumor sections associated with the cell proliferation marker-proliferating cell nuclear antigen (PCNA) clearly indicated that a greater number of actively proliferating tumor cells existed in tumor sections from the control and the GOFA/HACPN groups. In contrast, the tumor treated with DOX and GOFA-DOX showed weak PCNA immunoreactivity. The PCNA expression was the lowest in the GOFA-DOX/HACPN group than other groups (Figure 10B). Therefore, we conclude GOFA-DOX/HACPN can provide effective anticancer activity to effectively inhibit proliferation of cancer cells [48].

When the animals were euthanized, no gross abnormalities were observed in the treated mice. To further assess possible systemic toxicity, the major organs for the mice treated with GOFA-DOX/HACPN at day 21 were harvested for morphologic evaluation of H&E-stained sections and compared with those in the control group. As shown in Figure 11, the GOFA-DOX/HACPN group did not reveal any observable differences from the control group based on the histological examination of heart, lung, liver, spleen and kidney biopsy. H&E staining of the heart tissue sections showed striated cardiac muscles with the centrally placed nucleus. Normal alveoli without the sign of pulmonary fibrosis were seen in the lung sections. The histology of liver tissues revealed normal hepatocytes, central veins, portal triads and liver lobules. Red pulp and white pulp appeared in spleen samples. The kidney biopsy samples contained normal Bowman's capsule surrounding glomeruli as well as convoluted tubules. That the GOFA-DOX incorporated HACPN hydrogels exhibit reduced systemic toxicities could be due to the localized and delayed release of DOX encapsulated in HACPN at the tumor site for good biocompatibility and safety.

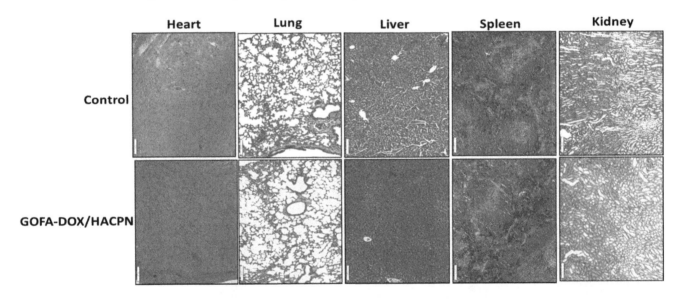

Figure 11. Histological examination of heart, lung, liver, spleen and kidney tissues by H&E stain after euthanization at day 21. Tissue biopsy did not reveal any observable differences between the control and the GOFA-DOX/HACPN group. Bar = 100 μm.

On blood sampling of animals after the experiment, the application of GOFA-DOX/HACPN did not significantly alter the level of blood counts and hepatic or renal functions from hematologic study when compared with the control group (Table 1). These results were consistent with the overall health of mice from histological analysis.

Clinical applications of anticancer drugs are limited by side effects such as cardiac toxicity [49]. From the safety evaluation data in Figure 11 and Table 1, the intratumoral delivery of GOFA-DOX/HACPN appeared to be well tolerated by the animals. This could be suggested to be stemmed from combined effects of intratumoral injection and in-situ forming drug delivery system. The intratumoral delivery of DOX using GOFA-DOX/HACPN could provide a high local concentration of the antitumor drug and the in-situ forming HACPN hydrogel together with GOFA-DOX would eliminate the initial burst release of DOX to reduce systemic toxicity [50].

Considering the toxicity of GO, it is generally considered to be safe for in vivo applications [51]. For HACPN, the biodegradable components chitosan and HA are safe science chitosan is biodegradable predominantly by lysozyme and by bacterial enzymes in the colon in vertebrates [52] while HA could be degraded through step-wise enzymatic or non-enzymatic reactions in vivo [53]. For the non-biodegradable PNIPAm component in HACPN, it was reported that low molecular weight PNIPAm showed good biocompatibility in vivo by undergoing renal clearance [54]. By using PNIPAm polymers with a low molecular weight (22 kDa) for HACPN synthesis [28], we did not expect the PNIPAm generated by HACPN degradation to exert any in vivo toxicity as it is below the renal cutoff [55].

Table 1. Blood analysis for evaluation of systemic toxicity.

Item	Unit	Control	GOFA-DOX/HACPN
Hematology			
WBC	10^3 cells/μL	5.78 ± 2.34	2.9 ± 0.6 *
RBC	10^6 cells/μL	8.57 ± 0.51	8.5 ± 0.2 *
HGB	g/dL	13.30 ± 0.87	13.2 ± 0.5 *
HCT	%	41.77 ± 2.23	39.1 ± 2.5 *
PLT	10^3 cells/μL	334.30 ± 29.8	279.5 ± 37.5 *
Clinical Chemistry			
AST	U/L	254.5 ± 19.1	294 ± 39.4 *
ALT	U/L	102.50 ± 0.71	113.8 ± 51.3 *
BUN	mg/dL	28.40 ± 3.54	32.1 ± 3.1 *
CREA	mg/dL	0.12 ± 0.01	0.13 ± 0.01 *

WBC: white blood cell; RBC: red blood cell; HGB: hemoglobin; HCT: hematocrit; PLT: platelet; AST: aspartate transaminase; ALT: alanine transaminase; BUN: blood urea nitrogen; CREA: creatinine Values are means ± standard deviation (SD) of six independent measurements. * $p > 0.05$ compared with control.

2.5.3. IVIS for Bioluminescence Imaging (BLI) Intensity

As residual hydrogel may influence the measurement of tumor volume, we further used a stably luciferase report gene-transfected MCF-7 cells (MCF-7/Luc) and in vivo imaging system (Xenogen IVIS-200, Caliper Life Sciences, Hopkinton, MA, USA) to determine the bioluminescence imaging (BLI) intensity of tumors formed from subcutaneous implanted MCF-7/Luc cells. It has been demonstrated that luciferase expression and bioluminescence does not affect tumor cell growth for MCF-7 cells [56]. For therapeutic effects from BLI imaging, the mean value of the normalized BLI signal intensity increased to 1738% in the control group after 21 days, reflecting an active tumor growth for MCF-7/Luc cells (Figure 12). Without any drug, the GOFA/HACPN treatment did not showed a significant difference in BLI signal from the control group, albeit with a lower mean BLI signal intensity of 1539%. In the DOX-treated group, the mean values decreased to 35.3% 21 days after single DOX administration, indicating that the cytotoxic effect of DOX affected tumor growth (Figure 12). In the GOFA-DOX group, the mean value further reduced to 25.0% with significant difference in BLI intensity from the DOX-treated group. However, a remarkable drop in normalized BLI signal intensity to 3.1% was observed for the combinatory GOFA-DOX/HACPN group and the BLI signal was significantly different from all DOX-treated groups. In general, the antitumor effect from different treatments with IVIS imaging was consistent with that from tumor volume change shown in Figure 9A.

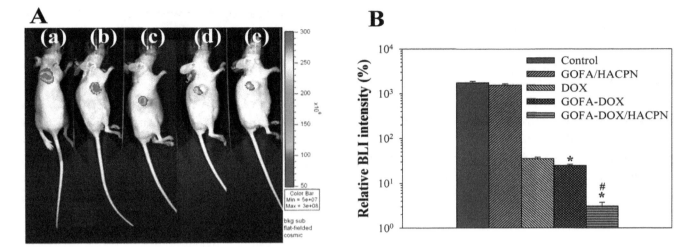

Figure 12. The bioluminescence imaging (BLI) of subcutaneously implanted MCF-7/Luc cells in nude mice. The BLI signal was measured at baseline (before treatment) and at day 21 after treatment. (**A**) Representative BLI obtained in the (**a**) control (saline), (**b**) GOFA/HACPN, (**c**) DOX, (**d**) GOFA-DOX and (**e**) GOFA-DOX/HACPN group by IVIS at day 21. (**B**) Plot of the relative BLI signal intensity at day 21 (mean ± SD, $n = 6$). The relative BLI signal intensity (%) was calculated from the total bioluminescent signal intensity at day 21 normalized by the total bioluminescent signal intensity at baseline. * $p < 0.05$ compared with DOX, # $p < 0.01$ compared with GOFA-DOX.

3. Materials and Methods

3.1. Materials

Graphene oxide (GO) (N002-PS) and quantum dots (QD) (QSA-490, CdSSe/ZnS core/shell QDs with amine group) were purchased from Angstron Materials (Dayton, OH, USA) and Ocean NanoTech (San Diego, CA, USA), respectively. N-isopropylacrylamide (NIPAM), azobisisobutyronitrile (AIBN), mercaptoacetic acid (MAA), chitosan (deacetylation degree = 98%, molecular weight = 1.5×10^5 Da), 2-morpholinoethane sulfonic acid (MES), 3-(4,5-dimethyl-2-thiazolyl)-2,5-diphenyl-2H-tetrazolium bromide, (MTT), 2,4,6-trinitrobenzene sulfonic acid (TNBS) and 4′,6-diamidino-2-phenylindole dihydrochloride (DAPI), folic acid (FA), doxorubicin (DOX) hydrochloride were purchased from Sigma-Aldrich (St. Louis, MO, USA). 1-ethyl-3-(3-dimethylaminopropyl) carbodiimide (EDC) and N-hydroxysuccinimide (NHS) were obtained from Acros (Geel, Belgium). Potassium salt of D-luciferin was obtained from Gold Biotechnology, Inc. (New Taipei City, Taiwan). Hyaluronic acid (HA, sodium hyaluronate) from *Streptococcus zooepidemicus* with an average molecular weight of 1.8×10^6 Da was purchased from Bloomage Freda Biopharm Co. (Jinan, China). Minimum Essential Medium (α-MEM, ThermoFisher Scientific, Waltham, MA, USA) and fetal bovine serum (FBS, HyClone, Logan, UT, USA) were used for cell culture.

3.2. Preparation and Characterization of GO and GOFA

3.2.1. Preparation of GO, GOFA and Quantum Dot (QD)-Labeled GO and GOFA

The preparation and modification of GO followed the modified Hummers' method [4,57]. Briefly, 1 g of GO was stirred in 23 mL sulfuric acid for 12 h, followed by slowly adding 3 g KMnO$_4$ below 20 °C. The temperature was increased to 40 °C while stirring for another 30 min. The temperature was increased to 80 °C and stirred for another 45 min. 46 mL of distilled deionized water (ddH$_2$O) was added and the solution was heated to 98–105 °C for 30 min, followed by cooling down to room temperature for 1 h. Additional ddH$_2$O (140 mL) and 10 mL of 30% H$_2$O$_2$ were added and reacted for 5 min at 40 °C. After the reaction, GO was washed three times with 5% hydrochloride acid by centrifugation and dialyzed against ddH$_2$O till the pH become neutral. Nano-sized GO was obtained by sonicating for 30 min at 800 W and filtered with a 0.2 μm filter and adjusted the final concentration of the GO solution to 0.2 mg/mL for future modification.

Folic acid (FA) molecules were conjugated to GO through carbodiimide-mediated covalent bonds formation between carboxyl groups in GO and amine groups in FA [9,58]. In short, 0.1 mg GO was mixed with 6 mM EDC and 6 mM NHS in 10 mL pH 6 phosphate buffered saline (PBS) for 1.5 h to activate the carboxyl groups in GO. One milliliter of FA solution (0.1 mg/mL) in pH 7.4 PBS was added to above solution and allowed to react at room temperature for 2 h to react the amine groups in FA with activated carboxyl groups in GO. After centrifugation at $14,000\times g$ for 30 min, the product was washed several times with ddH$_2$O to remove unreacted reagents and then dried at room temperature. The amount of FA immobilized to GO was determined by subtracting the amount of FA left in the reacting and washing solutions from the amount of FA initially added. The concentration of FA in the solution was determined by UV-Vis spectroscopy at 358 nm.

For preparing QD-labeled GO or GOFA, 0.5 mL of GO or GOFA (1 mg/mL) was reacted with 20 μL of 8 μM QDs and 0.05 mL of 60 mM EDC and 0.05 mL of 60 mM NHS for 90 min. After centrifugation at $14,000\times g$ for 30 min, the product was washed several times with PBS and dispersed in PBS for use.

3.2.2. Characterization of GO, GOFA and GOFA-DOX

An atomic force microscope (AFM) (XE-70, Park Systems, Santa Clara, CA, USA) was used to analyze the surface topography, size and thickness of samples. Diluted GO or GOFA in alcohol were deposited onto a freshly cleaved Mica substrate and imaged after alcohol evaporation. Transmission electron microscopy (TEM) images were taken using JEM-2000EXII TEM (JEOL, Tokyo, Japan). The Fourier transform infrared (FTIR) spectra were recorded on a FT-730 FTIR spectrometer (Horiba, Japan) by mixing samples with KBr and scanned from 400 to 4000 cm^{-1} at 2.5 mm/s.

3.3. Preparation and Characterization of HACPN Hydrogel

3.3.1. Synthesis of HACPN Hydrogel

The HACPN temperature-sensitive hydrogel was synthesized as described previously [28,59]. Briefly, NIPAM and AIBN were purified by recrystallization in n-hexane and methanol, respectively. PNIPAM end-capped with a carboxyl group (PNIPAM-COOH) was synthesized in benzene by free radical polymerization of NIPAM and MAA (chain transfer agent) in the presence of AIBN (initiator). PNIPAM-COOH was reacted with chitosan in 0.1 M MES buffer (pH 5.0) containing NHS and EDC to get chitosan-g-PNIPAM (CPN) copolymer. By thermally induced precipitation, the CPN copolymer was recovered by centrifugation. For HACPN synthesis, CPN copolymer was further reacted with HA in 0.1 M MES buffer (pH 5.0) containing EDC and NHS to get HACPN. Residual HA was removed by thermal precipitation of HACPN at 50 °C, followed by dialysis (molecular weight cut-off (MWCO) 300,000) at 4 °C and lyophilization.

3.3.2. Characterization of HACPN Hydrogel

To determine the LCST, 10% (w/v) polymer solutions (5% or 10% (w/v)) were prepared in ddH$_2$O. The sol-gel phase transition of the polymer solution was measured using an UV-Vis spectrophotometer (Spectronic 200, Thermo Scientific, Waltham, MA, USA) equipped with a circulator bath for temperature control. A semi-micro cuvette (10 mm light path) containing 2 mL of polymer solution was used. The absorbance of the polymer solution at 470 nm was recorded from 25 to 33 °C. The polymer solution was equilibrated at each test temperature for 60 min. From the thermo-precipitation curve by plotting the absorbance at 470 nm (OD$_{470}$) vs. temperature, the LCST of the polymer was defined as the temperature when the absorbance was half of the maximum value.

For sol-gel phase transition kinetics, 2 mL of 5% or 10% (w/v) of polymer solutions in ddH$_2$O were put in a semi-micro cuvette and sealed with Parafilm. The samples were equilibrated in a

25 °C incubator for 60 min and then placed in an UV-Vis spectrophotometer pre-equilibrated at 37 °C. The turbidity of polymer solution was recorded as a function of time up to 6 min.

For differential scanning calorimetry (DSC) analysis, 10 mg polymer solutions prepared in ddH$_2$O were placed in a DSC aluminum pan and analyzed with a Q20 DSC (TA Instruments, New Castle, DE, USA). The scan rate was 1 °C/min from 10 to 40 °C under 30 mL/min nitrogen.

For degradation of HACPN, 0.2 mL of 10% (*w/v*) HACPN hydrogel (20 mg HACPN) was placed in a pre-weighed Millicell® cell culture insert (Millipore) and immediately gelled at 37 °C. Five milliliters of PBS (pH 7.4, 37 °C) was added to the HACPN gel and the cell insert was shaken at 50 rpm in a 37 °C incubator. At different time points, samples were removed and rapidly frozen at −80 °C, followed by freeze-drying and weighing to obtain the residual weight of HACPN. The in vitro degradation of HACPN was calculated from the following equation,

$$\text{Residual weight}(\%) = (\frac{W_t}{W_i}) \times 100\% \tag{1}$$

where W_i is the initial weight of HACPN and W_t is the weight of HACPN at time t.

3.4. DOX Loading and Release

3.4.1. Loading of DOX on GOFA

A solution containing DOX (0.1–3.0 mg) and 0.1 mg of GOFA was prepared in 1 mL PBS (pH 7.4) and stirred at 4 °C for 24 h in dark. The GOFA-DOX were collected by ultracentrifugation (14,000× *g* for 15 min) and washed three times with PBS until the supernatant became color-free. The amount of unbound DOX in the solution was determined by measuring the absorbance at 490 nm (OD$_{490}$). The drug loading efficiency (%) and the drug loading content is defined as,

$$\text{Loading effcienct} (\%) = \frac{\text{Weight of loaded DOX (mg)}}{\text{Weight of initial DOX (mg)}} \times 100\% \tag{2}$$

$$\text{Loading content} = \frac{\text{Weight of loaded DOX (mg)}}{\text{Weight of GOFA (mg)}} \tag{3}$$

3.4.2. In Vitro DOX Release from GOFA-DOX and GOFA-DOX/HACPN

For drug release, 0.1 mg/mL GOFA-DOX was prepared in 1 mL of phosphate buffered saline (PBS) at pH 5.7 (endosomal pH) or at pH 7.4 (physiological pH) at 1.8 mg/mL DOX. The solution was shaken at 50 rpm and 37 °C, followed by ultracentrifugation to separate GOFA-DOX at pre-determined times [60]. All supernatant was removed and replenished with an equal volume of PBS of the same pH for further drug release studies. The concentration of DOX in the supernatant was quantified using an enzyme-linked immunosorbent assay (ELISA) reader at 490 nm. The DOX release results were calculated in a cumulative manner by the following equation [43],

$$\text{Cumulative Dox released} (\%) = (\frac{\text{Cumulative amout of DOX released}}{\text{Initial amount of DOX}}) \times 100\% \tag{4}$$

The DOX release from GOFA-DOX/HACPN hydrogel was determined for 10% (*w/v*) HACPN by dissolving 0.1 g HACPN in 1 mL GOFA-DOX solution (0.1 mg/mL in pH 7.4 PBS). 0.5 mL of HACPN solution was placed in Millicell® cell culture inserts fitted in a 6-well cell culture plate. 5 mL of PBS buffer (pH = 7.4) was added to each well to totally immerse the copolymer hydrogel in the insert and the plate was incubated at 37 °C by shaking at 50 rpm. At predetermined times, all solution in each well was removed for determination of the DOX concentration using an ELISA reader at 490 nm and an equal volume of PBS buffer (pH 7.4) was added to calculate the cumulative DOX release by Equation (4).

3.5. In Vitro Cell Culture

3.5.1. Cell Line and Cell Culture Condition

The MCF-7 human breast adenocarcinoma cell line (BCRC 60436) was obtained from the Bioresource Collection and Research Center (Hsinchu, Taiwan). The cells were cultured in α-MEM medium supplemented with 10% FBS at 37 °C in a humidified CO_2 incubator containing 5% CO_2. MCF-7 cells were sub-cultured routinely by using trypsin-ethylenediaminetetraacetic acid (EDTA) (Gibco, Thermo Fisher Scientific, Waltham, MA, USA) when cells reached 80–90% confluence.

The MCF-7/Luc cell line that could stably expresses firefly luciferase and neomycin-resistant genes was constructed from pGL4.51[*luc2*/CMV/Neo] plasmid vector (Promega, Madison, WI, USA) [56]. MCF-7 cells were transfected with the Luc-reporter vector and liposome (E2431, Promega) using standard protocols. Transfected cells were selected with 1 mg/mL G418 (Sigma-Aldrich, St. Louis, MO, USA) selection antibiotic for two weeks and the resistant colonies were isolated and tested for luciferase activity.

3.5.2. Intracellular Uptake

To evaluate the role of FA in cellular uptake of GOFA, MCF-7 cells were cultured in 0.5 mL α-MEM supplemented with 10% FBS in 24-well culture plates at 1×10^4 cells/well. Cells were grown overnight in a humidified CO_2 incubator at 37 °C under 5% CO_2 atmosphere, washed with sterilized PBS and incubated with 0.5 mL QD-labeled GO or GOFA suspension (0.1 mg/mL) for 1 h. Each testing samples were washed with PBS three times and fixed with 4% paraformaldehyde for 15 min, followed by nuclear staining with DAPI. In a separate experiment, the cells were pre-treated with free FA (1 mg/mL) for 1 h to block the folate receptor on cell surface before incubated with QD-labeled GOFA. Possible fluorescence signals from extracellular QD-labeled GOFA bound to the surfaces of MCF-7 cells were quenched by trypan blue dye solution for 15 min. Since trypan blue is excluded from entering live cells, all fluorescence signals observed will be only from GOFA taken intracellularly. The green fluorescence from QD and blue fluorescence from DAPI were examined under a confocal laser scanning microscope (Zeiss LSM 510 Meta, Oberkochen, Germany) with excitation/emission wavelength of 488 nm/500–550 nm and 364 nm/407–482 nm, respectively.

To determine intracellular uptake of GOFA-DOX and release of DOX, MCF-7 cells were cultured in 0.5 mL α-MEM supplemented with 10% FBS in 24-well culture plates at 1×10^4 cells/well. Cells were grown overnight in a humidified CO_2 incubator at 37 °C under 5% CO_2 atmosphere, washed with sterilized PBS and incubated with 0.5 mL DOX solution or GOFA-DOX suspension (0.1 mg/mL) for 1 h. Each testing samples were washed with PBS three times and fixed with 4% paraformaldehyde for 15 min, followed by nuclear staining with DAPI (blue) and examination under a confocal laser scanning microscope. The uptake of GOFA-DOX and release of DOX could be visualized by the green fluorescence of QD-labeled GOFA and the red fluorescence of DOX. The excitation wavelength is 543/488/364 nm (red/green/blue) and the emission wavelength is 550–650/500–550/407–482 nm (red/green/blue).

For transmission electron microscope (TEM) analysis, 1×10^5 of MCF-7 cells were grown on ThermoNox (Nunc, Roskilde, Denmark) coverslips and treated with GOFA for 24 h. The cells were fixed in a mixture of 2.5% paraformaldehyde and 2% glutaraldehyde solution for 2 h. Cells were rinsed in 0.1 M sodium cacodylate buffer (pH 7.4) and post-fixed in 1.0% osmium tetroxide for 30 min. The cells were then dehydrated in a graded ethanol series (30%, 50%, 70% with 3% uranyl acetate, 80%, 95% and 100%) for 10 min at each concentration and followed by two changes in 100% propylene oxide. After infiltration and embedding in epoxy resins at 60 °C for 48 h, ultrathin sections (approximately 80 nm) were examined under a FEI/Philips CM 120 TEM (Hillsboro, OR, USA).

3.5.3. In Vitro Cytotoxicity Assessment

For in vitro cytotoxicity tests, MCF-7 cells were cultured in α-MEM supplemented with 10% FBS in a 96-well culture plate at a seeding density of 1×10^4 cells/well and incubated overnight at 37 °C in a humidified 5% CO_2 atmosphere. After being rinsed with PBS (pH 7.4), the cells were incubated with 200 µL of DOX solutions, GO-DOX or GOFA-DOX suspensions prepared in culture medium containing different DOX concentrations to determine the IC50 (half-maximum inhibitory concentration) value. Cell viability after 24 h was determined using MTT assays by adding 50 µL MTT reagent to each well and incubated for 3 h at 37 °C. After removing the medium and MTT reagent, 200 µL of dimethylsulfoxide was added to the well to dissolve the crystal produced and the absorbance was measured at 540 nm using a Synergy HT microplate reader (BioTek, Winooski, VT, USA). Each experiment was repeated six times. All procedures were finished in conditions devoid of light. Cell viability using cell culture medium and GO (GOFA) were taken as 100% for DOX and GO-DOX (GOFA-DOX), respectively. Control cytotoxicity experiments to confirm the biocompatibility of the drug-free carrier were carried out using MCF-7 cells by following the same procedure as described above within a concentration range of 0.01–100 µg/mL GOFA.

The cytotoxicity of GOFA-DOX/HACPN was determined in a double-chamber dish with MCF-7 cells cultured in α-MEM supplemented with 10% FBS in a 24-well culture plate at a seeding density of 1×10^4 cells/well and incubated overnight at 37 °C in a humidified 5% CO_2 atmosphere. The GOFA/HACPN solution was prepared by dissolving 0.1 g HACPN in 1 mL GOFA-DOX solution (0.1 mg GOFA in pH 7.4 PBS) with 0, 0.001 or 0.025 mg/mL DOX). 0.2 mL of the GOFA-DOX/HACPN solution was placed in Millicell® cell culture inserts and fitted in the 24-well cell culture plate. The relative cell viability was determined by MTT assays at 24 and 72 h by MTT assays as described above with cell culture medium as control.

3.5.4. Analysis of Apoptosis Using Annexin V and Propidium Iodide Staining

Apoptotic MCF-7 cells were identified with fluorescein isothiocyanate-labeled Annexin V (Annexin V-FITC, BD Biosciences, Franklin Lakes, NJ, USA). Propidium iodide (PI) was also used as a dead cell marker. MCF-7 (5×10^5 cells per well) were seeded in a six-well plate and cultured for 24 h. After treatment with free DOX, GO-DOX and GOFA-DOX for 24 h, the cells were harvested, trypsinized, washed with PBS and incubated with Annexin V-FITC and PI for 15 min at room temperature in the dark. The samples were immediately analyzed with the FACSCalibur flow cytometer (BD Biosciences, Franklin Lakes, NJ, USA) with the CellQuest software.

3.6. Animal Studies

3.6.1. Xenograft Tumor Mouse Model

All animal procedures were approved by the Institutional Animal Care and Use Committee of Chang Gung University (IACUC Approval No. CGU14-092). Female nude mice (BALB/cAnN.Cg-Foxn1nu/CrlNarl, 4–6 weeks old, weighed between 20 and 25 g) were purchased from the National Laboratory Animal Center (Taipei, Taiwan) and used for the in vivo animal studies. Mice were cared, housed and maintained in specific sterile environment in the Laboratory Animal Center, Chang Gung University. Estrogen-responsive MCF-7 xenograft tumor model was established and maintained by injecting 5×10^6 MCF-7 cells (in 0.1 mL of Matrigel Matrix High Concentration, BD Biosciences, Franklin Lakes, NJ, USA) subcutaneously into the backs of the 6-week-old mice after anesthetized with 5 mg/kg xylazine (Rompum, Bayer) and 0.8 mg/kg Tiletamin + Zolezepam (Zoletil 50, Virbac) [61]. Animals were used in experiments after 14 days when the tumor volumes reached 60~100 mm^3.

3.6.2. In Vivo Antitumor Efficacy

Thirty tumor-bearing mice were randomly divided into 5 groups with 6 mice in each group. Group 1, intratumoral injection with 200 µL of saline (control); group 2, intratumoral injection with 200 µL of 10% (w/v) GOFA/HACPN; group 3, intratumoral injection with 200 µL of DOX solution (30 mg/kg of DOX); group 4, intravenous injection with 200 µL of GOFA-DOX (30 mg/kg of DOX); group 5, intratumoral injection with 200 µL of 10% (w/v) GOFA-DOX/HACPN (30 mg/kg of DOX). After administration, the tumor size and body weight was monitored continuously for 21 days. Tumor volumes were calculated based on the length and width of tumor (length $\times$ (width)^2/2). The relative of tumor volume (%) was calculated from V_t/V_0, where V_t indicated the tumor volume at time t and V_0 indicated the tumor volume at day 0. The relative body weight (%) was calculated according to W_t/W_0, where W_t indicated the weight at time t and W_0 indicated the weight at day 0.

3.6.3. Histological, Immunohistochemical, Hematologic and Biochemical Analysis

After sacrificing, tumor tissues were immediately harvested and fixed in 10% phosphate buffered formalin. The tissues were embedded in paraffin and sectioned (8 µm), followed by hematoxylin and eosin (H&E) staining. Paraffin-embedded tumor tissues were stained for proliferating cell nuclear antigen (PCNA) using N-Histofine® MOUSESTAIN KIT (Nichirei Biosciences Inc., Tokyo, Japan) following the manufacturer's protocol [62]. The primary antibody was mouse monoclonal anti-PCNA antibody (Abcam ab29).

To evaluate the systemic toxicity of GOFA-DOX/HACPN, major organs including hearts, livers, spleens, lungs and kidneys were harvested before euthanasia and embedded in paraffin and sectioned for H&E staining. Blood samples were collected for hematologic analysis (white blood cell count, red blood cell count, hemoglobin and hematocrit) and biochemical analysis (aspartate aminotransferase, alanine aminotransferase, blood urea nitrogen and creatinine) of major organ functions. The mice in the control group (saline) were used as comparison.

3.6.4. Bioluminescence Imaging (BLI) for In Vivo Evaluation of Anti-Tumor Efficacy

MCF-7/Luc cells were injected subcutaneously into the backs of the 6-week-old mice following and animal were grouped as described for MCF-7 cells. The bioluminescence imaging (BLI) was performed using noninvasive in vivo imaging system (IVIS) (Xenogen IVIS-200, Caliper Life Sciences, Hopkinton, MA, USA). Mice were anesthetized with 1% isoflurane in room air. D-Luciferin (Gold Biotechnology, New Taipei City, Taiwan) in PBS (15 mg/mL) was injected intraperitoneally at a dose of 150 mg/kg and images were acquired to determine the peak bioluminescence. The BLI intensity was determined at baseline (i.e., before treatment) and 21 days after treatment by measuring the total peak bioluminescent signal intensity through standardized regions of interest (ROIs) in tumor by using the Living Image® 4.0 software (PerkinElmer, Waltham, MA, USA). The relative BLI (%) was calculated from the total bioluminescent signal intensity at day 21 normalized by the total signal intensity at baseline.

3.7. Statistical Analyses

All data were reported as mean $\pm$ standard deviation (SD). Statistical significances were analyzed by Statistical Product and Service Solutions (SPSS) one-way ANOVA Least Significant Difference (LSD) test and differences were considered significant at $p < 0.05$.

4. Conclusions

In conclusion, we have confirmed the synthesis of the nano-sized anticancer drug carrier GOFA, the intracellular uptake of GOFA by endocytosis and the specific targeting effect of GOFA toward MCF-7 breast cancer cells. The high loading capacity of DOX on GOFA in addition to the pH-dependent drug release behavior could facilitate drug release after endocytosis and maintain a high drug concentration cytotoxic to MCF-7 cells. The temperature-sensitive in-situ forming hydrogel HACPN could provide fast sol-gel phase transition kinetics around the physiological temperature. The gelled HACPN could serve as a depot for continuous GOFA-DOX release during hydrogel degradation and offer a facile intratumoral delivery platform for the chemotherapeutic drug. Enhanced cytotoxicity of GOFA-DOX toward MCF-7 was confirmed through MTT assays and flow cytometry analysis, which could be ascribed to the FA-targeting effect. GOFA-DOX/HACPN also showed effective drug dosage and time-dependent cytotoxicity effects in vitro, suggesting its potential for in vivo anticancer therapy. From xenograft tumor mouse model with subcutaneously implanted MCF-7 (MCF-7/Luc) cells, tumor volume measurement and BLI signal intensity revealed the highest anticancer efficiency of GOFA-DOX/HACPN. H&E staining and immunohistochemistry of tumor tissues confirmed this treatment could result in the best effect to induce tumor necrosis and reduction of expression of the tumor cell proliferating marker (PCNA). In addition, no side effects were detected from biopsy of major organs and blood analysis to endorse the safety of this treatment. Taken together, we could conclude the intratumoral delivery of GOFA-DOX/HACPN could be suggested as a safe and effective drug delivery system for breast cancer chemotherapy or potentially also applicable to treatment of other local solid tumors.

Acknowledgments: We would like to express our appreciation of financial supports provided by Change Gung Memorial Hospital (CMRPD3E0272, CMRPD2G0081 and BMRP249) and the Ministry of Science and Technology (NERPD2C0461, MOST-106-2221-E-182-056-MY3). The Microscope Core Laboratory in Change Gung Memorial Hospital, Linkou, is acknowledged for the assistance in microscopic studies.

Author Contributions: Chih-Hao Chen and Jyh-Ping Chen conceived and designed the experiments; Yi Teng Fong and Chih-Hao Chen performed the experiments; Yi Teng Fong and Chih-Hao Chen analyzed the data; Yi Teng Fong and Jyh-Ping Chen wrote the paper.

References

1. Govindan, B.; Swarna Latha, B.; Nagamony, P.; Ahmed, F.; Saifi, M.A.; Harrath, A.H.; Alwasel, S.; Mansour, L.; Alsharaeh, E.H. Designed synthesis of nanostructured magnetic hydroxyapatite based drug nanocarrier for anti-cancer drug delivery toward the treatment of human epidermoid carcinoma. *Nanomaterials* **2017**, *7*, 138. [CrossRef] [PubMed]

2. Martínez-Carmona, M.; Colilla, M.; Vallet-Regí, M. Smart mesoporous nanomaterials for antitumor therapy. *Nanomaterials* **2015**, *5*, 1906–1937. [CrossRef] [PubMed]

3. Debbage, P. Targeted drugs and nanomedicine: Present and future. *Curr. Pharm. Des.* **2009**, *15*, 153–172. [CrossRef] [PubMed]

4. Lu, Y.-J.; Yang, H.-W.; Hung, S.-C.; Huang, C.-Y.; Li, S.-M.; Ma, C.; Chen, P.-Y.; Tsai, H.-C.; Wei, K.-C.; Chen, J.-P. Improving thermal stability and efficacy of BCNU in treating glioma cells using PAA-functionalized graphene oxide. *Int. J. Nanomed.* **2012**, *7*, 1737–1747.

5. Wang, Y.; Li, Z.; Wang, J.; Li, J.; Lin, Y. Graphene and graphene oxide: Biofunctionalization and applications in biotechnology. *Trends Biotechnol.* **2011**, *29*, 205–212. [CrossRef] [PubMed]

6. Yang, X.; Zhang, X.; Ma, Y.; Huang, Y.; Wang, Y.; Chen, Y. Superparamagnetic graphene oxide–Fe_3O_4 nanoparticles hybrid for controlled targeted drug carriers. *J. Mater. Chem.* **2009**, *19*, 2710–2714. [CrossRef]

7. Sun, X.; Liu, Z.; Welsher, K.; Robinson, J.T.; Goodwin, A.; Zaric, S.; Dai, H. Nano-graphene oxide for cellular imaging and drug delivery. *Nano Res.* **2008**, *1*, 203–212. [CrossRef] [PubMed]

8. Liu, Z.; Robinson, J.T.; Sun, X.; Dai, H. Pegylated nanographene oxide for delivery of water-insoluble cancer drugs. *J. Am. Chem. Soc.* **2008**, *130*, 10876–10877. [CrossRef] [PubMed]

9. Zhang, L.; Xia, J.; Zhao, Q.; Liu, L.; Zhang, Z. Functional graphene oxide as a nanocarrier for controlled loading and targeted delivery of mixed anticancer drugs. *Small* **2010**, *6*, 537–544. [CrossRef] [PubMed]

10. Yang, X.; Zhang, X.; Liu, Z.; Ma, Y.; Huang, Y.; Chen, Y. High-efficiency loading and controlled release of doxorubicin hydrochloride on graphene oxide. *J. Phys. Chem. C* **2008**, *112*, 17554–17558. [CrossRef]

11. Ma, N.; Zhang, B.; Liu, J.; Zhang, P.; Li, Z.; Luan, Y. Green fabricated reduced graphene oxide: Evaluation of its application as nano-carrier for pH-sensitive drug delivery. *Int. J. Pharm.* **2015**, *496*, 984–992. [CrossRef] [PubMed]

12. Wu, S.Y.; An, S.S.; Hulme, J. Current applications of graphene oxide in nanomedicine. *Int. J. Nanomed.* **2015**, *10*, 9–24.

13. Bae, K.H.; Chung, H.J.; Park, T.G. Nanomaterials for cancer therapy and imaging. *Mol. Cells* **2011**, *31*, 295–302. [CrossRef] [PubMed]

14. Cho, K.; Wang, X.; Nie, S.; Shin, D.M. Therapeutic nanoparticles for drug delivery in cancer. *Clin. Cancer Res.* **2008**, *14*, 1310–1316. [CrossRef] [PubMed]

15. Wu, B.; Zhao, N. A Targeted nanoprobe based on carbon nanotubes-natural biopolymer chitosan composites. *Nanomaterials* **2016**, *6*, 216. [CrossRef] [PubMed]

16. Sahu, S.K.; Mallick, S.K.; Santra, S.; Maiti, T.K.; Ghosh, S.K.; Pramanik, P. In vitro evaluation of folic acid modified carboxymethyl chitosan nanoparticles loaded with doxorubicin for targeted delivery. *J. Mater. Sci. Mater. Med.* **2010**, *21*, 1587–1597. [CrossRef] [PubMed]

17. Yang, C.L.; Chen, J.P.; Wei, K.C.; Chen, J.Y.; Huang, C.W.; Liao, Z.X. Release of doxorubicin by a folate-grafted, chitosan-coated magnetic nanoparticle. *Nanomaterials* **2017**, *7*, 85. [CrossRef] [PubMed]

18. Lu, Y.J.; Wei, K.C.; Ma, C.C.; Yang, S.Y.; Chen, J.P. Dual targeted delivery of doxorubicin to cancer cells using folate-conjugated magnetic multi-walled carbon nanotubes. *Colloids Surf. B Biointerfaces* **2012**, *89*, 1–9. [CrossRef] [PubMed]

19. Liow, S.S.; Dou, Q.; Kai, D.; Karim, A.A.; Zhang, K.; Xu, F.; Loh, X.J. Thermogels: In situ gelling biomaterial. *ACS Biomater. Sci. Eng.* **2016**, *2*, 295–316. [CrossRef]

20. Rzaev, Z.M.; Dincer, S.; Pişkin, E. Functional copolymers of *N*-isopropylacrylamide for bioengineering applications. *Prog. Polym. Sci.* **2007**, *32*, 534–595. [CrossRef]

21. Okano, T.; Yamada, N.; Sakai, H.; Sakurai, Y. A novel recovery system for cultured cells using plasma-treated polystyrene dishes grafted with poly(*N*-isopropylacrylamide). *J. Biomed. Mater. Res.* **1993**, *27*, 1243–1251. [CrossRef] [PubMed]

22. Gil, E.S.; Hudson, S.M. Stimuli-responsive polymers and their bioconjugates. *Prog. Polym. Sci.* **2004**, *29*, 1173–1222. [CrossRef]

23. Fakhari, A.; Subramony, J.A. Engineered in-situ depot-forming hydrogels for intratumoral drug delivery. *J. Control. Release* **2015**, *220*, 465–475. [CrossRef] [PubMed]

24. Wolinsky, J.B.; Colson, Y.L.; Grinstaff, M.W. Local drug delivery strategies for cancer treatment: Gels, nanoparticles, polymeric films, rods and wafers. *J. Control. Release* **2012**, *159*, 14–26. [CrossRef] [PubMed]

25. Kempe, S.; Mäder, K. In situ forming implants—An attractive formulation principle for parenteral depot formulations. *J. Control. Release* **2012**, *161*, 668–679. [CrossRef] [PubMed]

26. Loh, X.J.; Li, J. Biodegradable thermosensitive copolymer hydrogels for drug delivery. *Expert Opin. Ther. Pat.* **2007**, *17*, 965–977. [CrossRef]

27. Wu, W.; Chen, H.; Shan, F.; Zhou, J.; Sun, X.; Zhang, L.; Gong, T. A novel doxorubicin-loaded in situ forming gel based high concentration of phospholipid for intratumoral drug delivery. *Mol. Pharm.* **2014**, *11*, 3378–3385. [CrossRef] [PubMed]

28. Chen, J.-P.; Cheng, T.-H. Preparation and evaluation of thermo-reversible copolymer hydrogels containing chitosan and hyaluronic acid as injectable cell carriers. *Polymer* **2009**, *50*, 107–116. [CrossRef]

29. Huang, Y.-S.; Lu, Y.-J.; Chen, J.-P. Magnetic graphene oxide as a carrier for targeted delivery of chemotherapy drugs in cancer therapy. *J. Magn. Magn. Mater.* **2017**, *427*, 34–40. [CrossRef]

30. Zhi, F.; Dong, H.; Jia, X.; Guo, W.; Lu, H.; Yang, Y.; Ju, H.; Zhang, X.; Hu, Y. Functionalized graphene oxide mediated adriamycin delivery and miR-21 gene silencing to overcome tumor multidrug resistance in vitro. *PLoS ONE* **2013**, *8*, e60034. [CrossRef] [PubMed]

31. Lu, C.-H.; Zhu, C.-L.; Li, J.; Liu, J.-J.; Chen, X.; Yang, H.-H. Using graphene to protect DNA from cleavage during cellular delivery. *Chem. Commun.* **2010**, *46*, 3116–3118. [CrossRef] [PubMed]

32. Chen, J.P.; Cheng, T.H. Thermo-responsive chitosan-graft-poly(*N*-isopropylacrylamide) injectable hydrogel for cultivation of chondrocytes and meniscus cells. *Macromol. Biosci.* **2006**, *6*, 1026–1039. [CrossRef] [PubMed]

33. Fang, J.Y.; Chen, J.P.; Leu, Y.L.; Hu, J.W. Temperature-sensitive hydrogels composed of chitosan and hyaluronic acid as injectable carriers for drug delivery. *Eur. J. Pharm. Biopharm.* **2008**, *68*, 626–636. [CrossRef] [PubMed]

34. Feil, H.; Bae, Y.H.; Feijen, J.; Kim, S.W. Effect of comonomer hydrophilicity and ionization on the lower critical solution temperature of N-isopropylacrylamide copolymers. *Macromolecules* **1993**, *26*, 2496–2500. [CrossRef]

35. Gao, Y.; Yang, J.; Ding, Y.; Ye, X. Effect of urea on phase transition of poly(N-isopropylacrylamide) investigated by differential scanning calorimetry. *J. Phys. Chem. B* **2014**, *118*, 9460–9466. [CrossRef] [PubMed]

36. Kamath, K.R.; Park, K. Biodegradable hydrogels in drug delivery. *Adv. Drug Deliv. Rev.* **1993**, *11*, 59–84. [CrossRef]

37. Cho, J.K.; Hong, K.Y.; Park, J.W.; Yang, H.K.; Song, S.C. Injectable delivery system of 2-methoxyestradiol for breast cancer therapy using biodegradable thermosensitive poly(organophosphazene) hydrogel. *J. Drug Target.* **2011**, *19*, 270–280. [CrossRef] [PubMed]

38. Li, R.; Wu, R.A.; Zhao, L.; Hu, Z.; Guo, S.; Pan, X.; Zou, H. Folate and iron difunctionalized multiwall carbon nanotubes as dual-targeted drug nanocarrier to cancer cells. *Carbon* **2011**, *49*, 1797–1805. [CrossRef]

39. Zhou, T.; Zhou, X.; Xing, D. Controlled release of doxorubicin from graphene oxide based charge-reversal nanocarrier. *Biomaterials* **2014**, *35*, 4185–4194. [CrossRef] [PubMed]

40. Depan, D.; Shah, J.; Misra, R. Controlled release of drug from folate-decorated and graphene mediated drug delivery system: Synthesis, loading efficiency and drug release response. *Mater. Sci. Eng. C* **2011**, *31*, 1305–1312. [CrossRef]

41. Saul, J.M.; Annapragada, A.; Natarajan, J.V.; Bellamkonda, R.V. Controlled targeting of liposomal doxorubicin via the folate receptor in vitro. *J. Control. Release* **2003**, *92*, 49–67. [CrossRef]

42. Wong, H.L.; Rauth, A.M.; Bendayan, R.; Manias, J.L.; Ramaswamy, M.; Liu, Z.; Erhan, S.Z.; Wu, X.Y. A new polymer–lipid hybrid nanoparticle system increases cytotoxicity of doxorubicin against multidrug-resistant human breast cancer cells. *Pharm. Res.* **2006**, *23*, 1574–1585. [CrossRef] [PubMed]

43. Manaspon, C.; Viravaidya-Pasuwat, K.; Pimpha, N. Preparation of folate-conjugated Pluronic F127/chitosan core-shell nanoparticles encapsulating doxorubicin for breast cancer treatment. *J. Nanomater.* **2012**, *2012*, 22. [CrossRef]

44. Lee, D.-G.; Ponvel, K.M.; Kim, M.; Hwang, S.; Ahn, I.-S.; Lee, C.-H. Immobilization of lipase on hydrophobic nano-sized magnetite particles. *J. Mol. Catal. B Enzym.* **2009**, *57*, 62–66. [CrossRef]

45. Zunino, F.; Di Marco, A.; Zaccara, A.; Luoni, G. The inhibition of RNA polymerase by daunomycin. *Chem.-Biol. Interact.* **1974**, *9*, 25–36. [CrossRef]

46. Frederick, C.A.; Williams, L.D.; Ughetto, G.; Van der Marel, G.A.; Van Boom, J.H.; Rich, A.; Wang, A.-J. Structural comparison of anticancer drug-DNA complexes: Adriamycin and daunomycin. *Biochemistry* **1990**, *29*, 2538–2549. [CrossRef] [PubMed]

47. Meyn, M.S. Ataxia-telangiectasia and cellular responses to DNA damage. *Cancer Res.* **1995**, *55*, 5991–6001. [PubMed]

48. Kim, J.I.; Lee, B.S.; Chun, C.; Cho, J.-K.; Kim, S.-Y.; Song, S.-C. Long-term theranostic hydrogel system for solid tumors. *Biomaterials* **2012**, *33*, 2251–2259. [CrossRef] [PubMed]

49. Frishman, W.H.; Yee, H.C.M.; Keefe, D.; Sung, H.M.; Liu, L.L.; Einzig, A.I.; Dutcher, J. Cardiovascular toxicity with cancer chemotherapy. *Curr. Probl. Cancer* **1997**, *21*, 301–360. [CrossRef]

50. Luo, J.W.; Zhang, T.; Zhang, Q.; Cao, X.; Zeng, X.; Fu, Y.; Zhang, Z.R.; Gong, T. A novel injectable phospholipid gel co-loaded with doxorubicin and bromotetrandrine for resistant breast cancer treatment by intratumoral injection. *Colloids Surf. B Biointerfaces* **2016**, *140*, 538–547. [CrossRef] [PubMed]

51. Seabra, A.B.; Paula, A.J.; de Lima, R.; Alves, O.L.; Durán, N. Nanotoxicity of graphene and graphene oxide. *Chem. Res. Toxicol.* **2014**, *27*, 159–168. [CrossRef] [PubMed]

52. Kean, T.; Thanou, M. Biodegradation, biodistribution and toxicity of chitosan. *Adv. Drug Deliv. Rev.* **2010**, *62*, 3–11. [CrossRef] [PubMed]

53. Fakhari, A.; Berkland, C. Applications and emerging trends of hyaluronic acid in tissue engineering, as a dermal filler and in osteoarthritis treatment. *Acta Biomater.* **2013**, *9*, 7081–7092. [CrossRef] [PubMed]

54. Kohori, F.; Sakai, K.; Aoyagi, T.; Yokoyama, M.; Sakurai, Y.; Okano, T. Preparation and characterization of thermally responsive block copolymer micelles comprising poly(N-isopropylacrylamide-b-DL-lactide). *J. Control. Release* **1998**, *55*, 87–98. [CrossRef]

55. Patenaude, M.; Hoare, T. Injectable, degradable thermoresponsive poly(N-isopropylacrylamide) hydrogels. *ACS Macro Lett.* **2012**, *1*, 409–413. [CrossRef]

56. Tiffen, J.C.; Bailey, C.G.; Ng, C.; Rasko, J.E.; Holst, J. Luciferase expression and bioluminescence does not affect tumor cell growth in vitro or in vivo. *Mol. Cancer* **2010**, *9*, 299. [CrossRef] [PubMed]

57. Hummers, W.S., Jr.; Offeman, R.E. Preparation of graphitic oxide. *J. Am. Chem. Soc.* **1958**, *80*, 1339. [CrossRef]

58. Huang, P.; Xu, C.; Lin, J.; Wang, C.; Wang, X.; Zhang, C.; Zhou, X.; Guo, S.; Cui, D. Folic acid-conjugated graphene oxide loaded with photosensitizers for targeting photodynamic therapy. *Theranostics* **2011**, *1*, 240–250. [CrossRef] [PubMed]

59. Liao, H.-T.; Chen, C.-T.; Chen, J.-P. Osteogenic differentiation and ectopic bone formation of canine bone marrow-derived mesenchymal stem cells in injectable thermo-responsive polymer hydrogel. *Tissue Eng. Part C Methods* **2011**, *17*, 1139–1149. [CrossRef] [PubMed]

60. Grenha, A.; Seijo, B.; Remunán-López, C. Microencapsulated chitosan nanoparticles for lung protein delivery. *Eur. J. Pharm. Sci.* **2005**, *25*, 427–437. [CrossRef] [PubMed]

61. Wang, T.; Hartner, W.C.; Gillespie, J.W.; Praveen, K.P.; Yang, S.; Mei, L.A.; Petrenko, V.A.; Torchilin, V.P. Enhanced tumor delivery and antitumor activity in vivo of liposomal doxorubicin modified with MCF-7-specific phage fusion protein. *Nanomed. Nanotechnol. Biol. Med.* **2014**, *10*, 421–430. [CrossRef] [PubMed]

62. Xie, Y.; Long, Q.; Wu, Q.; Shi, S.; Dai, M.; Liu, Y.; Liu, L.; Gong, C.; Qian, Z.; Wei, Y. Improving therapeutic effect in ovarian peritoneal carcinomatosis with honokiol nanoparticles in a thermosensitive hydrogel composite. *RSC Adv.* **2012**, *2*, 7759–7771. [CrossRef]

13

Trends towards Biomimicry in Theranostics

Michael Evangelopoulos [1], Alessandro Parodi [2], Jonathan O. Martinez [1] and Ennio Tasciotti [1,3,*]

[1]   Center for Biomimetic Medicine, Houston Methodist Research Institute, Houston, TX 77030, USA;
      mevangelopoulos@houstonmethodist.org (M.E.); jomartinez@houstonmethodist.org (J.O.M.)
[2]   Department of Pharmacology, University of Illinois at Chicago, Chicago, IL 60607, USA; aparodi@uic.edu
[3]   Department of Orthopedics & Sports Medicine, Houston Methodist Hospital, Houston, TX 77030, USA
*   Correspondence: etasciotti@houstonmethodist.org;

Abstract: Over the years, imaging and therapeutic modalities have seen considerable progress as a result of advances in nanotechnology. Theranostics, or the marrying of diagnostics and therapy, has increasingly been employing nano-based approaches to treat cancer. While first-generation nanoparticles offered considerable promise in the imaging and treatment of cancer, toxicity and non-specific distribution hindered their true potential. More recently, multistage nanovectors have been strategically designed to shield and carry a payload to its intended site. However, detection by the immune system and sequestration by filtration organs (i.e., liver and spleen) remains a major obstacle. In an effort to circumvent these biological barriers, recent trends have taken inspiration from biology. These bioinspired approaches often involve the use of biologically-derived cellular components in the design and fabrication of biomimetic nanoparticles. In this review, we provide insight into early nanoparticles and how they have steadily evolved to include bioinspired approaches to increase their theranostic potential.

Keywords: biomimetic;   bioinspired;   cancer;   multistage   nanovectors;   nanomedicine; nanoparticles; theranostics

---

1. Introduction

Over the past several decades, medicine has benefitted significantly from the use of imaging modalities to help guide diagnosis and treatment. While our ability to look inside the body was initially largely limited to what could be felt, the introduction of more advanced imaging systems (e.g., X-ray imaging) helped revolutionize the field of imaging and is now among medicine's leading diagnostic tools. Since then, imaging modalities to treat diseases have evolved from simple X-rays to high resolution computer augmented virtual environments that allow physicians to navigate the various layers of the body in greater detail [1–4]. However, despite imaging systems evolving to generate great detail and delineate the complexity of the body, diagnosis and treatment algorithms continue to remain a two-step process, consequently limiting the onset of therapy [5]. More so, although nanotechnology has been introduced as an effective utility to concentrate a payload to a target site [6–8], thereby limiting toxicity to healthy tissue and other side effects, this approach continues to require two distinct steps to diagnose and treat disease. To mitigate these shortcomings, significant interest has been sparked towards the development of therapies that aim to combine diagnostic and therapeutic capabilities into a single agent.

This new class of treatment, referred to as theranostics, has led to the development of a large arsenal of therapeutic agents that offer a viable one-step treatment solution [9–11]. For example, nanomaterials capable of enhancing tumor imaging while concurrently delivering a therapy is only one application in which theranostic-based technologies are being exploited [12,13]. With the urgency required in the timely diagnosis and subsequent treatment of cancer, time-saving theranostic treatments have garnered tremendous support [5,14–16].

Recently, in an effort to further strengthen the effectiveness of theranostics, bioinspired approaches have been developed with a goal of providing biological-like behaviors to synthetic theranostic vectors. In this review, we outline the fundamental imaging modalities that have largely contributed to the development of theranostic-based therapies followed with a discussion on multi-step delivery vectors that have contributed to furthering efficacy for these imaging modalities. Lastly, a brief overview of bioinspired theranostic strategies is discussed.

2. Nanoparticle-Based Theranostics

2.1. Iron Oxide Nanoparticles

Iron Oxide nanoparticles (IONP) have generated tremendous momentum in nanomedicine due to their many beneficial properties [17]. Distinctive elements such as superparamagnetism, susceptibility to surface-modifications (e.g., polyethylene glycol, dextran, polypeptides, etc.), and high surface to volume ratios have proven highly useful, particularly for magnetic resonance imaging (MRI) and drug delivery [18–20]. Composed of ferrite nanocrystallites of magnetite and their oxidized counterpart maghemite, the last decade has witnessed considerable interest in these particles for theranostic applications. Specifically, it has been found that when IONP are reduced to a size of <20 nm, they become superparamagnetic in the presence of a magnetic field [21]. Conversely, when the magnetic field is turned off, the particles become highly dispersed [22]. In clinical applications, this feature is critical as the aggregation of particles can lead to detection and sequestration by the mononuclear phagocyte system (MPS), inhibiting IONP from reaching their target and significantly lowering their efficacy [23].

These features, coupled with the use of a magnetic field as a guiding mechanism, can be beneficial in a number of ways. For example, the total drug amount needed to achieve a clinical effect can be reduced, resulting in a decrease in the frequency of administration and minimal cytotoxic effects on healthy tissue [24]. Furthermore, when subjected to an alternating magnetic field, IONP have also been shown to dissipate heat, resulting in an increase in temperature in the surrounding area. This feature has been exploited in magnetic hyperthermia to kill cancer cells, resulting in an increase of over 10 °C at the injection site (Figure 1) [25]. Meanwhile, surface modifications (e.g., antibodies, dyes, chemotherapeutics) garnered beneficial properties for IONP by prolonging circulation [26] and increasing cancer-targeting abilities [27]. In one case, IONP were functionalized with cystine, the oxidized dimer of cysteine, to achieve improved biocompatibility and hydrophilicity [28]. In addition, cystine-functionalized IONP demonstrated versatility as a viable contrast agent for MRI, as well as ultrasonography, further exhibiting its potential for theranostic applications.

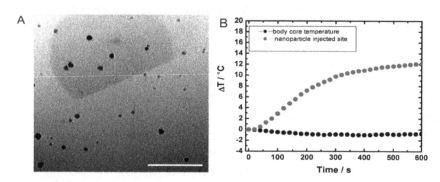

Figure 1. (**A**) Transmission electron microscope image of IONP fabricated with a dopamine-anchored shell, scale bar, 100 nm; (**B**) Quantitative analysis depicted the temperature changes at the nanoparticle injection site versus the body core as measured with a fiber optic temperature probe. Images reproduced from [25], with permission from BioMed Central Ltd., 2010.

While multifunctional nanoparticles have recently gained significant attention, improvements still need to be made in the loading ability of nanoparticles into the drug carrier. Yoon et al. reported that IONP co-loaded with the chemotherapeutic, paclitaxel, into micelles, showed promising results as a candidate for the combined imaging and treatment of cancer [29]. These results show micelles, encapsulated with both a chemotherapeutic payload and imaging agent, were able to inhibit the growth of a tumor in vivo by more than 50% compared to a control group, thereby demonstrating this coupled approach as a promising theranostic tool. Nevertheless, limitations of IONP continue to exist. For example, the physiological environment of the body causes drug-conjugated IONP to suddenly release the payload upon administration, thereby limiting its effectiveness at the intended site. Efforts to mitigate the adverse release of payloads have been achieved through the incorporation of layer-by-layer fabrication using oppositely charged polymers [30]. This attempt exhibited the development of a stabilized IONP formulation while also achieving the simultaneous loading of naturally-derived compounds.

In general, multi-modal systems incorporating IONP have drawn considerable attention for their magnetic and photothermal properties. In more recent efforts, merging polymer responsive materials with IONP have exhibited desirable properties through the manipulation of environmental factors to achieve therapeutic potency and imaging potential [31]. A more comprehensive analysis has recently been conducted by Pellegrino and coworkers discussing the current state of magnetic-based stimuli-responsive systems [32]. Nevertheless, the cytotoxicity of IONP is still debated, with some reports revealing increased toxicity (i.e., disruption of cell cytoskeleton) [33] and others demonstrating no toxicity (i.e., no increase of reactive oxygen species) [34]. Additionally, although IONP were successful in generating initial buzz under familiar names such as Feridex, they ultimately failed commercially due to adverse side effects and lack of diagnostic utility [35]. Despite this, a resurgence of their use has been found in the treatment of iron deficiency with more recent efforts exploiting the use of ferromagnetic IONP (i.e., permanent magnetism) for diagnostic imaging, thereby reaffirming the multitude of applications possible with IONP.

2.2. Gold Nanoparticles

Similar to IONP, gold-based nanoparticles have also gained significant popularity over the past decade, seeing applications ranging from optical bioimaging to detection of cancer. Features such as high surface area to volume ratio coupled with cytocompatibility and stability have made gold an ideal candidate for photothermal therapy [36]. In addition to these properties, ease of synthesis and conversion of heat using near-infrared (NIR) light have enabled the use of gold (e.g., nanoshells, nanorods, hollow gold) [37] for a variety of photo-triggered treatments. Specifically, using surface plasmon resonance for photodynamic therapy has drawn particular interest. In particular, exploitation of the combined resonant oscillation of free electrons present on the particle surface, thereby outputting a sharp absorption band, has led to the use of gold nanoparticles in a variety of imaging and therapeutic applications [38]. More so, the ability to conjugate antibodies onto the nanoparticle surface paved the way for direct electron microscopic visualization while minimal toxicity and light scattering efficiency opened the door for a multitude of biomedical applications. Khlebtsov et al. have shown promising results of multifunctional nanoparticles consisting of gold-loaded hematoporphyrin-doped silica particles as an antimicrobial therapeutic [39]. Others have also shown promising applications of gold-based nanoparticles as antibiotic [40] and vaccine [41] delivery systems.

Despite numerous advantageous features, concern over their cytotoxicity still remains. A study designed to evaluate the cytotoxic effects by Soenen et al. [42] revealed that high concentrations (200 nM) led to the formation of reactive oxygen species, resulting in a 20% decrease in cell viability after 24 h. Nevertheless, the same study exhibited that a concentration of 100 nM showed negligible toxicity. To mitigate toxicity, Choi et al. [43] designed a gold-loaded nanocarrier that was shown to increase circulation time and tumor accumulation while minimizing disruption of metabolic activity and cell viability. The ability to localize more gold to the tumor site through an increase in circulation enables a hyperthermia-based approach to be more effective and reveals a promising tool for translation into the clinic.

Although great success has been observed with gold nanoparticles using in vitro and in vivo models, lack of homogeneity in human cancer prevents gold from showing the same success in the clinic. In addition, the high cost associated with development of gold nanoparticles remains as another barrier preventing clinical translation [35,44]. For this reason, continued investigation in the scale-up for commercialization and clinical trials needs to be re-evaluated and optimized to meet the demand of the clinic. However, as is often the case with nanoparticles, delineation of nanoparticle accumulation at the target site can often be difficult to assess in clinical trials, serving as a barrier to their proper investigation.

2.3. Quantum Dots

Showing similar rise in popularity are non-metal theranostics such as quantum dots (QD), colloidal particles that can range in size from 1 to 10 nm in diameter [45,46]. These semiconductor nanocrystals, synthesized using a cadmium selenide (CdSe) core with a zinc sulfide layer to maintain desirable crystallinity and homogeneity, are able to emit light and exhibit distinctive optical qualities that are not found in organic dyes or florescent probes [47]. These qualities include exhibiting high luminescence, a more stable and restricted emission spectrum, and a broader excitation field [45,48]. This is helpful in monitoring long-term studies such as the interactions of multi-labeled biological markers in cells. Additionally, the ability to fine-tune the fluorescence emission of QD from ultraviolet to near-infrared wavelengths has exhibited beneficial properties for studying the extravasation of cancer cells in vivo. For example, conjugating antibodies that target different tumor markers onto QD allows for the real-time imaging of cancer cells as they metastasize [47].

Additionally, surface modification of QD can provide further benefits. To create water-stabilized QD with increased photostability and enhanced functionality, Medintz et al. were able to use ligand exchange to replace hydrophobic capping ligands with hydrophilic bifunctional ligands [49]. These aqueous QD can be used for fluorescence imaging or to trace receptor mediated trafficking in live cells and for long term labeling of endosomes without any drastic harmful effects [50]. After successful in vitro studies, Gao et al. developed a copolymer coated QD to target and image prostate cancer in vivo [51]. Using this method, the tumor could be actively probed by the antibody conjugated QDs and imaged in live animals. Further tuning the size to favor rapid clearance from the body and applications calling for high sensitivity have the potential to make QD an integral part of imaging the human body.

Nevertheless, caution must be taken when using QD in vivo. Many studies indicate that the use of cadmium is toxic and that it possesses DNA-damaging properties. Other groups suggest that the use of cadmium in the cellular environment also results in the formation of reactive oxygen species that contributes to cell death. Thus to prevent or reduce these harmful effects, passivation can be used to protect the core from oxidation and lower the toxic effects [52]. Nevertheless, more recent efforts have aimed to harness the diagnostic potential of QD and couple them with a chemotherapeutic such as doxorubicin, a commonly used anthracycline drug. In a study performed by Bagalkot et al., QD were used to develop a QD-aptamer-doxorubicin conjugate capable of targeting cancer cells (Figure 2) [53]. This approach harnesses the targeting potential of the aptamer specifically selected to localize at prostate cancer cells expressing the antigen. Following binding to the target, the conjugated doxorubicin is released, resulting in the activation of the QD core, consequently allowing for the simultaneous imaging of the cancer cells. However, to be properly translated into the clinic, significant work still needs to be performed investigating the toxicity of QD. As it currently stands, QD translation into in vivo models often portrays difficulty in identifying the dominant and compensation mechanism employed [54], spurring a need for a multi-modal QD system. In addition, further evaluation of toxicity is needed before QD can reach clinical translation status.

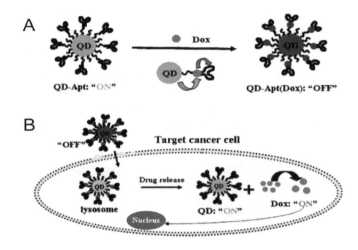

Figure 2. (**A**) Schematic illustration demonstrating the Bi-FRET-based QD-aptamer-doxorubicin nanoparticle. This approach results in the simultaneous quenching of QD and doxorubicin; QD fluorescence is quenched by doxorubicin while doxorubicin fluorescence is quenched by QD; (**B**) Schematic illustration depicting the internalization via the PSMA endocytosis pathway. Internalization results in the release of doxorubicin from the conjugated nanoparticle, thereby resulting in cell death and the triggering of QD fluorescence. Images reproduced from [53], with permission from American Chemical Society, 2007.

3. Multistage Nanovectors

Despite all the advantages first-generation nanoparticles provide [55,56], the many biological obstacles they are required to overcome have led to the development of several delivery vectors designed to decouple the multitude of tasks required to bypass these barriers [57–59]. Previously, our group introduced multistage nanovectors (MSV) [60,61], engineered to systemically shield, transport and reliably deliver therapeutic and imaging agents, thereby making them ideal for theranostics applications [62,63]. Designed using porous silicon due to its biocompatibility and degradability [64,65], well-established fabrication techniques make it possible to uniquely control parameters such as shape, size, and porosity that can aid in the strategic negotiation of biological barriers [56,57,66]. As one example, mathematical modeling has revealed that MSV exhibit superior margination and adhesion during systemic circulation, favoring the release of a payload into the extracellular space [67,68]. In addition, functionalization of the MSV surface with biological moieties (e.g., antibodies, aptamers, phages) can further aid in the negotiation of biological barriers such as avoidance of MPS and targeting of inflamed vasculature [8,69]. This versatility, combined with the ability to control the release kinetics of a payload [70], makes MSV a promising tool for theranostics applications [71,72]. Furthermore, porous silicon as a material has been extensively studied for various medical applications including diagnostics, drug delivery, implantables, and tissue engineering [73,74].

Nanoparticle Loading into Multistage Nanovectors

The nano-sized pores of MSV facilitate the loading and retention of several types of nanoparticles that effectively bestow MSV with novel therapeutic and diagnostic functions [75]. For example, loading MSV with liposomes containing small interfering RNA (siRNA) directed against the EphA2 oncoprotein resulted in the sustained delivery of siRNA and silencing of the protein in ovarian tumors for up to three weeks, substantially extending the silencing impact of free liposomes that previously required biweekly administration to achieve a similar response [76]. This work was further expanded to demonstrate an enhanced tumor response by combining chemotherapy (e.g., Paclitaxel and Docetaxel) with sustained EphA2 siRNA delivery using MSV [77]. This approach resulted in a significant reduction in tumor burden with complete inhibition of tumor growth when combined with chemotherapy in two different tumor models, including a highly aggressive and chemoresistant model (i.e., HeyA8-MDR). In addition, this approach of MSV/siRNA was validated in treating breast cancer by delivering siRNA-targeting ataxia telangiectasia mutated (ATM) genes using liposomes [78] or by modifying the surface of MSV with polyethyleneimine to form nanocomplexes within the pores to deliver ATM [79], STAT3, and GRP78 siRNA [80] inducing significant reduction in cancer stem cells. MSV loading with paclitaxel micelles exhibited a similar sustained delivery and suppressed tumor growth with a single administration, confirming the sustained release characteristics of MSV upon loading with nanoparticles [81].

Lastly, a cooperative thermal therapy approach for breast cancer was demonstrated by loading NIR responsive hollow gold nanoparticles into MSV [82]. This approach enabled a two-fold increase in heat generation and more efficient cell killing independent of genetic mutations expressed by the breast cancer cells (i.e., HER2 vs triple-negative) (Figure 3). This cooperative effect was generated due to the collective electromagnetic dipole-dipole coupling of gold nanoparticles within MSV, resulting in a coherent thermal spot-source allowing for more efficient heat dissipation and increased energy transfer and heat production.

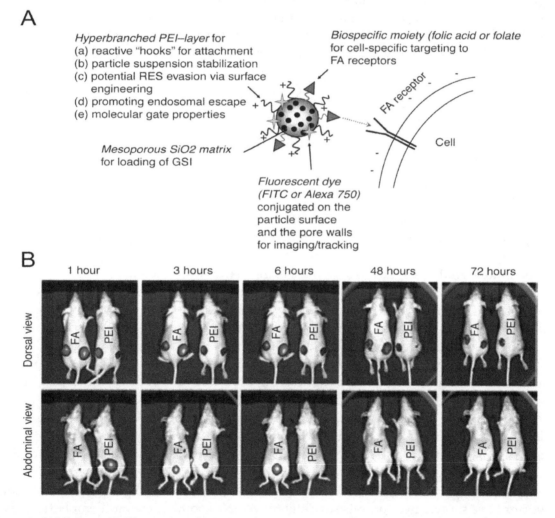

Figure 3. (**A**) Schematic illustration depicting the mesoporous silica nanoparticle matrix functionalized with a folate targeting moieties and fluorescent dyes; (**B**) Dorsal (top) and abdominal (bottom) in vivo images of tumor-bearing mice treated with non-conjugated mesoporous silica nanoparticles (PEI) and folate conjugated nanoparticles (FA) over a 72 h time period. Dorsal images depict nanoparticle accumulation in the tumor while abdominal images depict accumulation in the bladder. Mice were each inoculated with two tumors. Images reproduced from [82], with permission from Cell Press, 2011.

The diagnostic potential of MSV was further evaluated by investigating emerging properties upon loading with contrast agents. The loading of MSV with gadolinium-based contrast agents (Magnevist, spherical fullerenes and carbon nanotubes encapsulating gadolinium ions) revealed a 50-fold increase in the relaxivity of MRI compared to clinically available contrast agents and, thus, significantly enhanced the T_1 contrast possible [83]. This improved relaxivity and contrast enhancement was attributed to geometric confinement of the contrast agents within the pores of MSV. This confining effect resulted in an increased tumbling rate, thus inhibiting the ability of the contrast agents to rotate freely and effectively, reducing the mobility of the water molecules. The impact of confinement was studied by loading Magnevist in MSV with various pore sizes and demonstrated that smaller pores bestowed greater relaxivity enhancement [84].

In addition to gadolinium, MSV loaded with superparamagnetic iron oxide nanoparticles (SPION) demonstrated increased negative contrast suitable for T_2-weighted MRI compared to free SPION [85]. Furthermore, MSV have been successfully loaded with fluorescent QD [86] and carbon nanotubes [87] with their surface allowing for the covalent attachment of NIR fluorescent dyes, radioactive molecules, and therapeutic agents [88]. The flexible and versatile nature of MSV has the potential to generate theranostic agents by co-loading nanoparticles that individually provide therapeutic (e.g., siRNA, micelles, gold) or diagnostic (e.g., gadofullerenes, gadonanotubes, SPION, QD) action and thus whose combination would result in treatment and imaging. Alternatively, the surface of MSV could be used to attach diagnostic and therapeutic agents, permitting one to use the full porous matrix to load a nanoparticle payload. Furthermore, any current or future theranostic nanoparticle smaller than 100 nm can be incorporated into MSV with relative ease, enabling advanced generations of theranostic agents.

4. Bio-Inspired Theranostics

Recently, bio-inspired approaches have gained increasing popularity in overcoming the current limitations of drug delivery systems such as biocompatibility, toxicity, and targeting [89,90]. FDA-approved Abraxane, albumin-bound paclitaxel, represents the first example of a bio-inspired approach and has been shown to improve circulation time while reducing unwanted side effects of chemotherapy. Harnessing albumin's innate ability to transport hydrophobic molecules and interact with endothelial cells has led to Abraxane exhibiting increased efficacy of paclitaxel, thereby demonstrating itself as an effective adjuvant therapy. This manipulation of biological matter and its incorporation into synthetic carriers and payloads was proposed to both improve the delivery of drugs and assist in accumulation of imaging agents. As such, theranostics based on the mimicry or incorporation of biological components were developed to exploit all levels of biological complexity.

It is therefore not only important to select a material that works compatibly when administered but to also consider rational design when engineering drug delivery vectors. Although nanoparticle design has traditionally centered on the use of spherically-shaped particles due to ease of synthesis, more recent efforts have been biologically inspired, leading to the design of vehicles that are strategically shaped to optimally travel within the blood stream and overcome biological barriers. In the preceding case (Section 3), MSV were designed to mimic the size and shape of red blood cells to increase margination towards vessel walls. Similarly, other efforts have drawn inspiration from bacteria's worm-like structure (e.g., filomicelles) [91]. Specifically, the elongated shape of filomicelles and nanoworms have shown great promise as delivery vehicles both for chemotherapeutic delivery [92] and imaging applications [93]. In addition, hyper-branched polymeric structures have also been designed to covalently link drug molecules to a substrate, providing controlled drug release mediated through degradable linkages [94]. Nevertheless, although shape has played a pivotal role in drug delivery carrier design, other efforts have leveraged physical incorporation of biological components. As such, this section will highlight some key aspects of bio-inspired theranostics such as enzymatic substrates, natural-derived transporters, viruses, and cells.

4.1. Proteases

Proteases (e.g., caspases, metalloproteases (MMP), furin) have been identified as a component of the tumor environment that is commonly overexpressed and, thus, is a prime tool to exploit for the development of bio-inspired strategies. Recently, nanoformulated protease substrates were proposed as a new research tool to investigate proteolytic activity in the intra- and extra-cellular space. These substrates work by taking advantage of the cleavage of monomeric units that polymerize after cleavage, functioning as an enhanced fluorescent signal or theranostic agent [95,96]. Another strategy designed by Kim et al. involved the use of MMP and cathepsin B as an activation mechanism for fluorescent nanoprobes [97]. In this way, the imaging of a tumor area can be enhanced knowing that proteolitic enzymes are readily present in the tumor microenvironment, thereby leading to the cleavage of the imaging probe and higher specificity of imaging agents. Wong et al. developed a QD-loaded gelatin multistage nanoparticle designed to degrade in the presence of MMP-2, a protease highly expressed in the tumor microenvironment, thereby releasing smaller sized QD that readily diffuse into the tumor [98].

Cathepsins, monomeric proteases, have also been identified as viable targets to be employed in targeted-based therapies. Typically activated in low pH environments such as lysosomes, cathepsins have been abundantly expressed in various malignant tumors and are known to increase cancer cell recruitment. In one strategy, PEG was combined with cathepsin B to form a liposomal nanoparticle that facilitates the targeting of cathepsin B expressing cancer cells, allowing the release of a therapeutic payload at a target site [99]. Cathepsin was similarly used in an effort to mitigate the unwanted side effects of chemotherapeutic camptothecin derivatives [100]. When cathepsin B was conjugated onto a camptothecin derivative, similar anti-tumor effects were observed without any toxic effects. This method demonstrates considerable promise in the use of proteases to develop viable bioinspired strategies.

4.2. Lipoproteins

Similar to proteases, lipoprotein-based nanoparticles have also been extensively evaluated as a suitable bioinspired approach for the transport of theranostic payloads [101]. This class of nanoparticles is biochemically synthesized by the body and governs the transport of lipids, enabling fats to be carried in the blood stream. Additionally, lipoproteins possess innate biocompatibility properties, inspiring the design of long circulating particles aimed at improving the transport of hydrophobic payloads. Unique properties such as their small size (<40 nm) and amphiphilic nature favor their diffusion, in addition to their payload, deeper into the tumor mass. As such, low-density (LDL) and high-density (HDL) lipoprotein-based carriers have been developed to exploit these properties and increase the delivery of therapeutic and imaging agents through weak chemical interactions (i.e., covalent bonds) and the exchange of a hydrophobic core with a payload of interest.

For example, LDL conjugated with radiolabelled tracers was shown to accumulate in the tumor within 24 h of injection, shedding light to the abnormal traffic of these molecules and lipid metabolism during cancer [102]. Furthermore, LDL has been shown to possess great propensity in accommodating a variety of agents for photodynamic therapy (e.g., NIR-molecules [103–105]) and can further be modified to target cancer cells. For example, Zheng et al. showed that by conjugating a tumor-homing molecule through a lysine substitution and coupling LDL with folate, accumulation of LDL in cancer cells is improved [106]. Conversely, HDL-based delivery systems rely on the over expression of their natural receptor, scavenger receptor class B type I, in many cancer cells [107,108]. It was hypothesized that HDL could represent a major source of cholesterol for growing neoplastic lesions [109]. This led to increased interest in HDL-based carriers and the loading of chemotherapeutics (e.g., paclitaxel) [110] and NIR agents capable of generating reactive oxygen species under light irradiation, resulting in the killing of cancer cells.

4.3. Viral & Cellular Vesicles

Further inspiration for suitable bioinspired approaches was found by imitating the working mechanism of viruses. Their enhanced ability to target and integrate their genome into the DNA of human cells makes them a promising tool for drug delivery. In particular, adenoviral particles were investigated as ideal carriers for gene therapy in vivo with recent efforts focused on coupling these carriers with metallic particles for improved imaging and curative properties. Specifically, iron particles were shown to readily absorb onto the adenovirus surface resulting in a hybrid particulate with promising theranostic properties. To further refine and standardize the hybridization process, Everts et al. modified the surface of adenoviral vectors with gold nanoparticles [111]. This led to the ability to use the adenoviral vector for its tumor-associated antigen homing ability and the gold nanoparticles for their ablation properties.

Conversely, inspiration drawn directly from cells found in the body (i.e., erythrocytes, leukocytes, mesenchymal stem cells) have also gained increasing prominence. Over the past two decades, erythrocytes have been investigated for their biocompatibility, prolonged circulation, and their desirable isolation and manipulation properties. In addition, the ability to load a payload into the cellular body through concentration gradients makes erythrocytes a promising carrier. Methotrexate, a chemotherapeutic used to treat inflammatory diseases, loaded into erythrocytes, represents one of the first examples to successfully inhibit cancer growth. The loading of photo-triggered hematoporphyrin derivatives into erythrocytes has also been shown to provide antibody-mediated delivery of the derivatives with increased efficacy [112]. For prolonged circulation and decreased clearance of IONP, Markov et al. designed a protocol that incorporates IONP into erythrocytes that demonstrated considerable improvements in imaging properties of IONP for MRI [113]. In a similar strategy, Hu et al. incorporated erythrocyte cellular membrane to coat poly (lactic-co-glycolic acid) (PLGA) particles (Figure 4) [114]. Following functionalization with an erythrocyte shell, it was reported that PLGA particles remained in circulation for three days following administration in vivo, demonstrating promising potential as a delivery vector. This approach was later further optimized to combine a hybrid erythrocyte/platelet-derived membrane to provide increased circulation and marry the two distinct functions of each donor cell source [115].

Similarly, cell-derived vesicles known as exosomes have also garnered significant interest due to their small size and protein function. As such, exosomes have been reported as vesicles that facilitate transport of biological materials (e.g., proteins, mRNA) to different tissues by utilizing vascular systems [116]. This has led to attempts to isolate exosomes and load them with therapeutic payloads (e.g., siRNA) to exploit their natural tropism, in addition to their biocompatibility and prolonged circulation, thereby making them a promising tool for theranostics [117]. Despite this, exosomes still lack many of the proteins needed for targeting cancer and overcoming biological barriers to actively target inflammation. Leukocytes, on the other hand, are decorated with many essential proteins needed for bypassing the MPS, communicating with the endothelial layer, and reaching an inflammatory site.

Mesenchymal stem cells (MSC), often favored due to their innate ability to home to inflammation, have also been considering as a unique tool for drug delivery and as a theranostic system. When previously doped with hyaluronic acid, MSC displayed a substantial increase in homing to inflammation when evaluated in vivo using an inflamed ear animal model [118]. To exploit the innate homing observed with MSC, our group functionalized MSV with a photosensitizer and allowed MSC to internalize our nanoparticles [119]. In a breast cancer animal model, MSC demonstrated successful homing to the tumor, thereby facilitating precise photodynamic therapy using a low power laser source. This method resulted in a 70% decrease in tumor cell viability following photodynamic activation, demonstrating cell-based drug delivery as a versatile therapeutic strategy.

Inspired by the innate biological properties of leukocytes, our group developed a tool designed to mimic leukocytes while exploiting the MSV as our foundation. By coating MSV with freshly isolated leukocyte membranes, our group was able to prolong circulation, avoid MPS uptake, and communicate with the endothelium through critical surface markers [72]. Specifically, it was demonstrated that over 150 transmembrane proteins were successfully grafted onto the MSV particle [120] while still maintaining the bioactivity necessary to facilitate vascular permeability [121]. In addition, it was demonstrated that when MSV were functionalized with cellular membrane derived from a syngeneic cell source, prolonged circulation was achieved with a delay in sequestration in vivo [122].

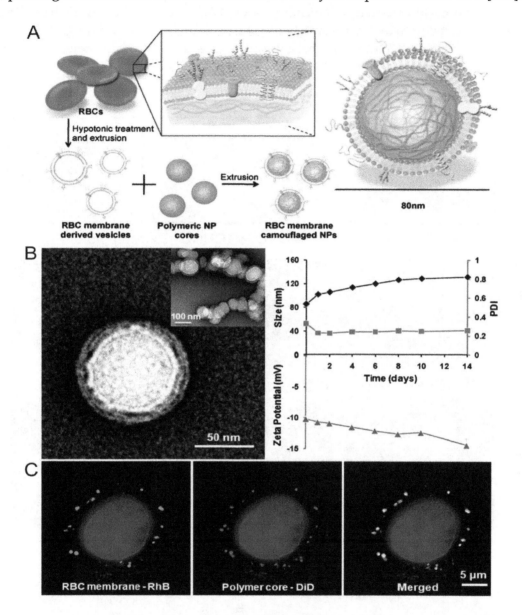

Figure 4. **(A)** Schematic illustration demonstrating the fabrication of erythrocyte-coated PLGA nanoparticles; **(B)** Transmission electron microscope images of erythrocyte-functionalized PLGA nanoparticles and DLS measurements depicted nanoparticle size (black), PDI (red), and zeta potential over 14 d; **(C)** Fluorescent microscope images depicting the colocalization of erythrocyte membranes (green) and PLGA cores (red) following internalization by cervical cancer HeLa cells after 6 h. Images reproduced from [114], with permission from National Academy of Sciences, 2011.

More recent efforts have incorporated leukocyte proteins directly into a proteolipid formulation, resulting in proteoliposomal vesicles dubbed leukosomes [123]. In this approach, the targeting potential and extended circulation of leukocytes can be granted to all classes of drugs capable of being loaded into liposomal core or within the liposomal bilayer (i.e., hydrophobic, hydrophilic, and amphiphilic). Using leukosomes, a 5-fold increase in targeting inflamed vasculature was displayed when compared to liposomes in as little as 1 h following intravenous administration, with an 8-fold increase being observed at 24 h (Figure 5). These features ultimately allow for greater accumulation at the inflammation site with minimal cytotoxicity to healthy cells, making them promising tools for further evaluation for theranostic-based therapy. Further evaluation of this bioinspired tool revealed a 16-fold increase in breast cancer accumulation relative to liposomes with similar significance also observed in an atherosclerotic plaque animal model [124]. In an effort to evaluate the potential imaging applications using MRI, leukosome bilayers were functionalized with gadolidium chelating phospholipids. This revealed a linear increase in contrast as the leukosome concentration increased, representing promise as an imaging modality and theranostic tool.

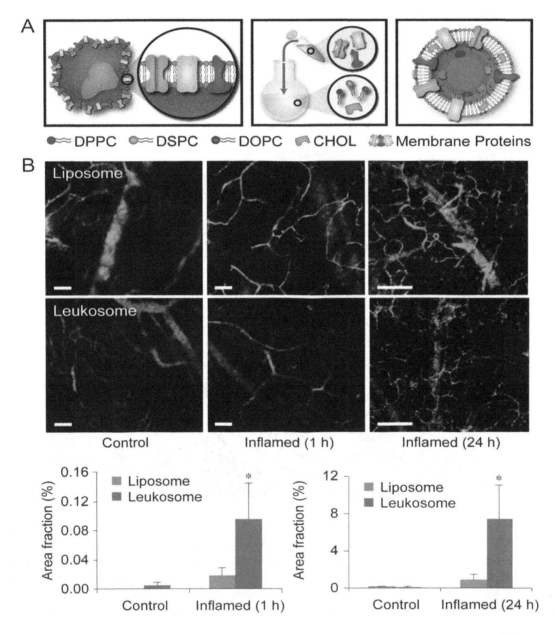

Figure 5. (**A**) Schematic illustration representing the synthesis and formulation of leukosome nanoparticles; (**B**) Intravital microscope images comparing liposome and leukosome accumulation in a lipopolysaccharide-inflamed mouse ear at 1 h and 24 h. Quantitative analysis was performed by calculating the area fraction covered by nanoparticles. Error bars represent the mean ± SD of a minimum of ten fields of view from three mice. Images reproduced from [123], with permission from Springer Nature, 2016.

As with many clinical therapeutics, ease of translation and scalability remains a valid concern. As such, our group exhibited development of leukosome particles using a commercially available microfluidic system did not hinder production and provided similar grafting compared to traditional thin layer evaporation [125]. Specifically, we demonstrated a comparable transfer of proteins onto the liposomal surface with more efficiency in protein integration observed (i.e., 90% protein integration). In addition, leukosomes were found to remain stable up to one month following fabrication, highlighting the validity of the micro-fluidic system in nanoparticle generation. Particularly, the use of the NanoAssemblr micro-fluidic system was showcased as a promising tool to be used in the fabrication of biomimetic nanoparticles up to 5 mL with scalability to larger micro-fluidic systems (i.e., 1 L batches) made possible with relative ease. Although further studies are still needed, bioinspired theranostics have displayed great promise as therapeutic and diagnostic tools, supplementing an already vast arsenal.

5. Conclusions and Future Perspectives

Over the past several years, nanotechnology has spurred the development of a multitude of delivery vehicles and the exploration of a variety of imaging modalities. Theranostics have recently been introduced as a means to unify the dual-step process typically required to diagnose and treat disease. Through the development of one-step theranostic platforms, it is now possible to visualize the disease while simultaneously providing therapy, allowing for the ability to tailor a therapeutic regimen to accommodate the adaptations of the disease and minimize toxicity to healthy tissue. Herein, we briefly highlighted how inorganic nanoparticles have been employed in the use of theranostic-based application (for further reading on the subject see [126,127]). However, to further maximize the efficiency of these theranostic platforms, it is critical to incorporate bioinspired approaches that can be strategically optimized to provide even greater targeting potential and accumulation of a payload. As mentioned in this review, bioinspired approaches have been created to not only harness the innate properties typically presented by the cells of the body, but to offer unique approaches to delivery therapeutic cargoes that display hydrophobic characteristics such as in the case of Abraxane.

In addition, although this review has focused primarily on a select number of nanotechnologies, it is important to note that other materials have also shown promising results as theranostic and biomimetic systems. For example, graphene, carbon nanotubes, and polymeric nanoparticles have garnered significant interest from the scientific community, with trends on social media also highlighting their popularity [128]. In the case of graphene, much work has been performed showcasing the photothermal abilities along with various targeted delivery strategies [129,130]. In addition, the use of other inorganic nanoparticles (e.g., halloysites) have also seen promising use in the stabilization of otherwise agglomerate-prone nanoparticles [131,132]. Overall, with the convergence of theranostic technologies and bioinspired approaches, a new wave of one-step solutions that offer personalized and precision-based technologies can be realized.

Nevertheless, to effectively translate current biomimetic theranostics into the clinic, further investigation into several components is still needed. First and foremost, the issue of scalability remains the primary barrier for translation into the clinic. As the incorporation of biological matter into nanoparticles requires refined and intricate decoration, scalability may not always be a case of simply doubling the materials required for fabrication. In addition, an issue that currently plagues nanoparticle success is lack of homogeneity between patient to patient, opposite of what is commonly observed in small animal models. This is further complicated by the observation of phenomena which are observed in animal models (e.g., enhanced permeability and retention) yet lack sufficient proof in humans. Although significant strides have been made in the translation of the various nanoparticles discussed into preclinical and clinical trials [35], additional work is still needed. Specifically, it is imperative that to effectively continue investigation, careful selection and examination of animal models is employed.

Author Contributions: M.E., A.P. and J.O.M. wrote the manuscript; M.E. and A.P. edited the manuscript: M.E. reorganized and supervised the manuscript preparation process; E.T. provided funding and final review; All authors provided discussion and accepted the final manuscript.

Acknowledgments: The authors would like to thank Iman K. Yazdi, Joseph S. Fernandez-Moure, Shilpa Scaria, and Sarah Hmaidan for valuable feedback.

References

1. Hara, M.; Shokur, S.; Yamamoto, A.; Higuchi, T.; Gassert, R.; Bleuler, H. Virtual environment to evaluate multimodal feedback strategies for augmented navigation of the visually impaired. In Proceedings of the 2010 Annual International Conference of the IEEE Engineering in Medicine and Biology, Buenos Aires, Argentina, 31 August–4 September 2010; pp. 975–978.

2. Hamacher, A.; Kim, S.J.; Cho, S.T.; Pardeshi, S.; Lee, S.H.; Eun, S.J.; Whangbo, T.K. Application of virtual, augmented, and mixed reality to urology. *Int. Neurourol J.* **2016**, *20*, 172–181. [CrossRef] [PubMed]

3. Kim, K.H. The potential application of virtual, augmented, and mixed reality in neurourology. *Int. Neurourol J.* **2016**, *20*, 169–170. [CrossRef] [PubMed]

4. Sun, G.C.; Wang, F.; Chen, X.L.; Yu, X.G.; Ma, X.D.; Zhou, D.B.; Zhu, R.Y.; Xu, B.N. Impact of virtual and augmented reality based on intraoperative magnetic resonance imaging and functional neuronavigation in glioma surgery involving eloquent areas. *World Neurosurg.* **2016**, *96*, 375–382. [CrossRef] [PubMed]

5. Mujar, M.; Dahlui, M.; Yip, C.H.; Taib, N.A. Delays in time to primary treatment after a diagnosis of breast cancer: Does it impact survival? *Prev. Med.* **2013**, *56*, 222–224. [CrossRef] [PubMed]

6. Rosenblum, D.; Joshi, N.; Tao, W.; Karp, J.M.; Peer, D. Progress and challenges towards targeted delivery of cancer therapeutics. *Nat. Commun.* **2018**, *9*, 1410. [CrossRef] [PubMed]

7. Fernandez-Moure, J.S.; Evangelopoulos, M.; Colvill, K.; Van Eps, J.L.; Tasciotti, E. Nanoantibiotics: A new paradigm for the treatment of surgical infection. *Nanomedicine (Lond)* **2017**, *12*, 1319–1334. [CrossRef] [PubMed]

8. Peer, D.; Karp, J.M.; Hong, S.; Farokhzad, O.C.; Margalit, R.; Langer, R. Nanocarriers as an emerging platform for cancer therapy. *Nat. Nanotechnol.* **2007**, *2*, 751–760. [CrossRef] [PubMed]

9. Muthu, M.S.; Leong, D.T.; Mei, L.; Feng, S.S. Nanotheranostics-application and further development of nanomedicine strategies for advanced theranostics. *Theranostics* **2014**, *4*, 660–677. [CrossRef] [PubMed]

10. Penet, M.F.; Chen, Z.; Kakkad, S.; Pomper, M.G.; Bhujwalla, Z.M. Theranostic imaging of cancer. *Eur. J. Radiol.* **2012**, *81*, 124–126. [CrossRef]

11. Kelkar, S.S.; Reineke, T.M. Theranostics: Combining imaging and therapy. *Bioconj. Chem.* **2011**, *22*, 1879–1903. [CrossRef] [PubMed]

12. Fan, Z.; Fu, P.P.; Yu, H.; Ray, P.C. Theranostic nanomedicine for cancer detection and treatment. *J. Food Drug Anal.* **2014**, *22*, 3–17. [CrossRef] [PubMed]

13. Sumer, B.; Gao, J. Theranostic nanomedicine for cancer. *Nanomedicine (Lond)* **2008**, *3*, 137–140. [CrossRef] [PubMed]

14. Ruddy, K.J.; Gelber, S.; Tamimi, R.M.; Schapira, L.; Come, S.E.; Meyer, M.E.; Winer, E.P.; Partridge, A.H. Breast cancer presentation and diagnostic delays in young women. *Cancer* **2014**, *120*, 20–25. [CrossRef] [PubMed]

15. Radzikowska, E.; Roszkowski-Sliz, K.; Chabowski, M.; Glaz, P. Influence of delays in diagnosis and treatment on survival in small cell lung cancer patients. *Adv. Exp. Med. Biol.* **2013**, *788*, 355–362. [PubMed]

16. Evangelopoulos, M.; Tasciotti, E. Bioinspired approaches for cancer nanotheranostics. *Nanomedicine (Lond)* **2017**, *12*, 5–7. [CrossRef] [PubMed]

17. Laurent, S.; Forge, D.; Port, M.; Roch, A.; Robic, C.; Vander Elst, L.; Muller, R.N. Magnetic iron oxide nanoparticles: Synthesis, stabilization, vectorization, physicochemical characterizations, and biological applications. *Chem. Rev.* **2008**, *108*, 2064–2110. [CrossRef] [PubMed]

18. Dilnawaz, F.; Singh, A.; Mohanty, C.; Sahoo, S.K. Dual drug loaded superparamagnetic iron oxide nanoparticles for targeted cancer therapy. *Biomaterials* **2010**, *31*, 3694–3706. [CrossRef] [PubMed]

19. Jun, Y.W.; Lee, J.H.; Cheon, J. Chemical design of nanoparticle probes for high-performance magnetic resonance imaging. *Angew. Chem. Int. Ed. Engl.* **2008**, *47*, 5122–5135. [CrossRef] [PubMed]

20. Yu, M.K.; Jeong, Y.Y.; Park, J.; Park, S.; Kim, J.W.; Min, J.J.; Kim, K.; Jon, S. Drug-loaded superparamagnetic iron oxide nanoparticles for combined cancer imaging and therapy in vivo. *Angew. Chem. Int. Ed. Engl.* **2008**, *47*, 5362–5365. [CrossRef] [PubMed]

21. Zou, P.; Yu, Y.; Wang, Y.A.; Zhong, Y.; Welton, A.; Galban, C.; Wang, S.; Sun, D. Superparamagnetic iron oxide nanotheranostics for targeted cancer cell imaging and ph-dependent intracellular drug release. *Mol. Pharm.* **2010**, *7*, 1974–1984. [CrossRef] [PubMed]

22. Wang, L.S.; Chuang, M.C.; Ho, J.A. Nanotheranostics—A review of recent publications. *Int. J. Nanomed.* **2012**, *7*, 4679–4695.

23. Lam, T.; Pouliot, P.; Avti, P.K.; Lesage, F.; Kakkar, A.K. Superparamagnetic iron oxide based nanoprobes for imaging and theranostics. *Adv. Colloid Interface Sci.* **2013**, *199–200*, 95–113. [CrossRef] [PubMed]

24. Indira, T.K.; Lakshmi, P.K. Magnetic nanoparticles—A review. *Int. J. Pharm. Sci. Nanotechnol.* **2010**, *3*, 1035–1042.

25. Balivada, S.; Rachakatla, R.S.; Wang, H.; Samarakoon, T.N.; Dani, R.K.; Pyle, M.; Kroh, F.O.; Walker, B.; Leaym, X.; Koper, O.B.; et al. A/C magnetic hyperthermia of melanoma mediated by iron(0)/iron oxide core/shell magnetic nanoparticles: A mouse study. *BMC Cancer* **2010**, *10*, 119. [CrossRef] [PubMed]

26. Sandiford, L.; Phinikaridou, A.; Protti, A.; Meszaros, L.K.; Cui, X.; Yan, Y.; Frodsham, G.; Williamson, P.A.; Gaddum, N.; Botnar, R.M.; et al. Bisphosphonate-anchored pegylation and radiolabeling of superparamagnetic iron oxide: Long-circulating nanoparticles for in vivo multimodal (t1 mri-spect) imaging. *ACS Nano* **2013**, *7*, 500–512. [CrossRef] [PubMed]

27. Rosen, J.E.; Chan, L.; Shieh, D.-B.; Gu, F.X. Iron oxide nanoparticles for targeted cancer imaging and diagnostics. *Nanomed. Nanotechnol. Biol. Med.* **2012**, *8*, 275–290. [CrossRef] [PubMed]

28. Dolci, S.; Domenici, V.; Vidili, G.; Orecchioni, M.; Bandiera, P.; Madeddu, R.; Farace, C.; Peana, M.; Tiné, M.R.; Manetti, R.; et al. Immune compatible cystine-functionalized superparamagnetic iron oxide nanoparticles as vascular contrast agents in ultrasonography. *RSC Adv.* **2016**, *6*, 2712–2723. [CrossRef]

29. Yoon, H.Y.; Saravanakumar, G.; Heo, R.; Choi, S.H.; Song, I.C.; Han, M.H.; Kim, K.; Park, J.H.; Choi, K.; Kwon, I.C.; et al. Hydrotropic magnetic micelles for combined magnetic resonance imaging and cancer therapy. *J. Control. Release* **2012**, *160*, 692–698. [CrossRef] [PubMed]

30. Mancarella, S.; Greco, V.; Baldassarre, F.; Vergara, D.; Maffia, M.; Leporatti, S. Polymer-coated magnetic nanoparticles for curcumin delivery to cancer cells. *Macromol. Biosci.* **2015**, *15*, 1365–1374. [CrossRef] [PubMed]

31. Espinosa, A.; Di Corato, R.; Kolosnjaj-Tabi, J.; Flaud, P.; Pellegrino, T.; Wilhelm, C. Duality of iron oxide nanoparticles in cancer therapy: Amplification of heating efficiency by magnetic hyperthermia and photothermal bimodal treatment. *ACS Nano* **2016**, *10*, 2436–2446. [CrossRef] [PubMed]

32. Mai, B.T.; Fernandes, S.; Balakrishnan, P.B.; Pellegrino, T. Nanosystems based on magnetic nanoparticles and thermo-or ph-responsive polymers: An update and future perspectives. *Acc. Chem. Res.* **2018**, *51*, 999–1013. [CrossRef] [PubMed]

33. Gupta, A.K.; Gupta, M. Cytotoxicity suppression and cellular uptake enhancement of surface modified magnetic nanoparticles. *Biomaterials* **2005**, *26*, 1565–1573. [CrossRef] [PubMed]

34. Muldoon, L.L.; Sandor, M.; Pinkston, K.E.; Neuwelt, E.A. Imaging, distribution, and toxicity of superparamagnetic iron oxide magnetic resonance nanoparticles in the rat brain and intracerebral tumor. *Neurosurgery* **2005**, *57*, 785–796. [CrossRef] [PubMed]

35. Anselmo, A.C.; Mitragotri, S. Nanoparticles in the clinic. *Bioeng. Transl. Med.* **2016**, *1*, 10–29. [CrossRef] [PubMed]

36. Chen, J.; Glaus, C.; Laforest, R.; Zhang, Q.; Yang, M.; Gidding, M.; Welch, M.J.; Xia, Y. Gold nanocages as photothermal transducers for cancer treatment. *Small* **2010**, *6*, 811–817. [CrossRef] [PubMed]

37. Young, J.K.; Figueroa, E.R.; Drezek, R.A. Tunable nanostructures as photothermal theranostic agents. *Ann. Biomed. Eng.* **2012**, *40*, 438–459. [CrossRef] [PubMed]

38. Amendola, V.; Pilot, R.; Frasconi, M.; Marago, O.M.; Iati, M.A. Surface plasmon resonance in gold nanoparticles: A review. *J. Phys. Condens. Matter* **2017**, *29*, 203002. [CrossRef] [PubMed]

39. Khlebtsov, B.N.; Tuchina, E.S.; Khanadeev, V.A.; Panfilova, E.V.; Petrov, P.O.; Tuchin, V.V.; Khlebtsov, N.G. Enhanced photoinactivation of staphylococcus aureus with nanocomposites containing plasmonic particles and hematoporphyrin. *J. Biophotonics* **2013**, *6*, 338–351. [CrossRef] [PubMed]

40. Rai, A.; Prabhune, A.; Perry, C.C. Antibiotic mediated synthesis of gold nanoparticles with potent antimicrobial activity and their application in antimicrobial coatings. *J. Mater. Chem.* **2010**, *20*, 6789–6798. [CrossRef]

41. Lin, A.Y.; Lunsford, J.; Bear, A.S.; Young, J.K.; Eckels, P.; Luo, L.; Foster, A.E.; Drezek, R.A. High-density sub-100-nm peptide-gold nanoparticle complexes improve vaccine presentation by dendritic cells in vitro. *Nanoscale Res. Lett.* **2013**, *8*, 72. [CrossRef] [PubMed]

42. Soenen, S.J.; Manshian, B.; Montenegro, J.M.; Amin, F.; Meermann, B.; Thiron, T.; Cornelissen, M.; Vanhaecke, F.; Doak, S.; Parak, W.J.; et al. Cytotoxic effects of gold nanoparticles: A multiparametric study. *ACS Nano* **2012**, *6*, 5767–5783. [CrossRef] [PubMed]

43. Choi, W.I.; Kim, J.Y.; Kang, C.; Byeon, C.C.; Kim, Y.H.; Tae, G. Tumor regression in vivo by photothermal therapy based on gold-nanorod-loaded, functional nanocarriers. *ACS Nano* **2011**, *5*, 1995–2003. [CrossRef] [PubMed]

44. Arvizo, R.; Bhattacharya, R.; Mukherjee, P. Gold nanoparticles: Opportunities and challenges in nanomedicine. *Expert Opin. Drug Deliv.* **2010**, *7*, 753–763. [CrossRef] [PubMed]

45. Madani, S.Y.; Shabani, F.; Dwek, M.V.; Seifalian, A.M. Conjugation of quantum dots on carbon nanotubes for medical diagnosis and treatment. *Int. J. Nanomed.* **2013**, *8*, 941–950.

46. Xu, G.; Mahajan, S.; Roy, I.; Yong, K.T. Theranostic quantum dots for crossing blood-brain barrier and providing therapy of hiv-associated encephalopathy. *Front. Pharm.* **2013**, *4*, 140. [CrossRef] [PubMed]

47. Shekhar, N.; Rao, M.E.B. Quantum dot: Novel carrier for drug delivery. *Int. J. Res. Pharm. Biomed. Sci.* **2011**, *2*, 448–458.

48. Pisanic, T.R., II; Zhang, Y.; Wang, T.H. Quantum dots in diagnostics and detection: Principles and paradigms. *Analyst* **2014**, *139*, 2968–2981. [CrossRef] [PubMed]

49. Medintz, I.L.; Clapp, A.R.; Mattoussi, H.; Goldman, E.R.; Fisher, B.; Mauro, J.M. Self-assembled nanoscale biosensors based on quantum dot FRET donors. *Nat. Mater.* **2003**, *2*, 630–638. [CrossRef] [PubMed]

50. Li, H.; Duan, Z.W.; Xie, P.; Liu, Y.R.; Wang, W.C.; Dou, S.X.; Wang, P.Y. Effects of paclitaxel on EGFR endocytic trafficking revealed using quantum dot tracking in single cells. *PLoS ONE* **2012**, *7*, e45465. [CrossRef] [PubMed]

51. Gao, X.; Xing, Y.; Chung, L.K.; Nie, S. Quantum dot nanotechnology for prostate cancer research. In *Prostate Cancer*, Chung, L.K., Isaacs, W., Simons, J., Eds.; Humana Press: New York, NY, USA, 2007; pp. 231–244.

52. Bae, W.K.; Joo, J.; Padilha, L.A.; Won, J.; Lee, D.C.; Lin, Q.; Koh, W.K.; Luo, H.; Klimov, V.I.; Pietryga, J.M. Highly effective surface passivation of pbse quantum dots through reaction with molecular chlorine. *J. Am. Chem. Soc.* **2012**, *134*, 20160–20168. [CrossRef] [PubMed]

53. Bagalkot, V.; Zhang, L.; Levy-Nissenbaum, E.; Jon, S.; Kantoff, P.W.; Langer, R.; Farokhzad, O.C. Quantum dot-aptamer conjugates for synchronous cancer imaging, therapy, and sensing of drug delivery based on bi-fluorescence resonance energy transfer. *Nano Lett.* **2007**, *7*, 3065–3070. [CrossRef] [PubMed]

54. Fang, M.; Peng, C.W.; Pang, D.W.; Li, Y. Quantum dots for cancer research: Current status, remaining issues, and future perspectives. *Cancer Biol. Med.* **2012**, *9*, 151–163. [PubMed]

55. Balasubramanian, K.; Evangelopoulos, M.; Brown, B.S.; Parodi, A.; Celia, C.; Iman, K.Y.; Tasciotti, E. Ghee butter as a therapeutic delivery system. *J. Nanosci. Nanotechnol.* **2017**, *17*, 977–982. [CrossRef] [PubMed]

56. Yazdi, I.K.; Ziemys, A.; Evangelopoulos, M.; Martinez, J.O.; Kojic, M.; Tasciotti, E. Physicochemical properties affect the synthesis, controlled delivery, degradation and pharmacokinetics of inorganic nanoporous materials. *Nanomedicine (Lond)* **2015**, *10*, 3057–3075. [CrossRef] [PubMed]

57. Blanco, E.; Shen, H.; Ferrari, M. Principles of nanoparticle design for overcoming biological barriers to drug delivery. *Nat. Biotechnol.* **2015**, *33*, 941–951. [CrossRef] [PubMed]

58. Khaled, S.Z.; Cevenini, A.; Yazdi, I.K.; Parodi, A.; Evangelopoulos, M.; Corbo, C.; Scaria, S.; Hu, Y.; Haddix, S.G.; Corradetti, B.; et al. One-pot synthesis of ph-responsive hybrid nanogel particles for the intracellular delivery of small interfering rna. *Biomaterials* **2016**, *87*, 57–68. [CrossRef] [PubMed]

59. Wolfram, J.; Shen, H.; Ferrari, M. Multistage vector (msv) therapeutics. *J. Control. Release* **2015**, *219*, 406–415. [CrossRef] [PubMed]

60. Tasciotti, E.; Liu, X.; Bhavane, R.; Plant, K.; Leonard, A.D.; Price, B.K.; Cheng, M.M.; Decuzzi, P.; Tour, J.M.; Robertson, F.; et al. Mesoporous silicon particles as a multistage delivery system for imaging and therapeutic applications. *Nat. Nanotechnol.* **2008**, *3*, 151–157. [CrossRef] [PubMed]

61. Martinez, J.O.; Brown, B.S.; Quattrocchi, N.; Evangelopoulos, M.; Ferrari, M.; Tasciotti, E. Multifunctional to multistage delivery systems: The evolution of nanoparticles for biomedical applications. *Chin. Sci. Bull.* **2012**, *57*, 3961–3971. [CrossRef] [PubMed]

62. Ferrari, M. Frontiers in cancer nanomedicine: Directing mass transport through biological barriers. *Trends Biotechnol.* **2010**, *28*, 181–188. [CrossRef] [PubMed]

63. Shen, J.; Wu, X.; Lee, Y.; Wolfram, J.; Yang, Z.; Mao, Z.W.; Ferrari, M.; Shen, H. Porous silicon microparticles for delivery of sirna therapeutics. *J. Vis. Exp.* **2015**, *95*, 52075. [CrossRef] [PubMed]

64. Martinez, J.O.; Evangelopoulos, M.; Chiappini, C.; Liu, X.; Ferrari, M.; Tasciotti, E. Degradation and biocompatibility of multistage nanovectors in physiological systems. *J. Biomed. Mater. Res. Part A* **2014**, *102*, 3540–3549. [CrossRef] [PubMed]

65. Martinez, J.O.; Boada, C.; Yazdi, I.K.; Evangelopoulos, M.; Brown, B.S.; Liu, X.; Ferrari, M.; Tasciotti, E. Short and long term, in vitro and in vivo correlations of cellular and tissue responses to mesoporous silicon nanovectors. *Small* **2013**, *9*, 1722–1733. [CrossRef] [PubMed]

66. Chiappini, C.; Tasciotti, E.; Fakhoury, J.R.; Fine, D.; Pullan, L.; Wang, Y.C.; Fu, L.; Liu, X.; Ferrari, M. Tailored porous silicon microparticles: Fabrication and properties. *Chemphyschem* **2010**, *11*, 1029–1035. [CrossRef] [PubMed]

67. Decuzzi, P.; Godin, B.; Tanaka, T.; Lee, S.Y.; Chiappini, C.; Liu, X.; Ferrari, M. Size and shape effects in the biodistribution of intravascularly injected particles. *J. Control. Release* **2010**, *141*, 320–327. [CrossRef] [PubMed]

68. Hossain, S.S.; Zhang, Y.; Liang, X.; Hussain, F.; Ferrari, M.; Hughes, T.J.; Decuzzi, P. In silico vascular modeling for personalized nanoparticle delivery. *Nanomedicine (Lond)* **2013**, *8*, 343–357. [CrossRef] [PubMed]

69. Martinez, J.O.; Evangelopoulos, M.; Karun, V.; Shegog, E.; Wang, J.A.; Boada, C.; Liu, X.; Ferrari, M.; Tasciotti, E. The effect of multistage nanovector targeting of vegfr2 positive tumor endothelia on cell adhesion and local payload accumulation. *Biomaterials* **2014**, *35*, 9824–9832. [CrossRef] [PubMed]

70. Martinez, J.O.; Evangelopoulos, M.; Bhavane, R.; Acciardo, S.; Salvatore, F.; Liu, X.; Ferrari, M.; Tasciotti, E. Multistage nanovectors enhance the delivery of free and encapsulated drugs. *Curr. Drug Targets* **2015**, *16*, 1582–1590. [CrossRef] [PubMed]

71. Shen, H.; Rodriguez-Aguayo, C.; Xu, R.; Gonzalez-Villasana, V.; Mai, J.; Huang, Y.; Zhang, G.; Guo, X.; Bai, L.; Qin, G.; et al. Enhancing chemotherapy response with sustained epha2 silencing using multistage vector delivery. *Clin. Cancer Ees.* **2013**, *19*, 1806–1815. [CrossRef] [PubMed]

72. Parodi, A.; Quattrocchi, N.; van de Ven, A.L.; Chiappini, C.; Evangelopoulos, M.; Martinez, J.O.; Brown, B.S.; Khaled, S.Z.; Yazdi, I.K.; Enzo, M.V.; et al. Synthetic nanoparticles functionalized with biomimetic leukocyte membranes possess cell-like functions. *Nat. Nanotechnol.* **2013**, *8*, 61–68. [CrossRef] [PubMed]

73. Tasciotti, E.; Cabrera, F.J.; Evangelopoulos, M.; Martinez, J.O.; Thekkedath, U.R.; Kloc, M.; Ghobrial, R.M.; Li, X.C.; Grattoni, A.; Ferrari, M. The emerging role of nanotechnology in cell and organ transplantation. *Transplantation* **2016**, *100*, 1629–1638. [CrossRef] [PubMed]

74. Scavo, M.P.; Gentile, E.; Wolfram, J.; Gu, J.; Barone, M.; Evangelopoulos, M.; Martinez, J.O.; Liu, X.; Celia, C.; Tasciotti, E.; et al. Multistage vector delivery of sulindac and silymarin for prevention of colon cancer. *Colloids Surf. B Biointerfaces* **2015**, *136*, 694–703. [CrossRef] [PubMed]

75. Godin, B.; Gu, J.; Serda, R.E.; Bhavane, R.; Tasciotti, E.; Chiappini, C.; Liu, X.; Tanaka, T.; Decuzzi, P.; Ferrari, M. Tailoring the degradation kinetics of mesoporous silicon structures through pegylation. *J. Biomed. Mater. Res. Part A* **2010**, *94*, 1236–1243. [CrossRef] [PubMed]

76. Tanaka, T.; Mangala, L.S.; Vivas-Mejia, P.E.; Nieves-Alicea, R.; Mann, A.P.; Mora, E.; Han, H.D.; Shahzad, M.M.; Liu, X.; Bhavane, R.; et al. Sustained small interfering rna delivery by mesoporous silicon particles. *Cancer Res.* **2010**, *70*, 3687–3696. [CrossRef] [PubMed]

77. Alvarez, S.D.; Derfus, A.M.; Schwartz, M.P.; Bhatia, S.N.; Sailor, M.J. The compatibility of hepatocytes with chemically modified porous silicon with reference to in vitro biosensors. *Biomaterials* **2009**, *30*, 26–34. [CrossRef] [PubMed]

78. Barnes, T.J.; Jarvis, K.L.; Prestidge, C.A. Recent advances in porous silicon technology for drug delivery. *Ther. Deliv.* **2013**, *4*, 811–823. [CrossRef] [PubMed]

79. Zhang, M.; Xu, R.; Xia, X.; Yang, Y.; Gu, J.; Qin, G.; Liu, X.; Ferrari, M.; Shen, H. Polycation-functionalized nanoporous silicon particles for gene silencing on breast cancer cells. *Biomaterials* **2014**, *35*, 423–431. [CrossRef] [PubMed]

80. Shen, J.; Xu, R.; Mai, J.; Kim, H.C.; Guo, X.; Qin, G.; Yang, Y.; Wolfram, J.; Mu, C.; Xia, X.; et al. High capacity nanoporous silicon carrier for systemic delivery of gene silencing therapeutics. *ACS Nano* **2013**, *7*, 9867–9880. [CrossRef] [PubMed]

81. Xu, W.; Ganz, C.; Weber, U.; Adam, M.; Holzhuter, G.; Wolter, D.; Frerich, B.; Vollmar, B.; Gerber, T. Evaluation of injectable silica-embedded nanohydroxyapatite bone substitute in a rat tibia defect model. *Int. J. Nanomed.* **2011**, *6*, 1543–1552. [CrossRef] [PubMed]

82. Mamaeva, V.; Rosenholm, J.M.; Bate-Eya, L.T.; Bergman, L.; Peuhu, E.; Duchanoy, A.; Fortelius, L.E.; Landor, S.; Toivola, D.M.; Linden, M.; et al. Mesoporous silica nanoparticles as drug delivery systems for targeted inhibition of notch signaling in cancer. *Mol. Ther.* **2011**, *19*, 1538–1546. [CrossRef] [PubMed]

83. Ananta, J.S.; Godin, B.; Sethi, R.; Moriggi, L.; Liu, X.; Serda, R.E.; Krishnamurthy, R.; Muthupillai, R.; Bolskar, R.D.; Helm, L.; et al. Geometrical confinement of gadolinium-based contrast agents in nanoporous particles enhances t1 contrast. *Nat. Nanotechnol.* **2010**, *5*, 815–821. [CrossRef] [PubMed]

84. Sethi, R.; Ananta, J.S.; Karmonik, C.; Zhong, M.; Fung, S.H.; Liu, X.; Li, K.; Ferrari, M.; Wilson, L.J.; Decuzzi, P. Enhanced mri relaxivity of gd(3+)-based contrast agents geometrically confined within porous nanoconstructs. *Contrast Media Mol. Imaging* **2012**, *7*, 501–508. [CrossRef] [PubMed]

85. Ferrati, S.; Mack, A.; Chiappini, C.; Liu, X.; Bean, A.J.; Ferrari, M.; Serda, R.E. Intracellular trafficking of silicon particles and logic-embedded vectors. *Nanoscale* **2010**, *2*, 1512–1520. [CrossRef] [PubMed]

86. Martinez, J.O.; Chiappini, C.; Ziemys, A.; Faust, A.M.; Kojic, M.; Liu, X.; Ferrari, M.; Tasciotti, E. Engineering multi-stage nanovectors for controlled degradation and tunable release kinetics. *Biomaterials* **2013**, *34*, 8469–8477. [CrossRef] [PubMed]

87. Godin, B.; Gu, J.; Serda, R.E.; Ferrati, S.; Liu, X.; Chiappini, C.; Tanaka, T.; Decuzzi, P.; Ferrari, M. Multistage mesoporous silicon-based nanocarriers: Biocompatibility with immune cells and controlled degradation in physiological fluids. *Newslett. Control. Release Soc.* **2008**, *25*, 9–11.

88. Tasciotti, E.; Godin, B.; Martinez, J.O.; Chiappini, C.; Bhavane, R.; Liu, X.; Ferrari, M. Near-infrared imaging method for the in vivo assessment of the biodistribution of nanoporous silicon particles. *Mol. Imaging* **2011**, *10*, 56–68. [CrossRef] [PubMed]

89. Parodi, A.; Molinaro, R.; Sushnitha, M.; Evangelopoulos, M.; Martinez, J.O.; Arrighetti, N.; Corbo, C.; Tasciotti, E. Bio-inspired engineering of cell- and virus-like nanoparticles for drug delivery. *Biomaterials* **2017**, *147*, 155–168. [CrossRef] [PubMed]

90. Molinaro, R.; Corbo, C.; Livingston, M.; Evangelopoulos, M.; Parodi, A.; Boada, C.; Agostini, M.; Tasciotti, E. Inflammation and cancer: In medio stat nano. *Curr. Med. Chem.* **2017**. [CrossRef]

91. Truong, N.P.; Whittaker, M.R.; Mak, C.W.; Davis, T.P. The importance of nanoparticle shape in cancer drug delivery. *Expert Opin Drug Deliv.* **2015**, *12*, 129–142. [CrossRef] [PubMed]

92. Truong, N.P.; Quinn, J.F.; Whittaker, M.R.; Davis, T.P. Polymeric filomicelles and nanoworms: Two decades of synthesis and application. *Polym. Chem.* **2016**, *7*, 4295–4312. [CrossRef]

93. Esser, L.; Truong, N.P.; Karagoz, B.; Moffat, B.A.; Boyer, C.; Quinn, J.F.; Whittaker, M.R.; Davis, T.P. Gadolinium-functionalized nanoparticles for application as magnetic resonance imaging contrast agents via polymerization-induced self-assembly. *Polym. Chem.* **2016**, *7*, 7325–7337. [CrossRef]

94. Fuchs, A.V.; Bapat, A.P.; Cowin, G.J.; Thurecht, K.J. Switchable 19f mri polymer theranostics: Towards in situ quantifiable drug release. *Polymer Chem.* **2017**, *8*, 5157–5166. [CrossRef]

95. Cao, C.-Y.; Chen, Y.; Wu, F.-Z.; Deng, Y.; Liang, G.-L. Caspase-3 controlled assembly of nanoparticles for fluorescence turn on. *Chem. Commun.* **2011**, *47*, 10320–10322. [CrossRef] [PubMed]

96. Chen, Y.; Liang, G. Enzymatic self-assembly of nanostructures for theranostics. *Theranostics* **2012**, *2*, 139–147. [CrossRef] [PubMed]

97. Yhee, J.Y.; Kim, S.A.; Koo, H.; Son, S.; Ryu, J.H.; Youn, I.C.; Choi, K.; Kwon, I.C.; Kim, K. Optical imaging of cancer-related proteases using near-infrared fluorescence matrix metalloproteinase-sensitive and cathepsin b-sensitive probes. *Theranostics* **2012**, *2*, 179–189. [CrossRef] [PubMed]

98. Wong, C.; Stylianopoulos, T.; Cui, J.; Martin, J.; Chauhan, V.P.; Jiang, W.; Popovic, Z.; Jain, R.K.; Bawendi, M.G.; Fukumura, D. Multistage nanoparticle delivery system for deep penetration into tumor tissue. In Proceedings of the National Academy of Sciences, Washington, DC, USA, 8 February 2011; Volume 108, pp. 2426–2431.

99. Mikhaylov, G.; Klimpel, D.; Schaschke, N.; Mikac, U.; Vizovisek, M.; Fonovic, M.; Turk, V.; Turk, B.; Vasiljeva, O. Selective targeting of tumor and stromal cells by a nanocarrier system displaying lipidated cathepsin b inhibitor. *Angew. Chem. Int. Ed.* **2014**, *53*, 10077–10081. [CrossRef] [PubMed]

100. Zhang, X.; Tang, K.; Wang, H.; Liu, Y.; Bao, B.; Fang, Y.; Zhang, X.; Lu, W. Design, synthesis, and biological evaluation of new cathepsin b-sensitive camptothecin nanoparticles equipped with a novel multifuctional linker. *Bioconj. Chem.* **2016**, *27*, 1267–1275. [CrossRef] [PubMed]

101. Ng, K.K.; Lovell, J.F.; Zheng, G. Lipoprotein-inspired nanoparticles for cancer theranostics. *Acc. Chem. Res.* **2011**, *44*, 1105–1113. [PubMed]

102. Corbin, I.R.; Li, H.; Chen, J.; Lund-Katz, S.; Zhou, R.; Glickson, J.D.; Zheng, G. Low-density lipoprotein nanoparticles as magnetic resonance imaging contrast agents. *Neoplasia* **2006**, *8*, 488–498. [CrossRef] [PubMed]

103. Li, H.; Marotta, D.E.; Kim, S.; Busch, T.M.; Wileyto, E.P.; Zheng, G. High payload delivery of optical imaging and photodynamic therapy agents to tumors using phthalocyanine-reconstituted low-density lipoprotein nanoparticles. *J. Biomed. Opt.* **2005**, *10*, 41203. [CrossRef] [PubMed]

104. Song, L.; Li, H.; Sunar, U.; Chen, J.; Corbin, I.; Yodh, A.G.; Zheng, G. Naphthalocyanine-reconstituted ldl nanoparticles for in vivo cancer imaging and treatment. *Int. J. Nanomed.* **2007**, *2*, 767–774.

105. Zheng, G.; Li, H.; Zhang, M.; Lund-Katz, S.; Chance, B.; Glickson, J.D. Low-density lipoprotein reconstituted by pyropheophorbide cholesteryl oleate as target-specific photosensitizer. *Bioconj. Chem.* **2002**, *13*, 392–396. [CrossRef]

106. Zheng, G.; Chen, J.; Li, H.; Glickson, J.D. Rerouting lipoprotein nanoparticles to selected alternate receptors for the targeted delivery of cancer diagnostic and therapeutic agents. In Proceedings of the National Academy of Sciences, Washington, DC, USA, 23 November 2005; Volume 102, pp. 17757–17762.

107. Mooberry, L.K.; Nair, M.; Paranjape, S.; McConathy, W.J.; Lacko, A.G. Receptor mediated uptake of paclitaxel from a synthetic high density lipoprotein nanocarrier. *J. Drug Target.* **2010**, *18*, 53–58. [CrossRef] [PubMed]

108. Cao, W.; Ng, K.K.; Corbin, I.; Zhang, Z.; Ding, L.; Chen, J.; Zheng, G. Synthesis and evaluation of a stable bacteriochlorophyll-analog and its incorporation into high-density lipoprotein nanoparticles for tumor imaging. *Bioconj. Chem.* **2009**, *20*, 2023–2031. [CrossRef] [PubMed]

109. Fiorenza, A.M.; Branchi, A.; Sommariva, D. Serum lipoprotein profile in patients with cancer. A comparison with non-cancer subjects. *Int. J. Clin. Lab. Res.* **2000**, *30*, 141–145. [CrossRef] [PubMed]

110. McConathy, W.J.; Nair, M.P.; Paranjape, S.; Mooberry, L.; Lacko, A.G. Evaluation of synthetic/reconstituted high-density lipoproteins as delivery vehicles for paclitaxel. *Anti-Cancer Drugs* **2008**, *19*, 183–188. [CrossRef] [PubMed]

111. Everts, M.; Saini, V.; Leddon, J.L.; Kok, R.J.; Stoff-Khalili, M.; Preuss, M.A.; Millican, C.L.; Perkins, G.; Brown, J.M.; Bagaria, H.; et al. Covalently linked au nanoparticles to a viral vector: Potential for combined photothermal and gene cancer therapy. *Nano Lett.* **2006**, *6*, 587–591. [CrossRef] [PubMed]

112. McHale, A.P.; McHale, M.L.; Blau, W. The effect of hematoporphyrin derivative and human erythrocyte ghost encapsulated hematoporphyrin derivative on a mouse myeloma cell line. *Cancer Biochem. Biophys.* **1988**, *10*, 157–164. [PubMed]

113. Markov, D.E.; Boeve, H.; Gleich, B.; Borgert, J.; Antonelli, A.; Sfara, C.; Magnani, M. Human erythrocytes as nanoparticle carriers for magnetic particle imaging. *Phys. Med. Biol.* **2010**, *55*, 6461–6473. [CrossRef] [PubMed]

114. Hu, C.M.; Zhang, L.; Aryal, S.; Cheung, C.; Fang, R.H.; Zhang, L. Erythrocyte membrane-camouflaged polymeric nanoparticles as a biomimetic delivery platform. In Proceedings of the National Academy of Sciences, Washington, DC, USA, 5 July 2011; Volume 108, pp. 10980–10985.

115. Dehaini, D.; Wei, X.; Fang, R.H.; Masson, S.; Angsantikul, P.; Luk, B.T.; Zhang, Y.; Ying, M.; Jiang, Y.; Kroll, A.V.; et al. Erythrocyte-platelet hybrid membrane coating for enhanced nanoparticle functionalization. *Adv. Mater.* **2017**, *29*, 1606209. [CrossRef] [PubMed]

116. Johnsen, K.B.; Gudbergsson, J.M.; Skov, M.N.; Pilgaard, L.; Moos, T.; Duroux, M. A comprehensive overview of exosomes as drug delivery vehicles-endogenous nanocarriers for targeted cancer therapy. *Biochim. Biophys. Acta-Rev. Cancer* **2014**, *1846*, 75–87. [CrossRef] [PubMed]

117. Tan, A.; Rajadas, J.; Seifalian, A.M. Exosomes as nano-theranostic delivery platforms for gene therapy. *Adv. Drug Deliv. Rev.* **2013**, *65*, 357–367. [PubMed]

118. Corradetti, B.; Taraballi, F.; Martinez, J.O.; Minardi, S.; Basu, N.; Bauza, G.; Evangelopoulos, M.; Powell, S.; Corbo, C.; Tasciotti, E. Hyaluronic acid coatings as a simple and efficient approach to improve msc homing toward the site of inflammation. *Sci. Rep.* **2017**, *7*, 7991. [PubMed]

119. Nakki, S.; Martinez, J.O.; Evangelopoulos, M.; Xu, W.; Lehto, V.P.; Tasciotti, E. Chlorin e6 functionalized theranostic multistage nanovectors transported by stem cells for effective photodynamic therapy. *ACS Appl. Mater. Interfaces* **2017**, *9*, 23441–23449. [PubMed]

120. Corbo, C.; Parodi, A.; Evangelopoulos, M.; Engler, D.A.; Matsunami, R.K.; Engler, A.C.; Molinaro, R.; Scaria, S.; Salvatore, F.; Tasciotti, E. Proteomic profiling of a biomimetic drug delivery platform. *Curr. Drug Targets* **2015**, *16*, 1540–1547. [PubMed]

121. Palomba, R.; Parodi, A.; Evangelopoulos, M.; Acciardo, S.; Corbo, C.; de Rosa, E.; Yazdi, I.K.; Scaria, S.; Molinaro, R.; Furman, N.E.; et al. Biomimetic carriers mimicking leukocyte plasma membrane to increase tumor vasculature permeability. *Sci. Rep.* **2016**, *6*, 34422. [CrossRef] [PubMed]

122. Evangelopoulos, M.; Parodi, A.; Martinez, J.O.; Yazdi, I.K.; Cevenini, A.; van de Ven, A.L.; Quattrocchi, N.; Boada, C.; Taghipour, N.; Corbo, C.; et al. Cell source determines the immunological impact of biomimetic nanoparticles. *Biomaterials* **2016**, *82*, 168–177. [CrossRef] [PubMed]

123. Molinaro, R.; Corbo, C.; Martinez, J.O.; Taraballi, F.; Evangelopoulos, M.; Minardi, S.; Yazdi, I.K.; Zhao, P.; De Rosa, E.; Sherman, M.B.; et al. Biomimetic proteolipid vesicles for targeting inflamed tissues. *Nat. Mater.* **2016**, *15*, 1037–1046. [CrossRef] [PubMed]

124. Martinez, J.O.; Molinaro, R.; Hartman, K.A.; Boada, C.; Sukhovershin, R.; De Rosa, E.; Kirui, D.; Zhang, S.; Evangelopoulos, M.; Carter, A.M.; et al. Biomimetic nanoparticles with enhanced affinity towards activated endothelium as versatile tools for theranostic drug delivery. *Theranostics* **2018**, *8*, 1131–1145. [CrossRef] [PubMed]

125. Molinaro, R.; Evangelopoulos, M.; Hoffman, J.R.; Corbo, C.; Taraballi, F.; Martinez, J.O.; Hartman, K.A.; Cosco, D.; Costa, G.; Romeo, I.; et al. Design and development of biomimetic nanovesicles using a microfluidic approach. *Adv. Mater.* **2018**, *30*, e1702749. [PubMed]

126. Xie, J.; Lee, S.; Chen, X. Nanoparticle-based theranostic agents. *Adv. Drug Deliv. Rev.* **2010**, *62*, 1064–1079. [CrossRef] [PubMed]

127. Medarova, Z.; Pham, W.; Farrar, C.; Petkova, V.; Moore, A. In vivo imaging of sirna delivery and silencing in tumors. *Nat. Med.* **2007**, *13*, 372–377. [CrossRef] [PubMed]

128. Sechi, G.; Bedognetti, D.; Sgarrella, F.; Van Eperen, L.; Marincola, F.M.; Bianco, A.; Delogu, L.G. The perception of nanotechnology and nanomedicine: A worldwide social media study. *Nanomedicine (Lond)* **2014**, *9*, 1475–1486. [CrossRef] [PubMed]

129. Zhang, Y.; Li, Y.; Ming, P.; Zhang, Q.; Liu, T.; Jiang, L.; Cheng, Q. Ultrastrong bioinspired graphene-based fibers via synergistic toughening. *Adv. Mater.* **2016**, *28*, 2834–2839. [CrossRef] [PubMed]

130. Orecchioni, M.; Cabizza, R.; Bianco, A.; Delogu, L.G. Graphene as cancer theranostic tool: Progress and future challenges. *Theranostics* **2015**, *5*, 710–723. [CrossRef] [PubMed]

131. Mingliang, D.; Baochun, G.; Demin, J. Newly emerging applications of halloysite nanotubes: A review. *Polym. Int.* **2010**, *59*, 574–582.

14

Inhibition of Glycolysis by Using a Micro/Nano-Lipid Bromopyruvic Chitosan Carrier as a Promising Tool to Improve Treatment of Hepatocellular Carcinoma

Nemany A. Hanafy [1,2,†,‡], Luciana Dini [3], Cinzia Citti [1,3], Giuseppe Cannazza [3,4] and Stefano Leporatti [1,*]

[1]   CNR NANOTEC-Istituto di Nanotecnologia, 73100 Lecce, Italy; nemany.hanafy@nanotec.cnr.it (N.A.H.); cinzia.citti@gmail.com (C.C.)
[2]   Department of Mathematics and Physics "E. De Giorgi", University of Salento, 73100 Lecce, Italy
[3]   Department of Biological and Environmental Sciences and Technologies (DiSTeBA), University of Salento, 73100 Lecce, Italy; luciana.dini@unisalento.it (L.D.); giuseppe.cannazza@unimore.it (G.C.)
[4]   Life Science Department, University of Modena e Reggio Emilia, 41121 Modena, Italy
*   Correspondence: stefano.leporatti@nanotec.cnr.it;
†   Present Address: Sohag Cancer Center, 82511 Sohag, Egypt.
‡   Present Address: Institute of Nanoscience and Nanotechnology, Kafrelsheikh University, 33516 Kafr ElSheikh, Egypt.

Abstract: Glucose consumption in many types of cancer cells, in particular hepatocellular carcinoma (HCC), was followed completely by over-expression of type II hexokinase (HKII). This evidence has been used in modern pharmacotherapy to discover therapeutic target against glycolysis in cancer cells. Bromopyruvate (BrPA) exhibits antagonist property against HKII and can be used to inhibit glycolysis. However, the clinical application of BrPA is mostly combined with inhibition effect for healthy cells particularly erythrocytes. Our strategy is to encapsulate BrPA in a selected vehicle, without any leakage of BrPA out of vehicle in blood stream. This structure has been constructed from chitosan embedded into oleic acid layer and then coated by dual combination of folic acid (FA) and bovine serum albumin (BSA). With FA as specific ligand for cancer folate receptor and BSA that can be an easy binding for hepatocytes, they can raise the potential selection of carrier system.

Keywords: nanocarrier; glycolysis; hepatocellular carcinoma (HCC); bromopyruvate

1. Introduction

Increase of glucose consumption in many types of cancer cells is supported mostly by overexpression of type II hexokinase (HKII) [1]. Hence, Hexokinase (ATP: D-hexose 6-phosphotransferase) is a key enzyme that catalyzes the first step in the glycolysis pathway. This enzyme transfers a phosphate group from ATP to glucose to form glucose-6-phosphate [2]. Moreover, HKII interacts with the outer membrane protein voltage dependent anion channel (VDAC). It blocks mitochondrial inter-membrane space protein release and prevents activation of the apoptotic process [3]. This unique property has gained attention from researchers to develop new chemotherapeutic strategies targeting the glycolysis pathway in cancer cells [4]. Various inhibitors affecting the key enzymes of the glycolysis pathway have been identified. Among the glycolytic inhibitors, bromopyruvate (BrPA) shows promising anticancer activity both in vitro and in vivo. Indeed, BrPA causes regression of solid tumors by ATP depletion [5]. It has, furthermore, been shown to be effective and, indeed, curative, as a single agent against hepatic tumors in animal models [5].

The crucial problem for using BrPA in clinical application is related to its interaction with normal cells, especially erythrocytes [6]. Thus, there is an urgent need to encapsulate BrPA inside smart carriers having efficient strategies from size, shape, and targeted for cancer cells. In our previous report, BrPA attached Poly(allylamine) hydrochloride was entrapped inside $CaCO_3$ rods during their fabrication. Encapsulated BrPA was absorbed by cancer cells and, furthermore, was released gradually with time as demonstrated by confocal microscopy and MTT assay [7]. However, non-specific, passive, targeting carriers can result in uptake by healthy cells. This can be minimized by the active targeting of the therapy, which has not been explored previously by this team. In our recent work, targeted hybrid lipid polymer is fabricated as an alternate assembly structure instead of liposomes. Their positive attributes (such as their tunable size, surface charge, high drug loading yield, sustained drug release profile, favorable stability in serum, good cellular targeting ability) make them a promising drug delivery vehicle for further in vivo tests. Hybrid polymeric protein carriers (HPPNCs) were assembled by using chitosan, oleic acid, and BSA-FA to produce a core-shell structure.

Chitosan is a copolymer of β-(1→4)-linked-2-acetamido-2-deoxy-D-glucopyranose and 2-amino-2-deoxy-D-glucopyranose [8]. Its unique properties, such as biodegradability, biocompatibility, nontoxicity, positively-charged, and rigid linear molecular structure make this macromolecule ideal as a drug carrier and delivery material [9]. Chitosan is soluble in aqueous solutions of various acids, but chitosan molecules have no amphiphilic property and cannot produce micelles in water. Thus, there are many reports on hydrophobic changes of chitosan, for example, palmitoyl glycol chitosan [10], deoxycholic acid-modified chitosan, [11], poly(N-isopropylacrylamide)-chitosan [12], linoleic acid-modified chitosan [13], linolenic acid modified chitosan [14], N-alkyl-O-sulfate chitosan [15], chitosanpolylactide graft copolymer [16], N-acetylchitosan, N-propionylchitosan, and N-butyrylchitosan, butanoylchitosan, hexanoy-chitosan, and benzoyl-chitosan [17]. Bovine serum albumin (BSA) is biodegradable, biocompatible, nontoxic, and not immunogenic [18], making it an ideal delivery carrier for drugs. In particular, BSA-based nanoparticles (NPs) might cause natural abundance in plasma, relative stability and inertness in biochemical pathways, availability, and a relatively benign in vivo biological fate [19]. A tumor-targeting agent, folic acid, was linked to BSA to increase the selective targeting ability of the conjugate [20]. Folic acid has been widely used as a ligand for folate receptor-mediated selective targeting and delivery of drugs into tumor cells [21]. The folate receptor has been found to be overexpressed in a wide range of tumors, and is known as a high-affinity membrane folate-binding protein, which mediates uptake of the vitamin by receptor-mediated endocytosis [22]. Recently, maximum entrapment efficiency investigation of similar systems was also performed [23] and use of SiRNA for following oral administration of chitosan/SiRNA nanoparticles was further investigated [24]. In a previous paper, we have investigated conjugation of folic acid with BSA. Whereas prior to the conjugation to BSA, FA was activated by using 1-ethyl-3-(3-dimethylaminopropyl) carbodiimide (EDAC) and NHS to trigger the binding of the carboxyl group (specifically the gamma-COOH) of FA to the free amino moieties of BSA [25]. The novelty of this work is to obtain nucleus made up of chitosan-oleic acid. Since the hydrophobic modification of chitosan that was done by coupling with fatty acid, can result in product with an amphiphilic behavior and self-aggregation. Then oleic acid grafted chitosan was inserted into a layer of albumin-FA to achieve higher drug levels in tumor tissue and to minimize side effects.

2. Results and Discussion

2.1. Characterization

Oleic acid is a mono-unsaturated fatty acid. It is able to generate reactive oxygen species (ROS) inside cells because it has free fatty acids with anti-neoplastic properties against cancer cells [26]. In this study, the active site of free fatty acid was blocked by dissolving oleic acid in alcohol [27] (e.g., in this study, ethanol was used). It was then heated for 2 h at 60 °C. Afterwards EDAC was added to activate the carboxylic group of oleic acid (see Figure 1) resulting in a homogenous esterified suspension [28]. Oleic acid (OA) was coupled to chitosan by the formation of amide linkages through the EDAC-mediated reaction with different degrees of amino substitution (DS) as described in a previous study [29] (see Figure 1, Step 1). Although chitosan molecules present no amphiphilic property and, therefore, cannot form micelles in water, chitosan chains can be modified by oleic acid by means of the introduction of carboxylic acid groups in the presence of water-soluble carbodiimide, which react with carboxyl groups of fatty acids, forming active ester intermediates. Consequently, the intermediates can react with primary amine groups of chitosan to create an amide bond. The final product of this assembly is a nano-sized self-aggregation in aqueous media [30]. These nuclei were made up of self-aggregated chitosan and oleic acid was coated by FA conjugated with BSA to target cancer cells and to minimize side effects [22].

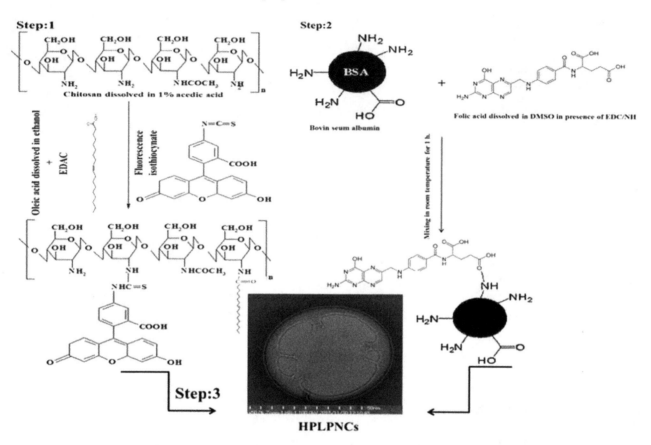

Figure 1. Scheme of hybrid polymer lipid protein nanocarrier structure. Step 1: self-assembly Structure of chitosan and oleic acid; step 2: conjugation folic acid with bovine serum albumin; and step 3: functionalization of chitosan grafted oleic acid surface by using BSA-FA.

The zeta potential of nanoparticles assembled by oleic acid-grafted chitosan showed good adsorption (81 ± 1.5 mV) (see Figure 2C) compared to chitosan alone and oleic acid alone. The results show a significant reduction of the potential surface of NPs after their fabrication, indicating that BSA-FAwas assembled up to surface of OA-grafted chitosan.

This result confirms the stability of this colloidal suspension for biological and environmental applications [31]. Additionally, it is a real indication for the combination of these dual structures compared to the zeta potential of both chitosan alone and oleic acid alone (see Figure 2A,B). Dynamic light scattering (DLS) investigation was also performed to gain evidence of the differences in the size of the materials used (see Figure S1 in the Supplementary Materials).

The distribution of used materials such as chitosan alone, oleic acid alone, oleic acid-grafted chitosan, and hybrid polymeric lipid protein micro/nano-particles on a scale bar were studied by DLS to describe the modification of the material size that was used during the experiment. The given result indicates that chitosan and oleic acid have high distributions before assembling and their complexes improve their uniformity. Hence, the polydispersity value (PDI) reflects the nanoparticle size distribution. In our study, PDI mostly ranged from 0.6 to 1. This wide range of values is closely related to the number of carboxyl groups of OA and the primary amino group of chitosan assembled together.

For the purpose of targeted delivery, the surface of NPs was also functionalized with FA conjugated to BSA. Their potential surface was modified after conjugation and measured at 18.6 ± 0.8 mV (see Figure 2D). This result indicates that the surface of OA-integrated chitosan was actually coated by a BSA-FA layer. Data of the BSA functionalized with FA was already published [25].

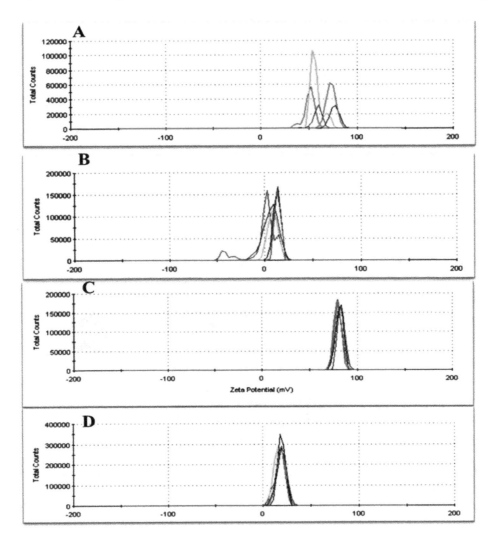

Figure 2. Zeta potential measurement: (**A**) chitosan solution alone; (**B**) oleic acid suspension alone; (**C**) chitosan grafted oleic acid; and (**D**) Hybrid Polymeric Lipid Protein Nanocarriers (HPLPNCs).

In order to characterize the structure of the hybrid nano-lipid, NPs were stained by uranyl acetate to enhance OA electron density and then imaged by Transmission Electron Microscopy (TEM). The results show a dim ring structure surrounding the core (see Figure 3) and three or four layers were completely attached having diameters of 30–60 nm [27]. These results indicated that the hydrophobic modified chitosan was well dispersed in aqueous media, with an increase in the amide linkage between chitosan and OA, and a denser hydrophobic core was formed [32]. These modifications can introduce hydrophobic groups into chitosan and form amphiphilic chitosan polymers. Some of these amphiphilic chitosan polymers can generate nano-sized self-aggregation in aqueous media [30]. In this study chitosan chains were modified by oleic acid through the introduction of the carboxylic acid group in the presence of water-soluble carbodiimide, which reacts with the carboxyl groups of fatty acids forming active ester intermediates. Consequently, the intermediates can react with primary amine groups of chitosan to form an amide bond (see scheme Figure 1).

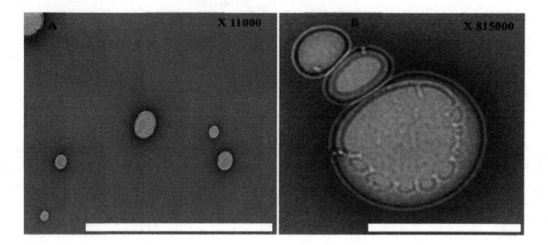

Figure 3. Transmission Electron Microscopy (TEM) characterization: (**A**) low magnification of HPLPNCs; and (**B**) high magnification view of HPLPNCs. Scale bars: 250 nm.

The NP furthermore comprises three distinct functional components: (i) a hydrophobic polymeric core where chitosan was successfully entrapped inside the core and it was the main place for drug encapsulation; (ii) a hydrophilic BSA-FA shell with a delivery targeting purpose and for good liver cell binding; and (iii) a lipid monolayer at the interface of the core and the shell that acts as a molecular fence to prevent drug leakage, thereby enhancing drug encapsulation efficiency, increasing drug loading yield, and controlling drug release [33]. Moreover, the fluorescein isothiocyanate (FITC) marker integrated inside carrier moieties shows good fluorescein intensity (see Figure 4A,B). However, the intensity of FITC-labeled HPPNCs was observed by fluorescence spectroscopy showing a peak at 520 nm. Similarly, the peak emerged by FITC integrated chitosan-oleic acid moieties. Figure 4C shows that intracellular nanoparticle uptake occurred after post-cell treatment. Hence, FITC-HPPNC was visualized as a green color distributed inside the cytoplasm. Cellular uptake study using FITC-labeled HPPNCs showed that cancer cells readily accumulate the nanoparticles within cells for up to 24 h post treatment. According to Equation (1), high-resolution mass spectrometry shows good results for the encapsulation of BrPA (see Figure 5) into the NPs. Quantitative calculations provide a loading efficiency of about 0.45 mg/mL and a percentage of loading of about 45%.

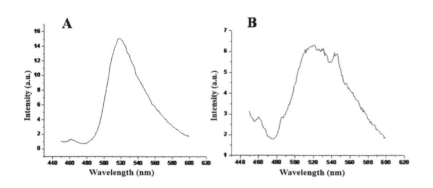
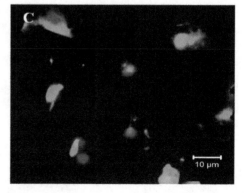

Figure 4. Fluorescence characterization: (**A**) Chitosan grafted oleic acid; (**B**) assembled structure of Hybrid Polymeric Lipid Protein Nano-carriers (HPLPNCs); and (**C**) cellular uptake.

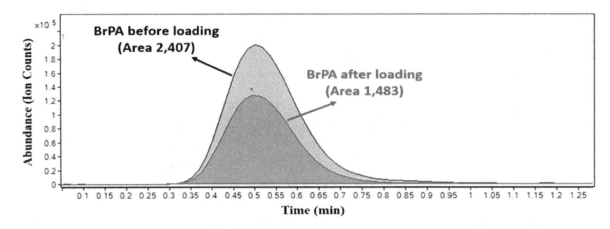

Figure 5. Overlapped high-resolution liquid chromatography coupled to mass spectrometry HPLC-HRMS chromatograms of BrPA before (black) and after (red) loading. The peak area was obtained from the extracted ion chromatogram (EIC) with m/z 164.9193 corresponding to the molecular ion $[M - H]^-$ of BrPA. The peak obtained after loading refers to BrPA concentration in the supernatant after centrifugation.

2.2. Cellular Experiments

The cellular internalization of hybrid polymeric lipid protein carriers was measured by fluorescence microscopy. Hence, FITC-labeled carriers are successfully localized inside cytoplasm and emitted green color (see Figure 4C). The optical density measurements give an indication of the relative viable cells present at the time the dye is added.

In this study, crystal violet was used to investigate the morphological characterization for all experimental conditions. Ethidium bromide was also used to show hyperchromatism and apoptotic bodies. Crystal violet (CV) is a triphenylmethane dye known as gentian violet, utilized widely to measure cell viability [34] or cell proliferation [35] under different conditions. Crystal violet can enter the cell membrane and reacts with cytoplasmic protein structures, distinguish between cytoskeleton and nuclear morphology. The morphological structure of either HLF cells incubated in normal conditions or that were incubated with free Hybrid Polymeric Lipid Protein Nanocarriers HPLPNCs appeared in well-organized structures with intact nuclei (see Figure 6). Most of the HLF cells incubated with free BrPA or encapsulated BrPA exhibited round and condensed structures with apoptotic morphology.

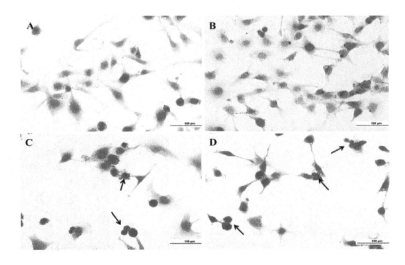

Figure 6. Crystal violet shows morphological characterization: (**A**) control HLF; (**B**) free HPLPNCs; (**C**) free BrPA; and (**D**) encapsulated BrPA. Arrows indicate apoptotic cells.

Ethidium bromide, a DNA binding dye, stains those cells that have lost their nuclear membrane integrity [36]. It is commonly used to visualize nuclear membrane disintegration and apoptotic body formations that are characteristic of apoptosis.

In Figure 7 control HLF cells and free HPLPNC showed rounded nucleus with one or more nucleoli. On the other side, hyper chromatic cells were characterized by the condensed yellow color in both free BrPA and encapsulated BrPA groups, in addition to apoptotic bodies, were seen in encapsulated BrPA slides.

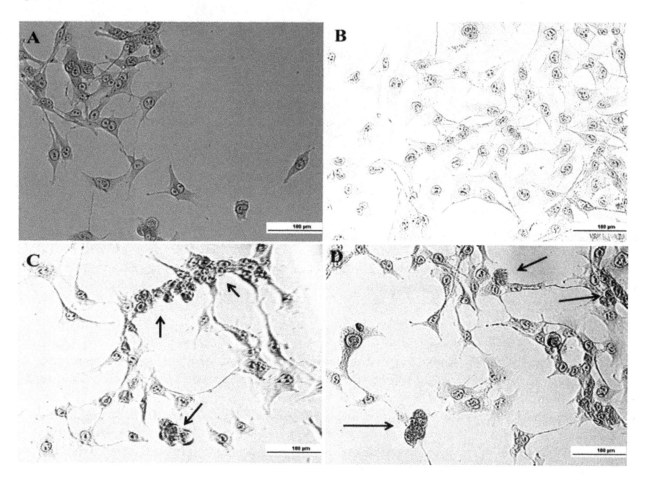

Figure 7. Hyperchromatism and apoptotic bodies: (**A**) control HLF; (**B**) free HPLPNCs; (**C**) free BrPA; and (**D**) encapsulated BrPA. Arrows indicate apoptotic bodies.

Trypan blue is one of the most commonly used methods for assessment of viability in a given cell population [37,38]. It is used in our study to quantify dead cells by spectrophotometry at 570 nm [31]. Optical analysis of the cultures revealed an admixture of live (trypan blue negative) and dead (trypan blue positive) in experimental condition. In Figure 8 the cell mortality measured by trypan blue assay was increased in case of free BrPA and also encapsulated BrPA, compared to control HLF cells and cells treated by free HPLPNC (capsules). Furthermore, upon increasing the treatment time (from 3 to 6 to 24 h) there is also a clear increase in cell death. In our previous work [25], and in this study, are reported the potential therapeutic effectiveness of targeted nanoparticles against cancer cells since they can allow smart chemotherapeutics to be accumulated in specific tumor sites, in order to minimize the potential side effects of chemotherapies on healthy cells, too. These advantages have received significant attention due to the overexpression of specific receptors, antigens, and molecules on cancer cell membrane. These molecules can be recognized by nanoparticles that were designed by folic acid [25], transferrin [39], short oligonucleotides of RNA or DNA that can fold into various conformations and engage in ligand binding [40], specific antibodies [41], and peptides [42].

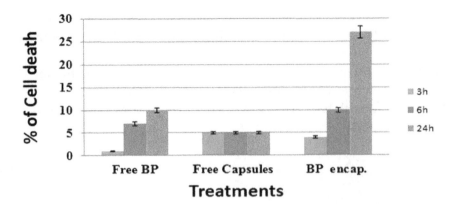

Figure 8. Trypan blue spectrophotometrical viability analysis against HLF cells. Percentage of dead cells upon increasing time (3–6–24 h) after treatment with free HPLPNC, free BrPA and encapsulated BrPA are reported. Data showed is an averaged value of three successive measurements with standard deviation (S.D.).

3. Materials and Methods

3.1. Chemicals

Chitosan oligosaccharide (Molecular Weight (MW) 5kDa), oleic acid, and 1-ethyl-3-(3-dimethylaminopropyl) carbodiimide (EDAC), dimethyl sulfoxide (DMSO), bromopyruvate, bovine serum albumin, folic acid, trypan blue, crystal violet, and ethiduim bromide were purchased from Sigma-Aldrich (Milan, Italy).

3.2. Carrier Fabrication

Step 1: 1 mL of oleic acid was dissolved in 10 mL of ethanol under sonication for 15 min, then heated in water bath at 60 °C for 2 h in the presence of EDAC and fluorescence isothiocyanate. Afterwards 0.5 mg chitosan was dissolved in 50 mL of 1% acetic acid. Then 5 mL of oleic acid was mixed with 25 mL of chitosan under rotation for 15 min.

Step 2: 65 mg of folic acid was dissolved in 2.5 mL of DMSO for 30 min. Then 30 mg of EDAC and 38 mg of NHS were added, completing rotation for 1 h. Afterwards 4 mg of BSA were dissolved in 50 mL of distilled water in the presence of EDAC for 30 min. At the end 0.5 mL of activated FA mixed with 25 mL of activated BSA under rotation for 30 min.

Step 3: Chitosan integrated oleic acid was coated by BSA conjugated with FA under rotation for 30 min. Then the mixture was centrifuged at 5000 rpm for 30 min at 20 °C. Afterwards the upper layer was separated and dissolved in 10 mL Milli Q water and the mixture was dialyzed against milli Q water overnight.

3.3. Characterization

3.3.1. Transmission Electron Microscopy (TEM)

Samples for TEM analysis were obtained by drop-casting a few microliters of solution onto standard TEM carbon-coated Cu-grids, and by allowing the solvent to fully evaporate. Samples were imaged by using a JEOL JEM 1011 TEM microscope (JEOL, Inc., Peabody, MA, USA) operating at 100 kV.

3.3.2. Fluorescence Spectrophotometry

The intensity of fluorescence markers was detected by Cary Eclipse fluorescence spectrophotometer (Agilent, Santa Clara, CA, USA). The analysis was performed on the following: chitosan integrated oleic acid-FITC and free hybrid assembly.

3.3.3. Zeta Potential Measurements

The zeta potential surface of carrier fabrication was measured by using a Malvern Nano ZS90 (Malvern Instruments, Malvern, UK). An average of five successful runs was considered for analysis.

3.3.4. Quantification of BrPA loaded HPLPNCs by Using HPLC-Mass Spectrometry (HPLC-MS)

Briefly, BrPA solution of known concentration was incubated overnight with HPLPNCs. Then, the supernatant was removed by centrifugation and it was analyzed by high-resolution liquid chromatography coupled to mass spectrometry (HPLC-HRMS). The loading percentage was defined as the residual BrPA moles in solution after loading divided by the moles of BrPA in solution before loading. In particular the encapsulation efficiency (% loading) was calculated as the relative difference between 3-BrPA concentrations before and after the incubation experiment (see Equation (1)).

$$\% \text{ Loading} = 100 \times ([\text{BrPA}]i - [\text{BrPA}]f)/[\text{BrPA}]i \qquad (1)$$

[BrPA]i is defined as the initial concentration of BrPA, [BrPA]f is defined as the final concentration of BrPA. HPLC-HRMS experiments were performed with an Agilent 6540 quadruple time-of-flight (QToF) mass spectrometer (Agilent, Santa Clara, CA, USA) equipped with an electrospray ionization (ESI) source and interfaced to an Agilent 1200 modular high-performance liquid chromatograph consisting of a binary pump, a vacuum degasser, a thermostated autosampler, and a thermostated column compartment. The following general conditions were adopted: ESI source operating in negative mode; solvent: 80% water (0.1% formic acid) and 20% acetonitrile; flow rate: 0.2 mL·min^{-1}; drying gas (N$_2$): 11 L·min^{-1}; nebulizer pressure: 45 psi; drying gas temperature: 350 °C; capillary voltage: 4000 V; fragmentor: 150 V; mass range: 50–1600 m/z. Mass spectrometry chromatograms were acquired and analyzed using Agilent Mass Hunter Qualitative Analyses version B.01.04 data processing software (Agilent, Santa Clara, CA, USA). A four non-zero point calibration curve was built for BrPA by plotting the concentration of the analytical standard in aqueous solution (0.1, 0.2, 0.5, and 1.0 mg/mL) against and the peak area of the m/z 164.9193 corresponding to the extracted ion chromatogram (EIC) of BrPA. The calibration equation was: $y = 5 \cdot 106 \, x + 495{,}851$ with a coefficient of determination $R^2 = 0.9979$.

3.4. Cellular Experiments

3.4.1. Cellular Studies

HLF cell lines were purchased as described in [43,44] and were maintained in DMEM medium supplemented with FBS (10%), penicillin (100 U·mL^{-1} culture medium), streptomycin (100 mg·mL^{-1} culture medium), and glutamine (5%). Cells were grown in an incubator at 37 °C, under 5% CO$_2$, and at 95% relative humidity. Cell lines were serum-starved for 24 h before any test.

3.4.2. Cellular Uptake

HLF Cell lines were seeded on sterilized glass coverslips into petri dishes, with a density of 2000 cells. They were grown under normal condition as previously described. After 24 h, 100 μL of hybrid assembly were added. Cellular uptake was measured after the next 24 h incubation by fluorescence microscopy.

3.4.3. Crystal Violet

Ten thousand HLF cells were seeded in 24 multi-wells and grown as previously described. After 24 h, cells were added with 100 μL of free hybrid lipid nanoparticles, or with free BrPA or with encapsulated BrPA and incubated for additional 24 h. Then, DMEM was discharged and cells were washed three times with phosphate buffered saline PBS (pH 7.2). Cells were fixed for 15 min with buffered formalin (3.7%), extensively washed with PBS (pH 7.3), and finally stained with 0.01% crystal violet in PBS. After removing excess stain, cells were incubated at PBS (pH 7.3). Optical images were captured in the bright field by using a fluorescence microscope (TCS SP5; Leica, Microsystem GmbH, Mannheim, Germany) equipped with a digital camera (Leica, Microsystem GmbH, Mannheim, Germany).

3.4.4. Ethidium Bromide (EB)

Cells were washed with $1\times$ PBS buffer (pH 7.4), fixed with absolute methanol for 10 min, and washed again with $1\times$ PBS buffer (pH 7.4). Cells were stained with 50 µL of EB (100 µg/mL) for 10–15 min and then they were immediately washed with PBS and observed under a light microscope.

3.4.5. Trypan Blue

According to procedure used by Uliasz and Hewett, 2007 [12], 50 mL of sterile 0.4% trypan blue solution (final concentration 0.05%) was added to each culture well and the plate placed back into the incubator (37 °C) for 15 min. Then dye-containing media was gently removed by washing (3×750 mL) with ice-cold phosphate buffered saline (0.01 M PBS). A slow, steady wash prevents loss of injured cells that may originate from mechanical handling. Visual analysis of the cultures showed a mixture of live (trypan blue negative) and dead (trypan blue positive) cells in each experimental condition. Cells were then lysed with 200 mL of sodium dodecyl sulfate (SDS; 1% w/v) and the contents gently fractured taking care not to introduce air bubbles. At the end, 175 mL of the SDS: trypan blue solution was transferred to a 96-well culture dish and measured spectrophotometrically at 590 nm.

4. Conclusions

Chitosan-grafted OA was used as a vehicle to encapsulate BrPA through electrostatic reaction of amino–hydroxyl groups. Hence, the OA layer acts as a molecular fence to prevent drug release. Finally HPLPNCs were fabricated with smart properties, such as nano-sized diameter, spherical shape, control drug release properties, good drug capacity, and dual combination targeting. Crystal violet and ethidium bromide results confirm efficiency of encapsulated BrPA, compared to HPLPNCs alone.

Acknowledgments: This work was supported by the REA research grant no. PITN-GA-2012-316549 (IT-LIVER) from the People Programme (Marie Curie Actions) of the European Union's Seventh Framework Programme (FP7/2007–2013).

Author Contributions: Nemany A. Hanafy designed and performed most of experiments, analyzed the results, generated the figures and tables, and wrote the manuscript; Luciana Dini performed and analyzed the SEM experiments and critically revised the manuscript; Cinzia Citti performed the HPLC-MS experiments and revised the manuscript; Giuseppe Cannazza analyzed HPLC-MS experiments and revised the manuscript; and Stefano Leporatti designed the experiments, supervised the study, discussed the data, and revised the manuscript. All authors read and approved the final manuscript.

References

1.   Chen, Z.; Zhang, H.; Lu, W.; Huang, P. Role of mitochondria-associated hexokinase II in cancer cell death induced by 3-bromopyruvate. *Biochim. Biophys. Acta* **2009**, *1787*, 553–560. [CrossRef] [PubMed]

2.   Macchioni, L.; Davidescu, M.; Sciaccaluga, M.; Marchetti, C.; Migliorati, G.; Coaccioli, S.; Roberti, R.; Corazzi, L.; Castigli, E. Mitochondrial dysfunction and effect of antiglycolytic bromopyruvic acid in GL15 glioblastoma cells. *J. Bioenerg. Biomembr.* **2011**, *43*, 507–518. [CrossRef] [PubMed]

3.   Pastorino, J.G.; Hoek, J.B.; Shulga, N. Activation of Glycogen Synthase Kinase 3β Disrupts the Binding of Hexokinase II to Mitochondria by Phosphorylating Voltage-Dependent Anion Channel and Potentiates Chemotherapy-Induced Cytotoxicity. *Cancer Res.* **2005**, *65*, 10545–10554. [CrossRef] [PubMed]

4.   Chen, Z.; Lu, W.; Garcia-Prieto, C.; Huang, P. The Warburg effect and its cancer therapeutic implications. *J. Bioenerg. Biomembr.* **2007**, *39*, 267–274. [CrossRef] [PubMed]

5.   Ko, Y.H.; Pedersen, P.L.; Geschwind, J.F. Glucose catabolism in the rabbit VX2 tumor model for liver cancer: Characterization and targeting hexokinase. *Cancer Lett.* **2001**, *173*, 83–91. [CrossRef]

6.   Sadowska-Bartosz, I.; Soszynski, M.; Ulaszewski, S.; Ko, Y.; Bartosz, G. Transport of 3-bromopyurvate across the human erytherocyte membrane. *Cell. Mol. Biol. Lett.* **2014**, *19*, 201–214. [CrossRef] [PubMed]

7.   Hanafy, N.A.N.; De Giorgi, M.L.; Nobile, C.; Cascione, M.F.; Rinaldi, R.; Leporatti, S. CaCO$_3$ rods as chitosan-polygalacturonic acid carriers for bromopyruvic acid delivery. *Sci. Adv. Mater.* **2016**, *8*, 514–523. [CrossRef]

8.   Rinaudo, M. Chitin and chitosan: Properties and applications. *Prog. Polym. Sci.* **2006**, *31*, 603–632. [CrossRef]

9.   Li, F.; Liu, W.G.; Yao, K.D. Preparation of oxidized glucose-crosslinked N-alkylated chitosan membrane and in vitro studies of pH-sensitive drug delivery behavior. *Biomaterials* **2002**, *23*, 343–347. [CrossRef]

10. Martin, L.; Wilson, C.G.; Koosha, F.; Tetley, L.; Gray, A.I.; Senel, S.; Uchegbu, I.F. The release of model macromolecules may be controlled by the hydrophobicity of palmitoyl glycol chitosan hydrogels. *J. Control. Release* **2002**, *80*, 87–100. [CrossRef]

11. Kim, Y.H.; Gihm, S.H.; Park, C.R.; Lee, K.Y.; Kim, T.W.; Kwon, I.C.; Chung, H.; Jeong, S.Y. Structural characteristics of size-controlled self-aggregates of deoxycholic acid-modified chitosan and their application as a DNA delivery carrier. *Bioconjug. Chem.* **2001**, *12*, 932–938. [CrossRef] [PubMed]

12. Wang, M.Z.; Fang, Y.; Hu, D.D. Preparation and properties of chitosan-poly(N-isopropylacrylamide) full-IPN hydrogels. *React. Funct. Polym.* **2001**, *48*, 215–221. [CrossRef]

13. Chen, X.G.; Lee, C.M.; Park, H.J. O/W emulsification for the selfaggregation and nanoparticle formation of linoleic acid-modified chitosan in the aqueous system. *J. Agric. Food Chem.* **2003**, *51*, 3135–3139. [CrossRef] [PubMed]

14. Liu, C.G.; Desai, K.G.H.; Chen, X.G.; Park, H.J. Linolenic acidmodified chitosan for formation of self assembled nanoparticles. *J. Agric. Food Chem.* **2005**, *53*, 437–441. [CrossRef] [PubMed]

15. Zhang, C.; Ping, Q.N.; Zhang, H.J.; Shen, J. Preparation of N-alkyl-O-sulfate chitosan derivatives and micellar solubilization of taxol. *Carbohydr. Polym.* **2003**, *54*, 137–141. [CrossRef]

16. Wu, Y.; Zheng, Y.L.; Yang, W.L.; Wang, C.C.; Hu, J.H.; Fu, S.K. Synthesis and characterization of a novel amphiphilic chitosan-polylactide graft copolymer. *Carbohydr. Polym.* **2005**, *59*, 165–171. [CrossRef]

17. Lee, D.W.; Powers, K.; Baney, R. Physicochemical properties and blood compatibility of acylated chitosan nanoparticles. *Carbohydr. Polym.* **2004**, *58*, 371–377. [CrossRef]

18. Xiao, J.B.; Wu, M.X.; Kai, G.Y.; Wang, F.J.; Cao, H.; Yu, X.B. ZnO-ZnS QDs interfacial heterostructure for drug/food delivery application: Enhancement of the binding affinities of flavonoid aglycones to bovine serum albumin. *Nanomedicine* **2011**, *7*, 850–858. [CrossRef] [PubMed]

19. Wang, G.; Uludag, H. Recent developments in nanoparticle-based drug delivery and targeting systems with emphasis on protein-based nanoparticles. *Expert Opin. Drug Deliv.* **2008**, *5*, 499–515. [CrossRef] [PubMed]

20. Du, C.; Deng, D.; Shan, L.; Wan, S.; Cao, J.; Tian, J.; Achilefu, S.; Gu, Y. A pH-sensitive doxorubicin prodrug based on folate-conjugated BSA for tumor-targeted drug delivery. *Biomaterials* **2013**, *34*, 3087–3097. [CrossRef] [PubMed]

21. Gruner, B.A.; Weitman, S.D. The folate receptor as a potential therapeutic anticancer target. *Investig. New Drugs* **1999**, *16*, 205–219. [CrossRef]

22. Sabharanjak, S.; Mayor, S. Folate receptor endocytosis and trafficking. *Adv. Drug Deliv. Rev.* **2004**, *56*, 1099–1109. [CrossRef] [PubMed]

23. Gandham, S.K.; Talekar, M.; Amit Singh, A.; Amiji, M.M. Inhibition of hexokinase-2 with targeted liposomal 3-bromopyruvate in an ovarian tumor spheroid model of aerobic glycolysis. *Int. J. Nanomed.* **2015**, *10*, 4405–4423.

24. Ballarín-González, B.; Dagnaes-Hansen, F.; Fenton, R.A.; Gao, S.; Hein, S.; Dong, M.; Kjems, J.; Howard, K.A. Protection and Systemic Translocation of siRNA Following Oral Administration of Chitosan/siRNA Nanoparticles. *Mol. Ther. Nucleic Acids* **2013**, *5*, e76. [CrossRef] [PubMed]

25. Hanafy, N.A.N.; Quarta, A.; Di Corato, R.; Dini, L.; Nobile, C.; Tasco, V.; Carallo, S.; Cascione, M.F.; Malfettone, A.; Soukupova, J.; et al. Hybrid Polymeric-Protein Nano-Carriers (HPPNC) for Targeted Delivery of TGFβ Inhibitors to Hepatocellular Carcinoma Cells. *J. Mater. Sci. Mater. Med.* **2017**, *28*, 120. [CrossRef] [PubMed]

26. Liu, J.; Shimizu, K.; Kondo, R. Anti-androgenic activity of fatty acids. *Chem. Biodivers.* **2009**, *6*, 503–512. [CrossRef] [PubMed]

27. Huang, L.; Cheng, X.; Liu, C.; Xing, K.; Zhang, J.; Sun, G.; Li, X.; Chen, X. Preparation, characterization, and antibacterial activity of oleic acid-grafted chitosan oligosaccharide nanoparticles. *Front. Biol. China* **2009**, *4*, 321–327. [CrossRef]

28. Marchetti, J.M.; Errazu, A.F. Esterification of free fatty acids using sulfuric acid as catalyst in the presence of triglycerides. *Biomass Bioenergy* **2008**, *32*, 892–895. [CrossRef]

29. Zhang, J.; Chen, X.G.; Huang, L.; Han, J.T.; Zhang, X.F. Self-assembled polymeric nanoparticles based on oleic acid-grafted chitosan oligosaccharide: Biocompatibility, protein adsorption and cellular uptake. *J. Mater. Sci. Mater. Med.* **2012**, *23*, 1775–1783. [CrossRef] [PubMed]

30. Janes, K.A.; Fresneau, M.P.; Marazuela, A.; Fabra, A.; Alonso, M.J. Chitosan nanoparticles as delivery systems for doxorubicin. *J. Control. Release* **2001**, *73*, 255. [CrossRef]

31. Uliasz, T.F.; Hewe, S.J. A microtiter trypan blue absorbance assay for the quantitative determination of excitotoxic neuronal injury in cell culture. *J. Neurosci. Methods* **2000**, *100*, 157–163. [CrossRef]

32. Esquenet, C.; Terech, P.; Boue, F.; Buhler, E. Structural and rheological properties of hydrophobically modified polysaccharide associative networks. *Langmuir* **2004**, *20*, 3583–3592. [CrossRef] [PubMed]

33. Chan, J.M.; Zhang, L.; Yuet, K.P.; Liao, G.; Rhee, J.W.; Langer, R.; Farokhzad, O.C. PLGA-lecithin-PEG core-shell nanoparticles for controlled drug delivery. *Biomaterials* **2009**, *30*, 1627–1634. [CrossRef] [PubMed]

34. Thomas, M.; Finnegan, C.E.; Rogers, K.M.; Purcell, J.W.; Trimble, A.; Johnston, P.G.; Boland, M.P. STAT1: A modulator of chemotherapy-induced apoptosis. *Cancer Res.* **2004**, *64*, 8357–8364. [CrossRef] [PubMed]

35. Zivadinovic, D.; Gametchu, B.; Watson, C.S. Membrane estrogen receptor-alpha levels in MCF-7 *breast cancer* cells predict cAMP and proliferation responses. *Breast Cancer Res* **2005**, *7*, R101–R112. [CrossRef] [PubMed]

36. Shukla, S.; Jadaun, A.; Arora, V.; Sinha, R.K.; Biyani, N.; Jain, V.K. In vitro toxicity assessment of chitosan oligosaccharidecoated iron oxide nanoparticles. *Toxicol. Rep.* **2015**, *2*, 27–39. [CrossRef] [PubMed]

37. Pappenheimer, A.J. Experimental studies upon lymphocytes: The reactions of lymphocytes under various experimental conditions. *J. Exp. Med.* **1917**, *25*, 25–31. [CrossRef]

38. Patterson, M.K., Jr. Measurement of growth and viability of cells in culture. *Methods Enzymol.* **1979**, *58*, 141–152. [PubMed]

39. Sahoo, S.K.; Ma, W.; Labhasetwar, V. Efficacy of transferrin-conjugated paclitaxel-loaded nanoparticles in a murine model of prostate. *Int. J. Cancer* **2004**, *112*, 335–340. [CrossRef] [PubMed]

40. Gu, F.X.; Karnik, R.; Wang, A.Z.; Alexis, F.; Levy-Nissenbaum, E.; Hong, S.; Langer, R.S.; Farokhzad, O.C. Targeted nanoparticles for cancer therapy. *Nano Today* **2007**, *2*, 14–21. [CrossRef]

41. Weiner, L.M.; Surana, R.; Wang, S. Monoclonal antibodies: Versatile platforms for cancer immunotherapy. *Nat. Rev. Immunol.* **2010**, *10*, 317–327. [CrossRef] [PubMed]

42. Pasqualini, R.; Ruoslahti, E. Organ targeting in vivo using phage display peptide libraries. *Nature* **1996**, *380*, 364–366. [CrossRef] [PubMed]

43. Giannelli, G.; Bergamini, C.; Fransvea, E.; Marinosci, F.; Quaranta, V.; Antonaci, S. Human hepatocellular carcinoma (HCC) cells require both $\alpha3\beta1$ integrin and matrix metalloproteinases activity for migration and invasion. *Lab. Investig.* **2001**, *81*, 613–627. [CrossRef] [PubMed]

44. Hanafy, N.A.; Ferraro, M.M.; Gaballo, A.; Dini, L.; Tasco, V.; Nobile, C.; De Giorgi, M.L.; Carallo, S.; Rinaldi, R.; Leporatti, S. Fabrication and characterization of ALK1fc-loaded fluoro-magnetic nanoparticles for inhibiting TGF β 1 in hepatocellular carcinoma. *RSC Adv.* **2016**, *6*, 48834–48842. [CrossRef]

Magnetic Graphene Oxide for Dual Targeted Delivery of Doxorubicin and Photothermal Therapy

Yu-Jen Lu [1], Pin-Yi Lin [2], Pei-Han Huang [1], Chang-Yi Kuo [2], K.T. Shalumon [2], Mao-Yu Chen [1] and Jyh-Ping Chen [2,3,4,5,*]

[1] Department of Neurosurgery, Chang Gung Memorial Hospital Linkuo Medical Center and College of Medicine, Chang Gung University, Taoyuan 33305, Taiwan; alexlu0416@gmail.com (Y.-J.L.); giselle.huang@gmail.com (P.-H.H.); mailtomaxi@gmail.com (M.-Y.C.)

[2] Department of Chemical and Materials Engineering, Chang Gung University, Taoyuan 33302, Taiwan; arrow06280@hotmail.com (P.-Y.L.); onesky1997@gmail.com (C.-Y.K.); shalumon@gmail.com (K.T.S.)

[3] Department of Plastic and Reconstructive Surgery and Craniofacial Research Center, Chang Gung Memorial Hospital, Linkou, Kwei-San, Taoyuan 33305, Taiwan

[4] Research Center for Food and Cosmetic Safety, Research Center for Chinese Herbal Medicine, College of Human Ecology, Chang Gung University of Science and Technology, Kwei-San, Taoyuan 33302, Taiwan

[5] Department of Materials Engineering, Ming Chi University of Technology, Tai-Shan, New Taipei City 24301, Taiwan

* Correspondence: jpchen@mail.cgu.edu.tw;

Abstract: To develop a pH-sensitive dual targeting magnetic nanocarrier for chemo-phototherapy in cancer treatment, we prepared magnetic graphene oxide (MGO) by depositing Fe_3O_4 magnetic nanoparticles on graphene oxide (GO) through chemical co-precipitation. MGO was modified with polyethylene glycol (PEG) and cetuximab (CET, an epidermal growth factor receptor (EGFR) monoclonal antibody) to obtain MGO-PEG-CET. Since EGFR was highly expressed on the tumor cell surface, MGO-PEG-CET was used for dual targeted delivery an anticancer drug doxorubicin (DOX). The physico-chemical properties of MGO-PEG-CET were fully characterized by dynamic light scattering, transmission electron microscopy, X-ray diffraction, Fourier transform Infrared spectroscopy, thermogravimetric analysis, and superconducting quantum interference device. Drug loading experiments revealed that DOX adsorption followed the Langmuir isotherm with a maximal drug loading capacity of 6.35 mg/mg, while DOX release was pH-dependent with more DOX released at pH 5.5 than pH 7.4. Using quantum-dots labeled nanocarriers and confocal microscopy, intracellular uptakes of MGO-PEG-CET by high EGFR-expressing CT-26 murine colorectal cells was confirmed to be more efficient than MGO. This cellular uptake could be inhibited by pre-incubation with CET, which confirmed the receptor-mediated endocytosis of MGO-PEG-CET. Magnetic targeted killing of CT-26 was demonstrated in vitro through magnetic guidance of MGO-PEG-CET/DOX, while the photothermal effect could be confirmed in vivo and in vitro after exposure of MGO-PEG-CET to near-infrared (NIR) laser light. In addition, the biocompatibility tests indicated MGO-PEG-CET showed no cytotoxicity toward fibroblasts and elicited minimum hemolysis. In vitro cytotoxicity tests showed the half maximal inhibitory concentration (IC50) value of MGO-PEG-CET/DOX toward CT-26 cells was 1.48 µg/mL, which was lower than that of MGO-PEG/DOX (2.64 µg/mL). The IC50 value could be further reduced to 1.17 µg/mL after combining with photothermal therapy by NIR laser light exposure. Using subcutaneously implanted CT-26 cells in BALB/c mice, in vivo anti-tumor studies indicated the relative tumor volumes at day 14 were 12.1 for control (normal saline), 10.1 for DOX, 9.5 for MGO-PEG-CET/DOX, 5.8 for MGO-PEG-CET/DOX + magnet, and 0.42 for MGO-PEG-CET/DOX + magnet + laser. Therefore, the dual targeting MGO-PEG-CET/DOX could be suggested as an effective drug delivery system for anticancer therapy, which showed a 29-fold increase in therapeutic efficacy compared with control by combining chemotherapy with photothermal therapy.

Keywords: graphene oxide; magnetic nanoparticles; doxorubicin; cetuximab; photothermal therapy

1. Introduction

Claiming the lives of 8.8 million people in 2015 alone, cancer is always a serious leading cause of death worldwide [1]. Currently, there are several different treatment techniques, including surgery, radiation, chemotherapy, targeted therapy, and immunotherapy [2]. Among these, chemotherapy has remained as one of the most common therapy methods for the treatment of different kinds of cancers. However, to be successful, chemotherapy may be dependent on several factors, including optimization of drug delivery to a specific targeting site, hence minimizing undesirable side effects to normal cells [3].

Advanced drug delivery systems are able to overcome the problems in conventional chemotherapy by offering carrier systems the possibility to hold sufficient amount of drug, prolong the circulation time, and provide controlled release of drug within tumor cells [4]. In particular, the application of nanotechnology in chemotherapeutics has huge potential to overcome the problems faced in drug delivery, and also provides a platform for the development of a multi-functional drug delivery nano-system for theranostic nanomedicine [5]. Although several nanomaterial-based chemotherapeutics have been successfully translated to clinical applications, the successful clinical translation of promising nanotherapy from benchside to bedside still faces plenty of hurdles. The inconsistency between the pre-clinical and clinical studies and the heterogeneity found in tumors may be suggested as two of the major challenges that nanomaterial-based anti-tumor therapies are facing for translational medicine [6].

Nanoparticles provide ample means of enforcing targeted therapy via passive targeting that refers to efficient localization of nanoparticles within the tumor microenvironment, as well as active targeting that represents the active uptake of nanoparticles by tumor cells. The miniscule size of nanoparticles not only enables far greater intracellular uptake as compared with micron-sized particles [7], it also allows for an inherent passive targeting by means of the enhanced permeability and retention (EPR) effect across tumor tissue's leaky microvasculature [8–10]. Furthermore, new classes of carbon-based nanomaterials, such as carbon nanotube [11] and graphene [12], augment the passive targeting mechanism by releasing their therapeutic moieties in response to a given external environment pH. As epidermal growth factor receptor (EGFR) is highly expressed on the surface of tumor cells, active targeting could be achieved through the surface modification of nanoparticles with a targeting ligand, the EGFR monoclonal antibody (cetuximab, CET), to increase the bindings of drug-loaded nanocarriers with surface receptors of cancer cells and to significantly enhance their intracellular uptake by targeted cancer cells [13,14]. On the other hand, there have been numerous studies exploring the conjugation of magnetic nanoparticles with chemotherapeutic agents, which can then be specifically targeted to localized tumors by guidance with an external magnetic field, hence further increasing the efficiency of anti-cancer therapy through magnetic targeting [15–17].

Graphene is currently the thinnest material in existence with a thickness of only 0.35 nm [18]. It has a two-dimensional planar structure composed of a sp^2 mixed-layer orbital with a considerably large specific surface area, making it suitable for carrying large quantities of substances (e.g., metal, biomolecules, and drugs) [19]. When used as a drug carrier, graphene is typically converted into graphene oxide (GO) to increase hydrophilicity by the introduction of oxygen-containing functional groups and bind with chemotherapeutic drugs, such as doxorubicin (DOX), by physical adsorption [20,21]. With loading capacities of up to 2.35 mg/mg of DOX, GO has a substantially greater loading capacity than other conventional drug carriers, such as polymeric micelle, hydrogel microparticles, and liposomes [22]. Furthermore, the adsorption between GO and DOX is pH-sensitive, which offers controlled drug release after intracellular uptake of DOX-loaded GO by cancer cells through endocytosis into the endosomes for release of its cargo in the low pH (~5) endosomal environment. Indeed, the blood's physiological pH (pH 7.4) is expected to prevent burst DOX release in the circulation after intravenous injection of DOX-loaded GO, whereas the lower pH environment after endocytosis into cancer cells would trigger the release of the drug intracellularly for enhanced chemotherapeutic efficacy [22–24].

It should be noted that current literature proposes that GO may induce the generation of reactive oxygen species in target cancer cells, which was deemed as one of the most important nanotoxicity mechanisms of GO [25]. Nonetheless, the nanotoxicity depends on the number of layers, size, surface properties, and methods of the synthesis of GO, in addition to the dose, time of exposure, cell type, and administration method [26]. Thus, generalizations of GO nanotoxicity should be avoided due to the presence of several parameters affecting the toxicity profile of GO. For cellular responses to sheet-like GO, discrepancies were reported for different cell types [27]. However, GO of greatly different sizes (350 nm vs. 2200 mm) was selectively internalized by two macrophages by phagocytosis and showed equal uptake amount in macrophages [28].

Another advantage that is offered by GO is its strong optical absorption in the near-infrared (NIR) tissue transparency window that may allow its potential use as a photothermal therapy agent. Photothermal therapy involves the use of light absorbents so as to absorb 808 nm NIR light and convert the light energy into thermal energy for the killing of cancer cells and the ablation of tumor tissue [29,30]. In recent years, researchers have successfully demonstrated that GO exposed to NIR could destroy cancer cells in vitro and shrink tumor size from animal experiments [31]. Thus, irradiating GO with NIR light after its intracellular uptake by cancer cells could be employed as a noninvasive method for cancer treatment in conjunction with its advantages as a nanocarrier for DOX.

Taken together, all of the considerations mentioned above, we aim to utilize GO's unique properties, pH-sensitive drug release, high drug loading, and strong optical NIR absorption, to develop a multi-functional DOX-carrying drug delivery system that incorporates dual-targeting drug delivery with photothermal therapy. We focus on using magnetic graphene oxide (MGO) by chemical co-precipitation of Fe_3O_4 magnetic nanoparticles on GO nano-platelets [32], which was further modified with polyethylene (PEG) and CET (MGO-PEG-CET), for magnetic and the receptor-mediated dual targeted delivery of DOX. We thoroughly characterize the properties of the nanocarriers and evaluate the anti-cancer therapeutic efficacy both in vitro and in vivo using high EGFR-expressing CT-26 murine colorectal cells.

2. Results and Discussion

2.1. Preparation and Characteriazation of MGO, MGO-PEG-CET and MGO-PEG-CET/DOX

The nanocarriers were synthesized according to the scheme in Figure 1. Modification using $ClCH_2COOH$ introduced abundant –COOH groups on MGO surface, which reacted with the –NH_2 groups of avidin through carbodiimide-mediated amide bond formation catalyzed by 1-(3-dimethylaminopropyl)-3-ethylcarbodiimide hydrochloride (EDC) and N-hydroxysuccinimide (NHS). Using biotin-PEG-NHS that has a terminal –NHS groups to react spontaneously with the –NH_2 groups of CET (or quantum dots, QDs), we prepared biotinylated PEG-CET (or PEG-QDs). Finally, MGO-PEG-CET (or MGO-PEG-CET-QDs) could be facially prepared by taking advantage of the high affinity of avidin toward biotin ($K_d = 10^{-15}$ M) and the capacity to bind up to four biotin molecules per avidin [33]. Also, as the bond formation between avidin and biotin is very rapid and is not unaffected by pH and temperature, which further facilitate the approach adopted here to conjugate CET to PEGylated MGO.

This method also provides a simple method for PEGylation of MGO, which is expected to decrease the aggregation of MGO by diminishing its interaction with serum proteins to modulate the EPR effect, reduce the reticuloendothelial system (RES) uptake, and increase the circulation time of MGO-PEG [34]. It was demonstrated that after coating with PEG, drug-loaded nanocarriers could accumulate less in the liver to result in higher tumor accumulation than unmodified ones without PEGylation [35]. From chemical analysis, the toluidine blue O (TBO) dye adsorption assay confirmed that each milligram of MGO contained $2.38 \times 10^{-4} \pm 5.04 \times 10^{-5}$ mmol of –COOH for conjugation with avidin. Quantitative analysis with protein assays indicated that the amount of avidin and CET conjugated to MGO is 1.938 ± 0.102 mg of avidin and 2.52 ± 0.212 mg of CET per mg of MGO, respectively.

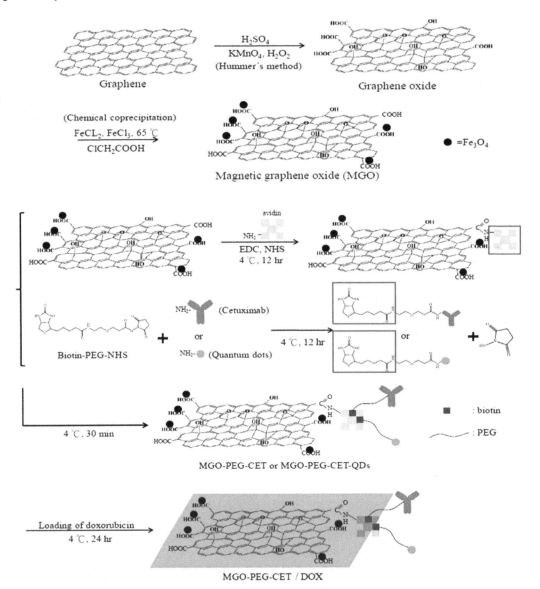

Figure 1. The flow diagram for producing doxorubicin (DOX)-loaded Magnetic Graphene Oxide (MGO)-polyethylene glycol (PEG)-cetuximab (CET) (MGO-PEG-CET/DOX). Fe_3O_4 magnetic nanoparticles were deposited on GO by chemical co-precipitation to prepare MGO. Avidin was bound to MGO by covalent binding while biotin-PEG N-hydroxysuccinimide (NHS) was conjugated to cetuximab (CET) or quantum dots (QDs). Mixing of avidin-modified MGO with biotin-PEG-CET and biotin-PEG-QDs could produce MGO-PEG-CET and MGO-PEG-CET-QDs for doxorubicin (DOX) loading and fluorescent tracking after intracellular uptake.

The structure of GO, MGO and MGO-PEG-CET were observed under transmission election microscope (TEM). Figure 2a shows the laminar stacking form of GO with size less than 300 nm, while Figure 2b depicts the appearance of black nanoparticles in MGO from the electron dense magnetite after chemical co-precipitation of Fe_3O_4 magnetic nanoparticles. After negative staining with 2% phosphotungstic acid that selectively binds to the basic groups (lysine and arginine residues) of proteins [36], magnetic nanoparticles appeared black while the light grey zones revealed the presence of avidin and CET in the TEM image of MGO-PEG-CET (Figure 2c). Figure 2d illustrates the crystal lattices of Fe_3O_4 on the MGO detected through selected area electron diffraction of the circled area of MGO, which further confirms the presence of well-crystallized Fe_3O_4 magnetic nanoparticles in MGO. For suspension stability, 1% MGO is stable in deionized (DI) water for 24 h, but not in phosphate buffered saline (PBS) (Figure 2e). Consistent with a previous report that surface modification with PEG and proteins (avidin and CET) could substantially improve the stability of GO [37], MGO-PEG-PET was confirmed to be free from agglomeration and sedimentation in PBS and cell culture medium after 24 h (Figure 2e).

Form Table 1, the average hydrodynamic diameter obtained from dynamic light scattering (DLS) indicated that the particle size was significantly increased from GO to MGO after decorating GO with Fe_3O_4. However, the particle size showed no significant difference between MGO and MGO-PEG-CET after grafting with soft polymer chains. As nanoparticles with hydrophilic surfaces and threshold size ~200 nm will show improved EPR effect by increasing residence time in blood [38], MGO-PEG-CET falls within this size range and is expected to reach the tumor and endocytosed by cancer cells. For zeta potentials, GO showed a highly negative value due to the presence of abundant oxygen-containing functional groups on GO surface. The zeta potential of MGO slightly increased to −35.1 mV as Fe_3O_4 showed a positive zeta potential (28.8 ± 0.3 mV) from the $-NH_2$ groups in ammonia used during chemical co-precipitation. When CET was conjugated to MGO, the zeta potential of MGO-PEG-CET further increased to ~20 mV as CET is a chimeric antibody with an isoelectric point of about 8.5 [39]. Nonetheless, the zeta potential is still high enough to confer dispersion stability by resisting aggregation.

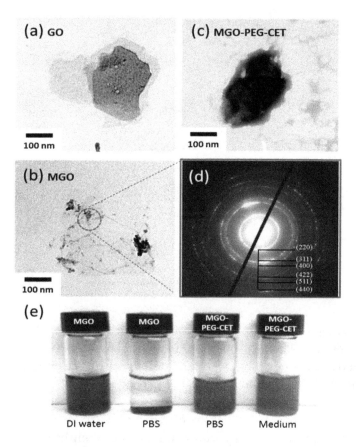

Figure 2. Transmission electron images of graphene oxide (GO) (**a**); MGO (**b**); and, MGO-PEG-CET after staining with 2% phosphotungstic acid (**c**); (**d**) The selected area electron diffraction patterns of MGO in the circled area in (**b**); (**e**) The suspension stability of 0.1 mg/mL MGO and MGO-PEG-CET in deionized (DI) water, phosphate buffered saline (PBS) and cell culture medium after 24 h.

Table 1. The particle size and polydispersity index (PDI) by dynamic light scattering (DLS) and zeta potential of different nanocarriers.

Sample	Particle Size (nm)	Polydispersity Index	Zeta Potential (mV)
GO	136.4 ± 5.7	0.18 ± 0.05	−44.3 ± 2.8
MGO	205.5 ± 19.9 *	0.28 ± 0.03 *	−35.1 ± 0.9 *
MGO-PEG-CET	215.7 ± 18.4 *	0.29 ± 0.03 *	−19.8 ± 0.4 *,#

$* p < 0.05$ compared with GO; $^{\#} p < 0.05$ compared with MGO.

Figure 3a shows X-ray diffraction (XRD) patterns of Fe_3O_4 and MGO. GO will show a typical diffraction peak at $2\theta = 11.6°$ due to the (0 0 2) reflection with spacing d = 0.91 nm [40,41]. For MGO, new diffraction peaks were found at $2\theta = 30.1°, 35.4°, 43.1°, 53.2°, 56.9°$, and $62.5°$, and identified as the cubic spinel crystal planes of Fe_3O_4 from JCPDS database [42]. In addition, the crystallite size of Fe_3O_4 could be estimated to be 10.9 nm from the strongest (3 1 1) reflection using the Debye-Scherrer equation [43].

From Fourier transform infrared (FTIR) analysis in Figure 3b, GO reveals characteristic bands at 1265 and 1074 cm^{-1} due to C–OH and C–O stretching vibrations, while the characteristic bands at 1623 and 3400 cm^{-1} are due to C=C and –OH [44]. In addition, the band at 1725 cm^{-1} could be assigned to C=O stretching vibrations from carbonyl and carboxylic groups in GO. MGO shows an additional characteristic peak at 572 cm^{-1} from the stretching vibration of Fe–O bond, suggesting that Fe_3O_4 is bound to GO successfully. For MGO-PEG-CET, additional peaks at 843, 947, and 1106 cm^{-1} could be assigned to PEG [45].

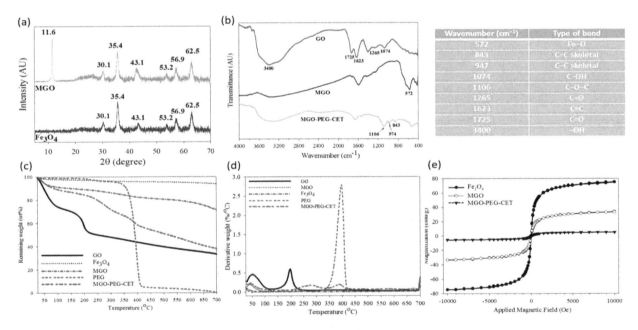

Figure 3. Characterization of MGO and MGO-PEG-CET by X-ray diffraction (XRD) (**a**); Fourier transform infrared (FTIR) (**b**); thermogravimetric analysis (TGA) (**c**); differential thermal analysis (DTA) (**d**); and superconducting quantum interference device (SQUID) (**e**). The table lists the wavenumbers of characteristic peak found in the FTIR spectra in (**b**).

Thermogravimetric analysis (TGA) was conducted on GO, Fe_3O_4, MGO, and MGO-PEG-CET (Figure 3c). After initial weight loss due to water, substantial weight loss (~21%) was shown by GO when heated from 130 to 250 °C with the decomposition of its oxygen-containing functional groups, which gave a peak decomposition temperature of 200 °C and 33% residual weight at 700 °C [46,47]. Fe_3O_4 had minimal weight loss of ~3% at 700 °C, corresponding to the loss of surface –OH functional groups [48]. PEG underwent ~90% weight loss between 330 °C and 420 °C with a peak decomposition temperature at ~400 °C from the differential thermal analysis (DTA) curve in Figure 3d, to give zero residual weight at 700 °C, as expected for an organic polymer [49]. For MGO, thermal decomposition was delayed and more residual weight (~72%) than GO was found at 700 °C. The difference in the residual weight between GO and MGO was used to calculate the mass percentage of Fe_3O_4 in MGO, which was ~42% after considering the weight loss of Fe_3O_4. When considering the TGA curve of PEG, MGO-PEG-CET showed additional weight loss from 340 to 440 °C and a peak decomposition temperature at ~400 °C, which correspond to the thermal decomposition of PEG and confirms the presence of PEG in the nanocarrier. The final residual weight was also consistent with MGO-PEG-CET (38%) < MGO (72%), as grafted PEG, in addition to avidin and CET, will contribute to additional weight loss. Using inductively coupled plasma-optical emission spectroscopy (ICP-OES), the weight percentage of Fe_3O_4 in MGO could be also confirmed to be 43%.

A superconducting quantum interference device (SQUID) magnetic field intensity analysis was conducted to obtain the hysteresis curves of the nanocarriers (Figure 3e). The saturation magnetization was 75.1 emu/g for Fe_3O_4, 33.4 emu/g for MGO, and 5.5 emu/g for MGO-PEG-CET. The reduced Fe_3O_4 weight percentage in the nanocarriers may lead to reduced saturation magnetization [50]. Thus, the saturation magnetization of MGO calculated from the saturation magnetization is 44% that of GO, which is close to the values from TGA (42%) and ICP-OES (43%). Further grafting with high molecular weight proteins (avidin molecular weight = ~67 kDa and CET molecular weight = ~152 kDa), and PEG is expected to substantially decrease the weight percentage of Fe_3O_4 in MGO-PEG-CET and influence the saturation magnetization. Nonetheless, calculation based on SQUID saturation magnetization indicated that MGO-PEG-CET contained 7% Fe_3O_4, which is less than that predicted by ICP-OES (12%). Thus, the reduced saturation magnetization value may originate from the diamagnetic natures of avidin, CET, and PEG on the MGO surface [50,51]. From the magnetization curve, the residue magnetization (remanence) was close to zero without applied external magnetic field (0.13 emu/g for Fe_3O_4, 0.6 emu/g for MGO, and 0.1 emu/g for MGO-PEG-CET) and no hysteresis loop was observed. Taken together, MGO-PEG-CET could be confirmed to be superparamagnetic from the SQUID magnetization curve, an important property for magnetic targeted delivery of DOX.

2.2. Drug Loading and Release

Figure 4a shows the effect of initial DOX concentration on the loading content (weight of DOX loaded per unit weight of MGO-PEG-CET) and the loading efficiency (weight percentage of DOX loaded) of DOX. As initial DOX concentration increased eight-fold from 0.05 to 0.4 mg/mL, the loading efficiency decreased only slightly from 89.8 to 82.1%, indicating high loading capacity of DOX on MGO-PEG-CET. However, the loading content increased continuously with increasing DOX concentration, in close to linear manner, and reached 3.26 mg/mg. With continuously increasing loading capacity, we also modeled the adsorption DOX to MGO-PEG-CET with the Langmuir adsorption isotherm, assuming MGO-PEG-CET to be an ideal adsorbent composed of series of distinct sites capable of binding DOX. Figure 4b indicated that the adsorption could be modeled satisfactory by the Langmuir adsorption isotherm with ($R^2 = 0.99$) and the maximal adsorption capacity could be obtained at 6.35 mg/mg [52]. Though initial DOX concentration could be theoretically increased to approach the maximum drug loading, the corresponding increase in solution viscosity hindered recovery of MGO by magnetic separation; therefore, the concentration ratio between MGO-PEG-CET and DOX was set at 1:4 (0.1 mg/mL MGO-PEG-CET with 0.4 mg/mL DOX) for future studies.

The release of DOX from MGO-PEG-CET/DOX was investigated from the cumulative percentage of DOX released at 37 °C in pH 7.4 or pH 5.7 PBS to simulate the extracellular and the intracellular environment (Figure 4c). Sustained release of DOX from MGO-PEG-CET/DOX was observed and the percentage of DOX released at pH 5.7 (54.6%) is about twice that released at pH 7.4 (29%) within one week, thus confirming the pH-sensitive DOX release. Moreover, the initial slope of the release curve at pH 5.7 demonstrates the effective and rapid release of drug in an acidic environment, fulfilling the requirement for intracellular DOX release in the endosome after intracellular uptake [53,54]. GO could adsorb DOX through π–π stacking and by hydrogen bonds between –OH (–COOH) groups of MGO-PEG-CET and –OH group of DOX [55]. Therefore, the pH-sensitive drug release may be due to the weakening of those hydrogen bonds when H$^+$ weakens hydrogen bond interactions and promotes drug release. By releasing its drug cargo in the acidic endosomal environment (pH < 6) after intracellular uptake, the cytotoxicity of MGO-PEG-CET/DOX toward cancer cells could be enhanced.

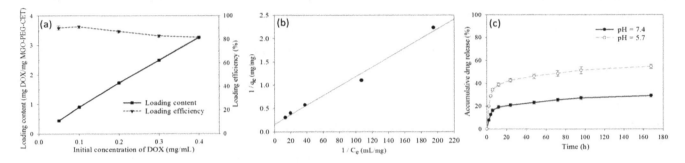

Figure 4. (a) Drug loading content and loading efficiency when a DOX solution with different initial concentration was mixed with an equal volume of 0.1 mg/mL MGO-PEG-CET; **(b)** The drug loading was satisfactorily modeled with the Langmuir adsorption isotherm where C_e is the equilibrium DOX concentration in the solution and q_e is the adsorbed DOX amount; and, **(c)** The release of DOX from MGO-PEG-CET/DOX in pH 7.4 and 5.7 PBS at 37 °C.

2.3. Intracelular Uptake

The high expression of EGFR on CT-26 surface is expected to facilitate ligand-targeting of CT-26 cancer cells using CET, an EGFR antibody [56]. This targeting effect could manifest itself through intracellular uptake of quantum dots (QDs)-tagged nanocarriers observed under a confocal microscope. Indeed, the confocal images in Figure 5 confirmed that CT-26 cells showed more intracellular uptake of MGO-PEG-CET than MGO-PEG from the signal intensity of QDs. Furthermore, the intracellular uptake of MGO-PEG-CET was inhibited when CT-26 cells were pre-treated with CET, thus confirming the receptor-mediated endocytosis of MGO-PEG-CET, as EGFR on cell surface could be blocked with excess CET. Therefore, we could confirm the enhanced intracellular uptake of CET-conjugated nanocarrier is governed by the binding of CET in MGO-PEG-CET to EGFR on CT-26 surface, which could provide an active targeting mechanism for targeted drug delivery.

The process of endocytosis was further confirmed by TEM. The TEM micrographs in Figure 6 clearly identified aggregates of MGO-PEG-CET within the endosomes after intracellular uptake, which are located in the cell cytoplasm and in close proximity to the cell nucleus. The endocytosis of MGO-PEG-CET is consistent with a previous report that studied the size-dependent intracellular uptake of protein-coated GO [57]. The authors reported that small GO (420 nm equivalent diameter) enter cells mainly through clathrin-mediated endocytosis, while large GO (860 nm equivalent diameter) enter through both phagocytosis and endocytosis.

Visualization of QDs-tagged MGO-PEG-CET/DOX after contacting with CT-26 cells revealed the green fluorescence of QDs-labeled MGO-PEG-CET in the cell cytoplasm, while the red fluorescence of DOX could only be identified in cell nuclei and merged with the blue fluorescence from the DAPI-stained cell nuclei (Figure 5). This implied DOX could be released from MGO-PEG-CET/DOX in the acidic intracellular environment after endocytosis, followed by releasing DOX into the nucleus to chelate with DNA molecules and exert cytotoxicity toward cancer cells [58]. Taken together, the confocal microscopy and TEM results strongly suggested that the cytotoxicity effects of DOX toward CT-26 could be facilitated by endocytosis of MGO-PEG-CET/DOX, followed by drug release at low endosomal pH value to enhance the anticancer activity of the drug.

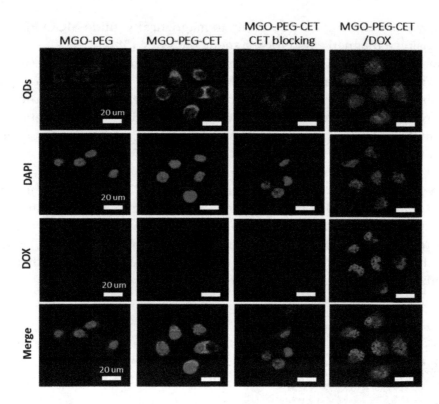

Figure 5. The confocal microscopy images of CT-26 cells after incubated with MGO-PEG, MGO-PEG-CET or MGO-PEG-CET/DOX for 1 h. Blocking of interaction between EGFR and CET (MGO-PEG-CET CET blocking) was carried out by pre-incubating CT-26 cells with CET (1 mg /mL) for 1 h to block EGFR receptors on cell surface followed by incubating with MGO-PEG-CET for 1 h. Bar = 20 μm.

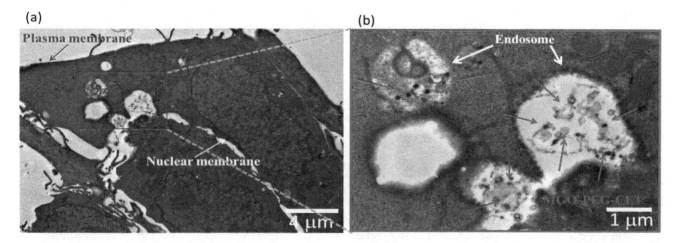

Figure 6. The transmission electron microscope (TEM) micrographs of CT-26 cells after contacting with MGO-PEG-CET for 1 h, bar = 4 μm. (**b**) is the magnified image of the red square shown in (**a**), bar = 1 μm.

2.4. Magnetic Targeting and Laser-Induced Hyperthermia

Through Live/Dead cell viability staining, we verified that an applied magnetic field in vitro could successfully guide MGO-PEG-CET/DOX to the magnetic targeting zone created by a magnet under the well in the cell culture dish. Within the magnetic targeting zone, there were hardly any live cells, while dead cells within this zone were likely to be detached from the well surface and removed during rinsing (Figure 7a). In contrast, abundant live cells (stained green) were detected outside the magnetic targeting zone, endorsing the possibility to magnetically guide MGO-PEG-CET/DOX to the tumor site in vivo using a magnetic field for magnetic targeting [58].

The photothermal effect was studied in vitro by measuring the temperature rise of solutions containing nanocarriers after irradiating with NIR laser at 2.5 W/cm^2 for 3 min (Figure 7b). Both GO and MGO showed a temperature rise, but the temperature increase was more pronounced for MGO. This is consistent with previous reports that both GO [59] and Fe$_3$O$_4$ magnetic nanoparticles [60] showed photothermal effects after absorbing light in the NIR region. The introduction of polymer and protein, such as PEG, avidin, and CET, may partially hamper the absorption of NIR light by MGO, resulting in a lower temperature rise for MGO-PEG-CET.

To observe the photothermal effect in vivo, MGO-PEG-CET was injected into healthy BALB/c mice (Figure 7c) or tumor-bearing BALB/c mice with CT-26 cells implanted subcutaneously (Figure 7d). Magnets were attached to the tumor for 2 h and both of the mice were exposed to NIR laser for 5 min at 2.5 W/cm^2. The regional temperature of the healthy mouse only rose to 42.5 °C, whereas the regional temperature of the tumor-bearing mouse rose to 60.1 °C. These results verified that MGO-PEG-CET is suitable for photothermal therapy in vivo [30].

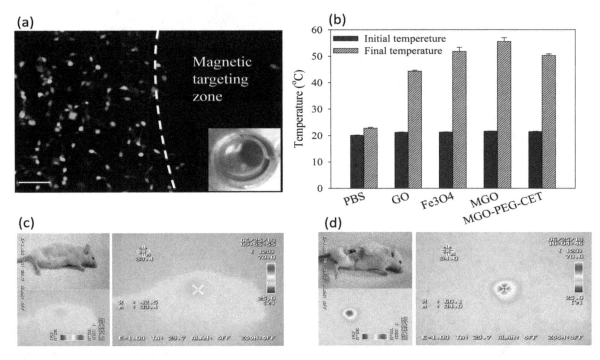

Figure 7. (a) Live/Dead staining of CT-26 cells after contacting with MGO-PEG-CET/DOX in a cell culture dish with a magnetic targeting zone created in a well of a culture dish by placing a magnet at the bottom of the well. The insert shows that MGO-PEG-CET/DOX was guided to the right corner of the well in the culture dish. Green: live cells; red: dead cells. Bar = 100 µm; (b) Temperature changes in vitro after exposure different nanocarriers (1 mg/mL in 0.2 mL of PBS) to NIR light at 2.5 W/cm^2 for 3 min. The in vivo temperature rise from thermal imaging of healthy BALB/c mouse (c) and tumor-bearing mouse (d) after intravenous injection of MGO-PEG-CET (7 mg/kg), followed by guidance with a magnetic field (1400 Gauss) for 2 h and exposure to NIR light (2.5 W/cm^2 for 5 min).

2.5. Biocompatibility of Nanocarriers

Biocompatibility tests were performed to assess the safety of the nanocarriers, including the cell viability test and hemolysis assay. The cell viability test was conducted on 3T3 fibroblast and CT-26 cells, which was incubated with different concentrations of MGO-PEG and MGO-PEG-CET. Both MGO-PEG and MGO-PEG-CET were non-toxic to fibroblasts in the concentration studies (Figure 8a). For CT-26, MGO-PEG was also biocompatible up to 100 µg/mL (Figure 8b). In contrast, MGO-PEG-CET shows mild toxicity from 10 to 100 μg/mL, and the relative cell viability was significantly significant different from those of MGO-PEG. It is well-documented that CET causes cytotoxicity to EGFR-expressing cancer cells, which renders CET to be a FDA approved drug for treating colon and head/neck cancers [61,62]. This feature is advantageous when considering that CET in the drug-free nanocarrier (MGO-PEG-CET) may also contribute to the killing of CT-26 cells.

An in vitro hemolysis assay was conducted to verify blood biocompatibility of MGO-PEG-CET. The absorption spectra (Figure 8c) of the supernatant of MGO-PEG-CET (31.25~250 μg/mL in PBS) after incubation with red blood cells (RBCs) at 37 °C for 2 h were conducted, with deionized (DI) water and PBS being, respectively, designated as the positive and negative controls. The osmotic pressure of DI water caused RBCs to rupture; thus, the absorbance spectrum of the DI water group showed absorbance values significantly higher than that of other groups. No visible hemolysis effect was observed after incubation with MGO-PEG-CET. The solution absorbance at 540 nm (OD_{540}) was the lowest for PBS, but slightly increased with increasing MGO-PEG-CET concentration, indicating that the nanocarrier caused slight but acceptable RBC damage (Figure 8d). That both of the solution colors and the absorbance of the MGO-PEG-CET solution were similar to that of the PBS endorsed minimum hemolysis due to MGO-PEG-CET and its safety for in vivo application as a drug carrier.

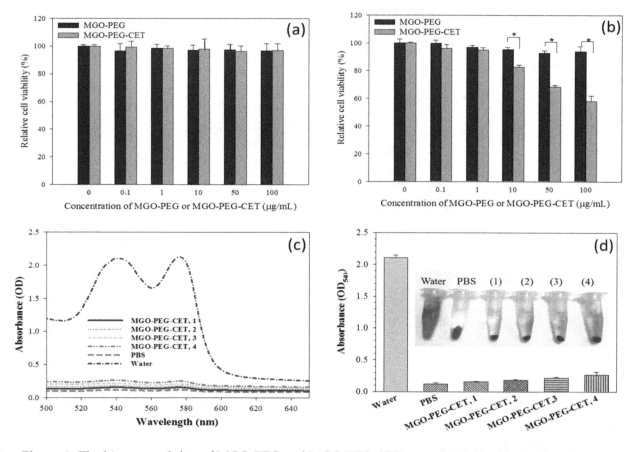

Figure 8. The biocompatibility of MGO-PEG and MGO-PEG-CET toward 3T3 fibroblasts (**a**) and CT-26 (**b**) by incubating cells with nanocarrier at different concentrations for 24 h and the relative cell viability was determined by MTT assays relative to culture medium (* $p < 0.05$); The hematological compatibility of MGO-PEG-CET was determined from the absorption spectra of the supernatant of MGO-PEG-CET after incubation with red blood cells in PBS for 2 h (**c**) for hemolytic assay and the optical density at 540 nm (OD_{540}) of the supernatant of MGO-PEG-CET was determined (**d**). Water and PBS were used as the positive and the negative controls, respectively. The temperature was at 37 °C. The concentrations of MGO-PEG-CET were 100 μg/mL (1), 200 μg/mL (2), 400 μg/mL (3) and 800 μg/mL (4) in (**d**).

2.6. The Efficacy of Combined Therapy In Vitro and In Vivo

Cell cytotoxicity assay was performed to assess the half maximal inhibitory concentration (IC50) of DOX after 24 h incubation with CT-26 cells in order to compare the efficacy of different treatments in vitro (Figure 9). The IC50 of DOX, MGO-PEG/DOX, MGO-PEG-CET/DOX, and MGO-PEG-CET/DOX + laser were 5.64, 2.64, 1.48, and 1.17 µg/mL, respectively. The results showed that MGO-PEG/DOX showed higher cytotoxicity than DOX, owing to the cellular uptake of MGO-PEG/DOX. The cytotoxicity could be further enhanced using MGO-PEG-CET/DOX with CET ligand-targeting to enhance the intracellular uptake of the nanocarrier and increase intracellular DOX concentration (Figure 5). Most importantly, MGO-PEG-CET/DOX treatment, followed by laser irradiation showed the highest cytotoxicity toward CT-26 cells with only one-fifth the IC50 of DOX, supporting the synergistic effects of chemotherapy and photothermal therapy.

The antitumor efficacy of MGO-PEG-CET/DOX was studied in vivo in a xenograft tumor model in mice. BALB/c mice with subcutaneous CT-26 tumors of 60–100 mm^3 were subjected to treatment with normal saline (control) and DOX in different ways. Gross images of the tumor-bearing mice taken on day 0 and 14 demonstrated the apparent tumor size differences in each group and the tumor removed from the animal on day 14 supported the anti-tumor effects with each treatment, but to a different degree (Figure 10a). Based on results of H&E staining of tumor tissue on day 14, necrosis of the cancer cells was most substantial in MGO-PEG-CET/DOX + magnet and MGO-PEG-CET/DOX + magnet + laser groups [59], but cell growth was observed in control, DOX and MGO-PEG-CET/DOX groups (Figure 10a).

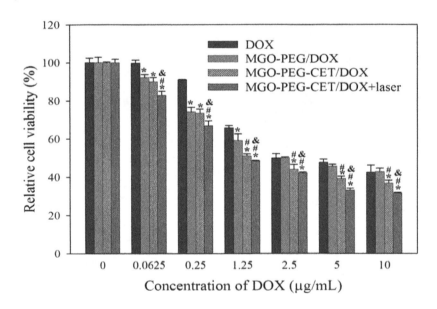

Figure 9. In vitro cytotoxicity of DOX, MGO-PEG/DOX, MGO-PEG-CET/DOX and MGO-PEG-CET/DOX + laser after contacted with CT-26 cells for 24 h. The laser group was subject to 2.5 W/cm^2 NIR light exposure for 3 min after treating with MGO-PEG-CET/DOX. * $p < 0.05$ compared with DOX. # $p < 0.05$ compared with MGO-PEG/DOX. & $p < 0.05$ as compared with MGO-PEG-CET/DOX.

The tumor volumes were recorded every other day up to 14 days and were expressed as relative tumor volume after normalizing the tumor volume at each time point with the tumor volume at day 0. At day 14, the average values of relative tumor volumes were 12.1 (control), 10.1 (free DOX), 9.5 (MGO-PEG-CET/DOX), 5.8 (MGO-PEG-CET/DOX + magnet) and 0.42 (MGO-PEG-CET/DOX + magnet + laser) (Figure 10b). When compared to the control, only MGO-PEG-CET/DOX + magnet and MGO-PEG-CET/DOX + magnet + laser groups showed substantial tumor suppression throughout the observation period (* $p < 0.05$). Although both free DOX and MGO-PEG-CET/DOX groups showed a general trend of tumor volume reduction as compared with the control with MGO-PEG-CET/DOX consistently performed better than DOX, both of the groups did not show significant difference in tumor volume from the control throughout the experiment. This underscores the importance of dual targeting with magnetic guidance in addition to ligand-targeting at the tumor site (MGO-PEG-CET/DOX + magnet) to bring about a significant difference from the control group in tumor volume. Nonetheless, the MGO-PEG-CET/DOX + magnet treatment failed to suppress tumor growth after day 8 with a rapid increase of tumor volume. This uncontrolled increase in tumor size could be alleviated by combining with photothermal therapy using laser light. Indeed, Only the MGO-PEG-CET/DOX + magnet + laser treatment could continuously suppress tumor growth and shrank the tumor size to a value less than the original value throughout the 14-day observation period. Undoubtedly, the significance of local hyperthermia for photothermal tumor ablation could be inferred for this remarkable enhancement in treatment efficacy [63]. As shown in Figure 10c, the mouse's body weight did not exhibit any significant difference between groups. However, mice in the control group showed a trend of better weight gain when compared to other groups under DOX treatment, which could be ascribed to the common adverse effect from chemotherapy. However, we did not observe any changes in appetite and behavior throughout the observation period for all of the mice under treatment.

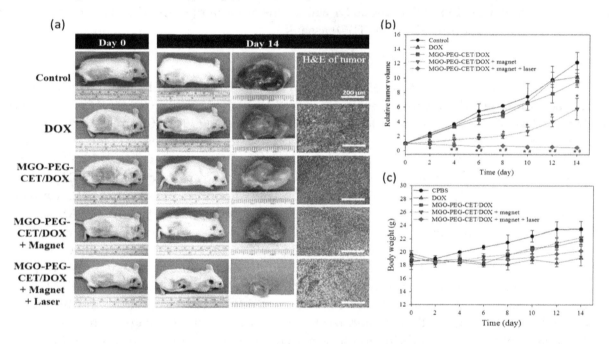

Figure 10. The anti-tumor efficacy in vivo with tumor-bearing BALB/C mice. BALB/c mice were subcutaneously implanted with CT-26 cells and were given different treatment by intravenous injection of normal saline (control), DOX, MGO-PEG-CET/DOX, MGO-PEG-CET/DOX + magnet, and MGO-PEG-CET/DOX + magnet + laser (30 mg/kg DOX). (a) The gross observation of tumor-bearing BALB/c mice on day 0 and 14, the gross view of incised tumor and the H&E staining of the incised tumor on day 14 (bar = 200 μm); The relative tumor volume (b) and body weight (c) were recorded. * $p < 0.05$ compared with control, DOX, and MGO-PEG-CET/DOX, # $p < 0.05$ as compared with MGO-PEG-CET/DOX + magnet.

3. Materials and Methods

3.1. Materials

Graphene oxide (N002-PDE) powder was obtained from Angstron Materials Inc. (Dayton, OH, USA). Potassium bromide (KBr) was purchased from Showa Chemical Co. (Tokyo, Japan). 1-(3-dimethylaminopropyl)-3-ethylcarbodiimide hydrochloride (EDC), and N-hydroxysuccinimide (NHS) were purchased from Acros Organics (Geel, Belgium). Avidin and cetuximab (CET) was purchased from Calbiochem (San Diego, CA, USA) and Merck (Darmstadt, Germany), respectively. Biotin-PEG-NHS (molecular weight = 3400 Da) was purchased from Nanocs Inc. (New York, NY, USA). Doxorubicin (DOX), 3-(4,5-Dimethyl-2-thiazolyl)-2,5-diphenyl-2H-tetrazolium bromide (MTT), 4',6-diamidine-2'-phenylindole dihydrochloride (DAPI), and RPMI-1640 medium for cell culture were all purchased from Sigma (St Louis, MO, USA). Live/Dead viability/cytotoxicity kit was purchased from Invitrogen (Carlsbad, CA, USA). Fetal bovine serum (FBS) purchased from Hyclone, GE Healthcare (Logan, UT, USA) was used for cell culture. All of the reagents were of analytical grade.

3.2. Preparation of Magnetic Graphene Oxide (MGO)

GO nano-platelets was prepared by a modified Hummers' method, as reported before [20]. Chemical co-precipitation was used to deposit Fe_3O_4 on GO surface by dispersing 25 mg of GO, 108 mg of $FeCl_3 \cdot 6H_2O$ and 40 mg of $FeCl_2 \cdot 4H_2O$ (mole ratio of $Fe^{2+}:Fe^{3+} = 1:2$) in 50 mL of deionized (DI) water by sonication for 30 min. The solution was purged with N_2 for 30 min (to prevent oxidation of Fe_3O_4) and was heated to 65 °C. Next, 1 g of $ClCH_2COOH$ was added to the solution to convert –OH to –COOH. After 1 h, 2 g of NaOH was added to the solution for reaction at a basic environment for an additional 30 min. A magnet was used to collect magnetic graphene oxide (MGO) from the solution, followed by washing with copious DI water. The amount of –COOH groups on MGO surface was determined by the toluidine blue O (TBO) assays.

3.3. Preparation of MGO-PEG-CET and MGO-PEG-CET-QDs

0.05 mL of 60 mM 1-ethyl-3-(3-dimethylaminopropyl) carbodiimide (EDC) and 0.05 mL of 60 mM N-hydroxysuccinimide (NHS) were prepared in phosphate-buffered saline (PBS, pH = 7.4) and mixed with 0.5 mL of MGO (1 mg/mL) solution prepared above at 4 °C for 30 min for activation of the –COOH groups of MGO. 1 mg of avidin was then added and the solution was left to react for 12 h at 4 °C for formation of amide bond between –COOH of MGO and –NH$_2$ of avidin (MGO-avidin). MGO-avidin was recovered from the solution with a magnet and washed with PBS. The amount of avidin in MGO-avidin was quantified from the amount of unbound avidin in the solution using the Coomassie (Bradford) Protein Assay Kit (Thermo Fisher Scientific, Waltham, MA, USA).

To synthesized biotin-PEG-CET and biotin-PEG-QDs, 0.2 mg of biotin-PEG-NHS was reacted with 4.2 mg of CET or 20 μL of quantum dots (QDs, QSA-490, with amine group from Ocean Nanotech, San Diego, CA, USA) in 1 mL PBS for 12 h at 4 °C through a spontaneous covalent bond formation between NHS esters and –NH$_2$ groups in CET or QDs. Biotin-PEG-CET was reacted with MGO-avidin prepared above and incubated at 4 °C for 30 min for binding between avidin and biotin to from MGO-PEG-CET. MGO-PEG-CET was separated from the solution with a magnet and its CET content was determined from the unbound CET in the supernatant using Coomassie (Bradford) Protein Assay Kit. Biotin-PEG-QDs were used to bind empty biotin binding sites of avidin on MGO-PEG-CET to prepare fluorescently labelled MGO-PEG-CET-QDs. MGO-PEG and MGO-PEG-QDs were prepared similarly by replacing CET with glycine to react with biotin-PEG-NHS.

3.4. Physico-Chemical Properties of Nanocarriers

The particles size, polydispersity (PDI) and zeta potential of nanocarriers were determined by dynamic light scattering (DLS) using a Nano ZA90 Zetasizer (Malvern Instruments Ltd., Worcestershire, UK) with particle suspensions that were prepared in DI water. For transmission electron microscopy (TEM), the particles was diluted to 0.01 mg/mL in DI water and then dropped onto a 200 mesh carbon-coated copper grid, followed by drying at 25 °C for one day before loading into the microscope. MGO-PEG-CET was stained with 2% phosphotungstic acid for 30 s before drying. The morphology and size of particle were observed by TEM (JEOL JEM-1230, Tokyo, Japan) at 100 kV. For Fourier transform infrared (FTIR) spectroscopy, the samples were blended with KBr, compressed to form a pellet and analyzed with a TENSOR II FTIR Spectrometer (Bruker Optics Inc., Billerica, MA, USA). The transmission spectra were obtained from 400 to 4000 cm^{-1} at 2.5 mm/s with a resolution of 4 cm^{-1}. The iron contents of samples were analyzed by inductively coupled plasma optical emission spectroscopy (ICP-OES, Optima 2100 DV, Perkin Elmer, Waltham, MA, USA). For X-ray diffraction (XRD) analysis of the crystal structures of samples, a D2 PHASER X-ray powder diffractometer (Bruker AXS Inc., Madison, WI, USA) was used by scanning dried power in the 2 θ range of 5°–70°. The step size was 0.04° and measurement time was 2 s per step. The phases were compared with the JCPDS database for identification. The crystallite size was determined using the Debye-Scherrer equation. Thermogravimetric analysis (TGA) was conducted with 8~10 mg of powder sample in nitrogen atmosphere from 25 to 750 °C, with a heating rate of 10 °C/min using a Q50 TGA from TA Instruments (New Castle, DE, USA). The magnetization curves were obtained with a superconducting quantum interference device (SQUID) magnetometer (MPMS XL-7, Quantum Design, San Diego, CA, USA) at 25 °C and applied magnetic field of 10,000 G.

3.5. Drug Loading and Release

Doxorubicin (DOX) loading onto MGO-PEG-CET was accomplished by mixing 0.1 mg MGO-PEG-CET with different amount of DOX in 1 mL PBS (pH 7.4) at 4 °C for 24 h. After separating MGO-PEG-CET/DOX by a strong magnet, the concentration of DOX in the supernatant was determined by a UV/Vis spectrophotometer (U3010, Hitachi, Tokyo, Japan) at 490 nm. The amount of DOX on MGO-PEG-CET/DOX was calculated from mass balance with the drug loading content (mg/mg) being defined as weight of DOX loaded/weight of MGO-PEG-CET and the drug loading efficiency (%) defined as (weight of DOX loaded/weight of DOX initially added) × 100.

For drug release, MGO-PEG-CET/DOX was placed in 1 mL of PBS (pH 5.7 or pH 7.4) and shaken at 120 rpm and 37 °C in dark. A magnet was used to separate MGO-PEG-CET/DOX at predetermined time points and the precipitate was re-suspended with 1 mL of fresh PBS of the same pH. The amount of DOX released from PEG-MGO-CET/DOX was determined from DOX concentration in the supernatant using a UV/Vis spectrophotometer at 490 nm in a cumulative manner with drug release (%), defined as (weight of DOX released/weight of DOX loaded) × 100.

3.6. Intracellular Uptake

CT-26 murine colonic carcinoma cells were obtained from Professor Chia-Rui Shen at the Graduate Institute of Medical Biotechnology of Chang Gung University, Taiwan. To observe the intracellular uptake of nanocarriers by CT-26 cells, 5×10^4 cells were seeded to 15-mm glass slides placed in a 24-well plate. After adding cell culture medium (RPMI-1640 with 10% FBS) and cultured for 24 h, MGO-PEG-QDs, MGO-PEG-CET-QDs, or MGO-PEG-CET-QDs/DOX was separately added to each well and incubated for another 1 h. After removing the cell culture medium and washing with PBS, cells was fixed with 4% paraformaldehyde for 15 min and were stained with 1 μg/mL DAPI for 10 min. To further confirm that the interaction between CET and EGFR molecules was the mechanism for enhancing the targeting efficacy of CET-conjugated nanocarriers, CT-26 cells were pre-treated with 1 mg/mL of CET for 1 h to block the EGFR molecules on cell surface before incubating with MGO-PEG-CET-QDs. The slides were observed under a confocal laser scanning microscope (Zeiss LSM 510 Meta, Oberkochen, Germany). The uptake of MGO and release of DOX could be visualized by the green fluorescence of QDs-labelled MGO-PEG or MGO-PEG-CET and the red fluorescence of DOX. The excitation wavelength is Red/Green/Blue = 543/488/364 nm and the emission wavelength is Red/Green/Blue = 550–650/500–550/407–482 nm.

The phenomenon of cell uptake was also observed through transmission electron microscope (TEM), where 5×10^4 CT-26 cells were grown on ThermoNox (Nunc, Thermo Fisher Scientific, Waltham, MA, USA) coverslips and were treated with MGO-PEG-CET for 24 h. After fixing with a mixture of 2% glutaraldehyde and 2.5% paraformaldehyde for 2 h, 0.1 M sodium cacodylate buffer (pH 7.4) was used to rinse the cells followed by post-fixing 30 min in 1.0% osmium tetroxide. Graded ethanol series (30%, 50%, 70%, 80%, 95%, and 100%) were used to dehydrate the cells for 10 min at each concentration, followed by two rinses in 100% propylene oxide. With infiltration and embedding in epoxy resins for

48 h at 60 °C, ~80 nm ultrathin specimen were sectioned and examined under a FEI/Philips CM 120 TEM (FEI, Hillsboro, OR, USA).

3.7. Photothermla Effect

In vitro photothermal effect was determined in 0.2 mL suspensions of GO, MGO, and MGO-PEG-PET (1 mg/mL in PBS) in 96-well cell culture plates by irradiating with an 808 nm continuous-wave near infrared (NIR) laser at a power of 2.5 W/cm^2 (0.4 cm^2 laser area) for 3 min. The temperature of the solution before and after exposure to NIR light was determined with a K-Type thermal couple thermometer (Hanna Instruments, Woonsocket, RI, USA).

In vivo photothermal effect was from thermal imaging of a tumor-bearing BALB/c mouse after the intravenous injection of MGO-PEG-CET. The tumor-bearing mouse was injected with MGO-PEG-CET (7 mg/kg), followed by guidance with a magnetic field (1400 Gauss) for 2 h and exposure to NIR light at 2.5 W/cm^2 (0.4 cm^2 laser area) for 5 min. Thermal images were captured with an infrared thermal imaging camera (Thermo GEAR G100EX, Avio, Tokyo, Japan) to measure the temperature distribution around the tumor area. A healthy BALB/c mouse was used as a control after exposure to the same NIR light for 5 min at similar same location.

3.8. Magnetic Guidance In Vitro

To examine the effect of magnetic guidance of MGO-PEG-CET, 0.5 mL cell culture medium containing CT-26 cells (5×10^4) was added to each well of a 24-well plate and was cultured for 24 h. After adding MGO-PEG-CET/DOX to each well to reach a final concentration of 0.1 mg/mL, the culture plate was placed on a magnetic separator, which had 7.5 mm diameter permanent magnets glued to the center of each well, followed by 24 h cell culture. After washing with PBS, a Live/Dead cell viability assay was conducted by examining with an inverted fluorescence microscope to determine live and dead cells around the magnetic targeting zone created by the magnet.

3.9. Blood Compatibility Analysis

The hemolysis assay was conducted to evaluate the whole blood compatibility of MGO-PEG-CET. The red blood cells (RBCs) from Sprague-Dawley (SD) rats (BioLASCO, Taipei, Taiwan) were obtained by removing the serum from the whole blood after centrifugation at 3500 rpm at 4 °C for 10 min. All of the animal experiments were conducted according to protocols approved by the Chang Gung University's Institutional Animal Care and Use Committee (IACUC Approval No.: CGU15-168). Following wash with PBS five times, the cells were diluted to ten times of the original volume with PBS. The diluted RBC (0.3 mL) suspension was mixed with 1.2 mL of DI water (positive control), 1.2 mL of PBS (negative control), or 1.2 mL of different concentration of MGO-PEG-CET in PBS. The mixtures were incubated at 37 °C for 30 min and centrifuged. The absorbance values of the supernatants were recorded from 500 to 650 nm using an ultraviolet-visible (UV/Vis) Spectrophotometer and compared at 540 nm (OD$_{540}$) for all the samples.

3.10. In Vitro Cytotoxicity

Approximately 5×10^3 CT-26 cells in 200 μL cell culture medium were placed in each well of a 96-well culture plate and cultured for 24 h. After removing the spent culture medium, different concentrations of DOX (free DOX, MGO-PEG/DOX, or MOG-PEG-CET/DOX) in 200 μL cell culture medium was added to each well and incubated at 37 °C for 24 h. The medium in each well was removed and each well was washed with PBS, followed by adding 200 μL diluted MTT solution (1 mg/mL in culture medium) and incubated for 2 h at 37 °C in dark. The MTT solution was removed and purple formazan crystals in each well was dissolved with 200 μL dimethyl sulfoxide and the solution absorbance was measured with a microplate reader at 570 nm (OD$_{570}$). The cytotoxicity to CT-26 cells was determined from the relative cell viability (%) relative to cells cultured in cell culture medium.

3.11. Mouse Subcutaneous Tumor Model

Female BALB/c mice weighing approximately 15–20 g (4–6 weeks old) were purchased from BioLASCO (Taipei, Taiwan). All of the animal experiments were conducted according to protocols that were approved by the Chang Gung University's Institutional Animal Care and Use Committee (IACUC Approval No.: CGU15-168). CT-26 cells were harvested by 0.1% trypsin-EDTA, washed once with PBS, re-suspended in serum-free RPMI-1640 (1×10^7 cells in 100 μL) and were subcutaneously injected into the right flank of each mouse. When the tumors had grown to approximately 60–100 mm^3 (about 14 days), the tumor-bearing mice were randomized into five groups ($n = 6$ in each group): group 1 (control) received 200 μL intravenous (IV) injection of normal saline; group 2 received 200 μL IV injection of DOX solution (30 mg/kg); group 3 received 200 μL IV injection of 9.2 mg/kg MGO-PEG-CET/DOX (containing 30 mg/kg DOX); group 4 was treated as in groups 3, but the tumor was exposed to a magnetic field of 1400 Gauss with a magnet for 2 h after IV injection; group 5 was treated as in group 4 but the tumor was exposed to additional NIR irradiation (808 nm wavelength, 2.5 W/cm^2) for 5 min every two days. Injections were carried out over 2 min through the tail vein, with withdrawal of needle over 1 min to prevent back leak. The animal body weight and tumor volume were continuously monitored on alternate days for two weeks post treatment [64]. For ethical reasons, animals were euthanized when the volume of the implanted tumor reached 2 cm^3. The tumor size was measured using a caliper and defined as: tumor volume = (length × width × width)/2. Tumors were collected on day 14 of the treatment, fixed in 10% buffered formalin, followed by paraffin-embedment and sectioning to 2–3 μm thickness for hematoxylin and eosin (H&E) staining.

3.12. Statistical Analyses

All data were reported as mean ± standard deviation (SD) and subject to one-way analysis of variance (ANOVA) analysis. Tukey's post-hoc test was used to determine the difference between any two groups with p-value < 0.05 considered to be statistically significant.

4. Conclusions

We presented a dual-targeting nanomedicine approach for cancer therapy using MGO-PEG-CET/DOX that combines co-precipitated Fe_3O_4 magnetic nanoparticles and CET (an EGFR antibody) for magnetic and receptor-mediated ligand-targeting of malignant CT-26 mouse colon carcinoma. The combinatory chemo-photothermal therapy comprises the antitumor drug DOX and laser-induced hyperthermia with contribution from the EGFR-specific antibody (CET). Through this comprehensive design, the MGO-PEG-CET/DOX showed enhanced cytotoxicity toward CT-26 in vitro and inhibited tumor propagation in vivo. The anti-tumor effects could be augmented using an NIR laser for photothermal therapy in vitro and in vivo. From the proof-of-concept report using magnetic targeting plus NIR laser irradiation, which successfully shrunk tumors to 42% of its original volume in 14 days, this study provides a new paradigm to evolve traditional chemotherapeutic drug (DOX) and to overcome its side effects. The dual targeting MGO-PEG-CET drug delivery system could be implied to offer an extraordinary platform in promoting the success of cancer therapy.

Acknowledgments: We would like to express our appreciation of financial supports provided by Change Gung Memorial Hospital (CMRPD2G0081, CMRPD2G0082, CMRPG3F1742 and BMRP249) and the Ministry of Science and Technology (MOST-106-2221-E-182-056-MY3). The authors thank the Microscopy Center at Chang Gung University and the Microscope Core Laboratory in Change Gung Memorial Hospital Linkuo Medical Center for technical assistance.

Author Contributions: Yu-Jen Lu and Jyh-Ping Chen conceived and designed the experiments; Yu-Jen Lu and Pin-Yi Lin performed the experiments; Pin-Yi Lin, Chang-Yi Kuo and Mao-Yu Chen analyzed the data; Yu-Jen Lu, Pei-Han Huang, K.T. Shalumon and Jyh-Ping Chen wrote the paper.

References

1. Organization, W.H. Cancer. Available online: http://www.who.int/cancer/en/ (accessed on 19 October 2017).
2. Feng, S.S.; Chien, S. Chemotherapeutic engineering: Application and further development of chemical engineering principles for chemotherapy of cancer and other diseases. *Chem. Eng. Sci.* **2003**, *58*, 4087–4114. [CrossRef]
3. Skalickova, S.; Loffelmann, M.; Gargulak, M.; Kepinska, M.; Docekalova, M.; Uhlirova, D.; Stankova, M.; Fernandez, C.; Milnerowicz, H.; Ruttkay-Nedecky, B.; et al. Zinc-modified nanotransporter of doxorubicin for targeted prostate cancer delivery. *Nanomaterials* **2017**, *7*, 435. [CrossRef] [PubMed]
4. Au, J.L.; Jang, S.H.; Zheng, J.; Chen, C.T.; Song, S.; Hu, L.; Wientjes, M.G. Determinants of drug delivery and transport to solid tumors. *J. Controll. Release* **2001**, *74*, 31–46. [CrossRef]
5. Lammers, T.; Aime, S.; Hennink, W.E.; Storm, G.; Kiessling, F. Theranostic nanomedicine. *Acc. Chem. Res.* **2011**, *44*, 1029–1038. [CrossRef] [PubMed]
6. Quader, S.; Kataoka, K. Nanomaterial-enabled cancer therapy. *Mol. Ther.* **2017**, *25*, 1501–1513. [CrossRef] [PubMed]
7. Goldberg, M.; Langer, R.; Jia, X. Nanostructured materials for applications in drug delivery and tissue engineering. *J. Biomater. Sci. Polym. Ed.* **2007**, *18*, 241–268. [CrossRef] [PubMed]
8. Duncan, R. The dawning era of polymer therapeutics. *Nat. Rev. Drug Discov.* **2003**, *2*, 347–360. [CrossRef] [PubMed]
9. Maeda, H. The enhanced permeability and retention (EPR) effect in tumor vasculature: The key role of tumor-selective macromolecular drug targeting. *Adv. Enzyme Regul.* **2001**, *41*, 189–207. [CrossRef]
10. Matsumura, Y.; Maeda, H. A new concept for macromolecular therapeutics in cancer chemotherapy: Mechanism of tumoritropic accumulation of proteins and the antitumor agent smancs. *Cancer Res.* **1986**, *46*, 6387–6392. [PubMed]
11. Lu, Y.J.; Wei, K.C.; Ma, C.C.; Yang, S.Y.; Chen, J.P. Dual targeted delivery of doxorubicin to cancer cells using folate-conjugated magnetic multi-walled carbon nanotubes. *Colloids Surf. B Biointerfaces* **2012**, *89*, 1–9. [CrossRef] [PubMed]
12. McCallion, C.; Burthem, J.; Rees-Unwin, K.; Golovanov, A.; Pluen, A. Graphene in therapeutics delivery: Problems, solutions and future opportunities. *Eur. J. Pharm. Biopharm.* **2016**, *104*, 235–250. [CrossRef] [PubMed]
13. Hong, S.; Leroueil, P.R.; Majoros, I.J.; Orr, B.G.; Baker, J.R.; Holl, M.M.B. The binding avidity of a nanoparticle-based multivalent targeted drug delivery platform. *Chem. Biol.* **2007**, *14*, 107–115. [CrossRef] [PubMed]
14. Montet, X.; Funovics, M.; Montet-Abou, K.; Weissleder, R.; Josephson, L. Multivalent effects of rgd peptides obtained by nanoparticle display. *J. Med. Chem.* **2006**, *49*, 6087–6093. [CrossRef] [PubMed]
15. Mejias, R.; Perez-Yague, S.; Gutierrez, L.; Cabrera, L.I.; Spada, R.; Acedo, P.; Serna, C.J.; Lazaro, F.J.; Villanueva, A.; Morales, M.P.; et al. Dimercaptosuccinic acid-coated magnetite nanoparticles for magnetically guided in vivo delivery of interferon gamma for cancer immunotherapy. *Biomaterials* **2011**, *32*, 2938–2952. [CrossRef] [PubMed]
16. Sanson, C.; Diou, O.; Thevenot, J.; Ibarboure, E.; Soum, A.; Brulet, A.; Miraux, S.; Thiaudiere, E.; Tan, S.; Brisson, A.; et al. Doxorubicin loaded magnetic polymersomes: Theranostic nanocarriers for mr imaging and magneto-chemotherapy. *ACS Nano* **2011**, *5*, 1122–1140. [CrossRef] [PubMed]
17. Yang, C.L.; Chen, J.P.; Wei, K.C.; Chen, J.Y.; Huang, C.W.; Liao, Z.X. Release of doxorubicin by a folate-grafted, chitosan-coated magnetic nanoparticle. *Nanomaterials* **2017**, *7*, 85. [CrossRef] [PubMed]
18. Shang, N.G.; Papakonstantinou, P.; McMullan, M.; Chu, M.; Stamboulis, A.; Potenza, A.; Dhesi, S.S.; Marchetto, H. Catalyst-free efficient growth, orientation and biosensing properties of multilayer graphene nanoflake films with sharp edge planes. *Adv. Funct. Mater.* **2008**, *18*, 3506–3514. [CrossRef]
19. Yang, X.Y.; Zhang, X.Y.; Ma, Y.F.; Huang, Y.; Wang, Y.S.; Chen, Y.S. Superparamagnetic graphene oxide-Fe_3O_4 nanoparticles hybrid for controlled targeted drug carriers. *J. Mater. Chem.* **2009**, *19*, 2710–2714. [CrossRef]
20. Sun, X.; Liu, Z.; Welsher, K.; Robinson, J.T.; Goodwin, A.; Zaric, S.; Dai, H. Nano-graphene oxide for cellular imaging and drug delivery. *Nano. Res.* **2008**, *1*, 203–212. [CrossRef] [PubMed]
21. Liu, J.; Cui, L.; Losic, D. Graphene and graphene oxide as new nanocarriers for drug delivery applications. *Act. Biomater.* **2013**, *9*, 9243–9257. [CrossRef] [PubMed]

22.   Li, Y.M.; Jiang, T.; Lv, Y.; Wu, Y.; He, F.; Zhuo, R.X. Amphiphilic copolymers with pendent carboxyl groups for high-efficiency loading and controlled release of doxorubicin. *Colloids Surf. B Biointerfaces* **2015**, *132*, 54–61. [CrossRef] [PubMed]

23.   Felber, A.E.; Dufresne, M.H.; Leroux, J.C. Ph-sensitive vesicles, polymeric micelles, and nanospheres prepared with polycarboxylates. *Adv. Drug Deliv. Rev.* **2012**, *64*, 979–992. [CrossRef] [PubMed]

24.   Simoes, S.; Moreira, J.N.; Fonseca, C.; Duzgunes, N.; de Lima, M.C. On the formulation of ph-sensitive liposomes with long circulation times. *Adv. Drug Deliv. Rev.* **2004**, *56*, 947–965. [CrossRef] [PubMed]

25.   Yan, T.; Zhang, H.; Huang, D.; Feng, S.; Fujita, M.; Gao, X.D. Chitosan-functionalized graphene oxide as a potential immunoadjuvant. *Nanomaterials* **2017**, *7*, 59. [CrossRef] [PubMed]

26.   Seabra, A.B.; Paula, A.J.; de Lima, R.; Alves, O.L.; Durán, N. Nanotoxicity of graphene and graphene oxide. *Chem. Res. Toxicol.* **2014**, *27*, 159–168. [CrossRef] [PubMed]

27.   Huang, J.; Zong, C.; Shen, H.; Liu, M.; Chen, B.; Ren, B.; Zhang, Z. Mechanism of cellular uptake of graphene oxide studied by surface-enhanced raman spectroscopy. *Small* **2012**, *8*, 2577–2584. [CrossRef] [PubMed]

28.   Yue, H.; Wei, W.; Yue, Z.; Wang, B.; Luo, N.; Gao, Y.; Ma, D.; Ma, G.; Su, Z. The role of the lateral dimension of graphene oxide in the regulation of cellular responses. *Biomaterials* **2012**, *33*, 4013–4021. [CrossRef] [PubMed]

29.   Yang, K.; Wan, J.M.; Zhang, S.; Tian, B.; Zhang, Y.J.; Liu, Z. The influence of surface chemistry and size of nanoscale graphene oxide on photothermal therapy of cancer using ultra-low laser power. *Biomaterials* **2012**, *33*, 2206–2214. [CrossRef] [PubMed]

30.   Zhang, W.; Guo, Z.; Huang, D.; Liu, Z.; Guo, X.; Zhong, H. Synergistic effect of chemo-photothermal therapy using pegylated graphene oxide. *Biomaterials* **2011**, *32*, 8555–8561. [CrossRef] [PubMed]

31.   Ma, X.X.; Tao, H.Q.; Yang, K.; Feng, L.Z.; Cheng, L.; Shi, X.Z.; Li, Y.G.; Guo, L.; Liu, Z. A functionalized graphene oxide-iron oxide nanocomposite for magnetically targeted drug delivery, photothermal therapy, and magnetic resonance imaging. *Nano Res.* **2012**, *5*, 199–212. [CrossRef]

32.   Huang, Y.S.; Lu, Y.J.; Chen, J.P. Magnetic graphene oxide as a carrier for targeted delivery of chemotherapy drugs in cancer therapy. *J. Magn. Magn. Mater.* **2017**, *427*, 34–40. [CrossRef]

33.   Park, J.W.; Mok, H.; Park, T.G. Epidermal growth factor (EGF) receptor targeted delivery of pegylated adenovirus. *Biochem. Bioph. Res. Commun.* **2008**, *366*, 769–774. [CrossRef] [PubMed]

34.   Jokerst, J.V.; Lobovkina, T.; Zare, R.N.; Gambhir, S.S. Nanoparticle pegylation for imaging and therapy. *Nanomedicine* **2011**, *6*, 715–728. [CrossRef] [PubMed]

35.   Gref, R.; Minamitake, Y.; Peracchia, M.T.; Trubetskoy, V.; Torchilin, V.; Langer, R. Biodegradable long-circulating polymeric nanospheres. *Science* **1994**, *263*, 1600–1603. [CrossRef] [PubMed]

36.   Höög, J.L.; Gluenz, E.; Vaughan, S.; Gull, K. Chapter 8—Ultrastructural investigation methods for trypanosoma brucei. In *Methods in Cell Biology*; Müller-Reichert, T., Ed.; Academic Press: Camgridge, MA, USA, 2010; Volume 96, pp. 175–196.

37.   Jokar, S.; Pourjavadi, A.; Adeli, M. Albumin-graphene oxide conjugates; carriers for anticancer drugs. *RSC Adv.* **2014**, *4*, 33001–33006. [CrossRef]

38.   Acharya, S.; Sahoo, S.K. PLGA nanoparticles containing various anticancer agents and tumour delivery by epr effect. *Adv. Drug Deliv. Rev.* **2011**, *63*, 170–183. [CrossRef] [PubMed]

39.   Tseng, S.H.; Chou, M.Y.; Chu, I.M. Cetuximab-conjugated iron oxide nanoparticles for cancer imaging and therapy. *Int. J. Nanomed.* **2015**, *10*, 3663–3685.

40.   Mahmoud, W.E. Morphology and physical properties of poly(ethylene oxide) loaded graphene nanocomposites prepared by two different techniques. *Eur. Polym. J.* **2011**, *47*, 1534–1540. [CrossRef]

41.   Murugan, A.V.; Muraliganth, T.; Manthiram, A. Rapid, facile microwave-solvothermal synthesis of graphene nanosheets and their polyaniline nanocomposites for energy strorage. *Chem. Mater.* **2009**, *21*, 5004–5006. [CrossRef]

42.   Liang, R.P.; Liu, C.M.; Meng, X.Y.; Wang, J.W.; Qiu, J.D. A novel open-tubular capillary electrochromatography using beta-cyclodextrin functionalized graphene oxide-magnetic nanocomposites as tunable stationary phase. *J. Chromatogr. A* **2012**, *1266*, 95–102. [CrossRef] [PubMed]

43.   He, H.; Gao, C. Supraparamagnetic, conductive, and processable multifunctional graphene nanosheets coated with high-density Fe_3O_4 nanoparticles. *ACS Appl. Mater. Interfaces* **2010**, *2*, 3201–3210. [CrossRef] [PubMed]

44.   Zhu, Y.; Murali, S.; Cai, W.; Li, X.; Suk, J.W.; Potts, J.R.; Ruoff, R.S. Graphene and graphene oxide: Synthesis, properties, and applications. *Adv. Mater.* **2010**, *22*, 3906–3924. [CrossRef] [PubMed]

45. Kolhe, P.; Kannan, R.M. Improvement in ductility of chitosan through blending and copolymerization with peg: Ftir investigation of molecular interactions. *Biomacromolecules* **2003**, *4*, 173–180. [CrossRef] [PubMed]

46. Shen, J.F.; Shi, M.; Ma, H.W.; Yan, B.; Li, N.; Ye, M.X. Hydrothermal synthesis of magnetic reduced graphene oxide sheets. *Mater. Res. Bull.* **2011**, *46*, 2077–2083. [CrossRef]

47. Xu, L.Q.; Wang, L.; Zhang, B.; Lim, C.H.; Chen, Y.; Neoh, K.G.; Kang, E.T.; Fu, G.D. Functionalization of reduced graphene oxide nanosheets via stacking interactions with the fluorescent and water-soluble perylene bisimide-containing polymers. *Polymer* **2011**, *52*, 2376–2383. [CrossRef]

48. Ghosh, S.; Badruddoza, A.Z.M.; Hidajat, K.; Uddin, M.S. Adsorptive removal of emerging contaminants from water using superparamagnetic Fe_3O_4 nanoparticles bearing aminated beta-cyclodextrin. *J. Environ. Chem. Eng.* **2013**, *1*, 122–130. [CrossRef]

49. Wang, C.; Feng, L.; Yang, H.; Xin, G.; Li, W.; Zheng, J.; Tian, W.; Li, X. Graphene oxide stabilized polyethylene glycol for heat storage. *Phys. Chem. Chem. Phys.* **2012**, *14*, 13233–13238. [CrossRef] [PubMed]

50. Chen, J.P.; Yang, P.C.; Ma, Y.H.; Tu, S.J.; Lu, Y.J. Targeted delivery of tissue plasminogen activator by binding to silica-coated magnetic nanoparticle. *Int. J. Nanomed.* **2012**, *7*, 5137–5149. [CrossRef] [PubMed]

51. Hsu, H.L.; Chen, J.P. Preparation of thermosensitive magnetic liposome encapsulated recombinant tissue plasminogen activator for targeted thrombolysis. *J. Magn. Magn. Mater.* **2017**, *427*, 188–194. [CrossRef]

52. Wang, Y.; Yang, S.T.; Wang, Y.; Liu, Y.; Wang, H. Adsorption and desorption of doxorubicin on oxidized carbon nanotubes. *Colloids Surf. B Biointerfaces* **2012**, *97*, 62–69. [CrossRef] [PubMed]

53. Oishi, M.; Hayashi, H.; Iijima, M.; Nagasaki, Y. Endosomal release and intracellular delivery of anticancer drugs using ph-sensitive PEGylated nanogels. *J. Mater. Chem.* **2007**, *17*, 3720–3725. [CrossRef]

54. Lee, M.; Jeong, J.; Kim, D. Intracellular uptake and ph-dependent release of doxorubicin from the self-assembled micelles based on amphiphilic polyaspartamide graft copolymers. *Biomacromolecules* **2015**, *16*, 136–144. [CrossRef] [PubMed]

55. Zhang, R.Y.; Olin, H. Carbon nanomaterials as drug carriers: Real time drug release investigation. *Mater. Sci. Eng. C Mater. Biol. Appl.* **2012**, *32*, 1247–1252. [CrossRef]

56. Cai, W.; Chen, K.; He, L.; Cao, Q.; Koong, A.; Chen, X. Quantitative PET of EGFR expression in xenograft-bearing mice using ^{64}Cu-labeled cetuximab, a chimeric anti-egfr monoclonal antibody. *Eur. J. Nucl. Med. Mol. Imaging* **2007**, *34*, 850–858. [CrossRef] [PubMed]

57. Mu, Q.; Su, G.; Li, L.; Gilbertson, B.O.; Yu, L.H.; Zhang, Q.; Sun, Y.P.; Yan, B. Size-dependent cell uptake of protein-coated graphene oxide nanosheets. *ACS Appl. Mater. Interfaces* **2012**, *4*, 2259–2266. [CrossRef] [PubMed]

58. Chertok, B.; David, A.E.; Yang, V.C. Polyethyleneimine-modified iron oxide nanoparticles for brain tumor drug delivery using magnetic targeting and intra-carotid administration. *Biomaterials* **2010**, *31*, 6317–6324. [CrossRef] [PubMed]

59. Yang, K.; Zhang, S.; Zhang, G.; Sun, X.; Lee, S.-T.; Liu, Z. Graphene in mice: Ultrahigh in vivo tumor uptake and efficient photothermal therapy. *Nano Lett.* **2010**, *10*, 3318–3323. [CrossRef] [PubMed]

60. Chu, M.; Shao, Y.; Peng, J.; Dai, X.; Li, H.; Wu, Q.; Shi, D. Near-infrared laser light mediated cancer therapy by photothermal effect of Fe_3O_4 magnetic nanoparticles. *Biomaterials* **2013**, *34*, 4078–4088. [CrossRef] [PubMed]

61. Maiello, E.; Gebbia, V.; Manzione, L.; Giuliani, F.; Morelli, F.; Arcara, C.; Grimaldi, A.; Colucci, G. Clinical results of EGFR-targeted therapies in advancedcolorectal cancer. *EJC Suppl.* **2008**, *6*, 64–69. [CrossRef]

62. Rivera, F.; Vega-Villegas, M.E.; Lopez-Brea, M.F. Cetuximab, its clinical use and future perspectives. *Anticancer Drugs* **2008**, *19*, 99–113. [CrossRef] [PubMed]

63. O'Neal, D.P.; Hirsch, L.R.; Halas, N.J.; Payne, J.D.; West, J.L. Photo-thermal tumor ablation in mice using near infrared-absorbing nanoparticles. *Cancer Lett.* **2004**, *209*, 171–176. [CrossRef] [PubMed]

64. Kirui, D.K.; Khalidov, I.; Wang, Y.; Batt, C.A. Targeted near-IR hybrid magnetic nanoparticles for in vivo cancer therapy and imaging. *Nanomedicine* **2013**, *9*, 702–711. [CrossRef] [PubMed]

Permissions

List of Contributors

Elka Touitou, Hiba Natsheh and Shaher Duchi
The Institute for Drug Research, School of Pharmacy, Faculty of Medicine, The Hebrew University of Jerusalem, Jerusalem 91120, Israel

Yongle Luo
School of Chemical Engineering and Energy Technology, Dongguan University of Technology, Dongguan 523808, China
Safety Evaluation Department, Guangdong safety production technology center Co. Ltd., Guangzhou 510075, China

Xujun Yin, Xi Yin, Anqi Chen, Lili Zhao, Gang Zhang, Wenbo Liao and Xiangxuan Huang
School of Chemical Engineering and Energy Technology, Dongguan University of Technology, Dongguan 523808, China

Juan Li and Can Yang Zhang
Advanced Research Institute for Multidisciplinary Science, Beijing Institute of Technology, Beijing 100081, China

Rohini Atluri
Nano-Bio Engineering Laboratory, Southeast Missouri State University, Cape Girardeau, MO 63701, USA
Mechanical and Energy Engineering Department, University of North Texas, Denton, TX 76207, USA

Rahul Atmaramani
Nano-Bio Engineering Laboratory, Southeast Missouri State University, Cape Girardeau, MO 63701, USA
Department of Bioengineering, The University of Texas at Dallas, Richardson, TX 75080, USA

Gamage Tharaka and Jian Peng
Department of Physics and Engineering Physics, Southeast Missouri State University, Cape Girardeau, MO 63701, USA

Thomas McCallister and Somesree GhoshMitra
Nano-Bio Engineering Laboratory, Southeast Missouri State University, Cape Girardeau, MO 63701, USA

David Diercks
Department of Metallurgical and Materials Engineering, Colorado School of Mines, Golden, CO 80401, USA

Santaneel Ghosh
Nano-Bio Engineering Laboratory, Southeast Missouri State University, Cape Girardeau, MO 63701, USA

Department of Physics and Engineering Physics, Southeast Missouri State University, Cape Girardeau, MO 63701, USA

Ana Santos-Rebelo and Catarina Garcia
Centro de Investigação em Biociências e Tecnologias da Saúde (CBIOS), Universidade Lusófona de Humanidades e Tecnologias, Campo Grande 376, 1749-024 Lisboa, Portugal
Department of Biomedical Sciences, Faculty of Pharmacy, University of Alcalá, Ctra. A2 km33,600 Campus Universitario, 28871 Alcalá de Henares, Spain

Carla Eleutério
Faculdade de Farmácia, Universidade de Lisboa (FFUL), Av. Prof. Gama Pinto, 1649-003 Lisboa, Portugal

Ana Bastos, João F. Pinto and Maria M. Gaspar
Faculdade de Farmácia, Universidade de Lisboa (FFUL), Av. Prof. Gama Pinto, 1649-003 Lisboa, Portugal
iMed.ULisboa-Faculdade de Farmácia, Universidade de Lisboa, Av. Prof. Gama Pinto, 1649-003 Lisboa, Portugal

Sílvia Castro Coelho and Manuel A. N. Coelho
Laboratory for Process Engineering, Environment (LEPABE), Department of Chemical Engineering, Faculty of Engineering, University of Porto, 4200-135 Porto, Portugal

Jesús Molpeceres
Department of Biomedical Sciences, Faculty of Pharmacy, University of Alcalá, Ctra. A2 km33,600 Campus Universitario, 28871 Alcalá de Henares, Spain

Ana S. Viana
Centro de Química e Bioquímica (CQB), Centro de Química Estrutural (CQE), Faculdade de Ciências, Universidade de Lisboa, Campo Grande 1749-016 Lisboa, Portugal

Lia Ascensão
Centre for Environmental and Marine Studies (CESAM), Faculdade de Ciências, Universidade de Lisboa, Campo Grande 1749-016 Lisboa, Portugal

Patrícia Rijo
Centro de Investigação em Biociências e Tecnologias da Saúde (CBIOS), Universidade Lusófona de Humanidades e Tecnologias, Campo Grande 376, 1749-024 Lisboa, Portugal
iMed.ULisboa-Faculdade de Farmácia, Universidade de Lisboa, Av. Prof. Gama Pinto, 1649-003 Lisboa, Portugal

Catarina P. Reis
Faculdade de Farmácia, Universidade de Lisboa (FFUL), Av. Prof. Gama Pinto, 1649-003 Lisboa, Portugal
iMed.ULisboa-Faculdade de Farmácia, Universidade de Lisboa, Av. Prof. Gama Pinto, 1649-003 Lisboa, Portugal
Institute of Biophysics and Biomedical Engineering (IBEB), Faculdade de Ciências, Universidade de Lisboa, 1749-016 Lisboa, Portugal

Eleonora Colombo, Michele Biocotino, Pierfausto Seneci and Daniele Passarella
Dipartimento di Chimica, Università degli Studi di Milano, Via Golgi 19, 20133 Milano, Italy

Giulia Frapporti and Giovanni Piccoli
CIBIO, Università di Trento, Via Sommarive 9, 38123 Povo (TN), Italy

Pietro Randazzo
Promidis Srl, San Raffaele Scientific Research Park, Torre San Michele 1, Via Olgettina 60, 20132 Milan, Italy

Michael S. Christodoulou
DISFARM, Sezione di Chimica Generale e Organica "A. Marchesini", Universitdegli Studi di Milano, via Venezian 21, 20133 Milano, Italy

Laura Polito
ISTM-CNR, via Fantoli 16/15, 20138 Milan, Italy

Anna V. Stavitskaya, Andrei A. Novikov, Mikhail S. Kotelev, Dmitry S. Kopitsyn, Evgenii V. Ivanov and Vladimir A. Vinokurov
Functional Aluminosilicate Nanomaterials Lab, Gubkin University, Moscow 119991, Russia

Elvira V. Rozhina, Ilnur R. Ishmukhametov and Rawil F. Fakhrullin
Bionanotechnology Lab, Institute of Fundamental Medicine and Biology, Kazan Federal University, Kazan, Republic of Tatarstan, Russian Federation

Yuri M. Lvov
Functional Aluminosilicate Nanomaterials Lab, Gubkin University, Moscow 119991, Russia

Institute for Micromanufacturing, Louisiana Tech University, Ruston, LA 71272, USA

Sara Palchetti, Luca Digiacomo and Giulio Caracciolo
Department of Molecular Medicine, Sapienza University of Rome, Viale Regina Elena 291, 00161 Rome, Italy

Damiano Caputo and Roberto Coppola
Department of General Surgery, University Campus-Biomedico di Roma, Via Alvaro del Portillo 200, 00128 Rome, Italy

Anna Laura Capriotti
Department of Chemistry, Sapienza University of Rome, P.le Aldo Moro 5, 00185 Rome, Italy

Daniela Pozzi
Department of Molecular Medicine, Sapienza University of Rome, Viale Regina Elena 291, 00161 Rome, Italy
Istituti Fisioterapici Ospitalieri, Istituto Regina Elena, Via Elio Chianesi 53, 00144 Rome, Italy

Simona Giarra, Virginia Campani, Laura Mayol and Giuseppe De Rosa
Department of Pharmacy, University of Naples Federico II, D. Montesano 49, 80131 Naples, Italy

Silvia Zappavigna, Marianna Abate, Alessia Maria Cossu and Michele Caraglia
Department of Biochemistry, Biophysics and General Pathology, Second University of Naples, L. De Crecchio 7, 80138 Naples, Italy

Carlo Leonetti and Manuela Porru
UOSD SAFU, IRCCS Regina Elena National Cancer Institute, E. Chianesi 53, 00144 Rome, Italy

Yuge Feng and Junfa Zhu
National Synchrotron Radiation Laboratory and Department of Chemical Physics, University of Science and Technology of China, Hefei 230029, China

Chengliang Wang and Jianye Zang
Hefei National Laboratory for Physical Sciences at Microscale, CAS Center for Excellence in Biomacromolecules, Collaborative Innovation Center of Chemistry for Life Sciences, and School of Life Sciences, University of Science and Technology of China, Hefei 230026, China

Fei Ke
Department of Applied Chemistry and State Key Laboratory of Tea Plant Biology and Utilization, Anhui Agricultural University, Hefei 230036, China

Ana Rita O. Rodrigues, Joana O. G. Matos, Armando M. Nova Dias, Bernardo G. Almeida, Elisabete M. S. Castanheira and Paulo J. G. Coutinho
Centro de Física da Universidade do Minho (CFUM), Campus de Gualtar, 4710-057 Braga, Portugal

Ana Pires, André M. Pereira and João P. Araújo
IFIMUP/IN — Instituto de Nanociência e Nanotecnologia, Universidade do Porto, R. Campo Alegre, 4169-007 Porto, Portugal

Maria-João R. P. Queiroz
Centro de Química da Universidade do Minho (CQUM), Campus de Gualtar, 4710-057 Braga, Portugal

Nikita A. Navolokin, Georgy S. Terentyuk and Galina N. Maslyakova
Remote Controlled Theranostic Systems Lab, Saratov State University, Saratov 410012, Russia
Scientific Research Institute of Fundamental and Clinical Uronephrology, Saratov Medical State University, Saratov 410000, Russia

Sergei V. German and Dmitry A. Gorin
Remote Controlled Theranostic Systems Lab, Saratov State University, Saratov 410012, Russia
Biophotonics Laboratory, Skoltech Center for Photonics and Quantum Materials, Skolkovo Institute of Science and Technology, Moscow 121205, Russia

Alla B. Bucharskaya, Olga S. Godage and Viktor V. Zuev
Scientific Research Institute of Fundamental and Clinical Uronephrology, Saratov Medical State University, Saratov 410000, Russia

Nikolaiy A. Pyataev, Pavel S. Zamyshliaev and Mikhail N. Zharkov
Laboratory of Pharmacokinetics and Targeted Drug Delivery, Medicine Institute, National Research Ogarev Mordovia State University, Saransk 430005, Russia

Gleb B. Sukhorukov
Remote Controlled Theranostic Systems Lab, Saratov State University, Saratov 410012, Russia
School of Engineering and Materials Science, Queen Mary University of London, London E1 4NS, UK

Yi Teng Fong
Department of Chemical and Materials Engineering, Chang Gung University, Taoyuan 33302, Taiwan
Department of Plastic and Reconstructive Surgery and Craniofacial Research Center, Chang Gung Memorial Hospital, Linkou, Kwei-San, Taoyuan 33305, Taiwan

Chih-Hao Chen
Department of Plastic and Reconstructive Surgery and Craniofacial Research Center, Chang Gung Memorial Hospital, Linkou, Kwei-San, Taoyuan 33305, Taiwan

Michael Evangelopoulos and Jonathan O. Martinez
Center for Biomimetic Medicine, Houston Methodist Research Institute, Houston, TX 77030, USA

Alessandro Parodi
Department of Pharmacology, University of Illinois at Chicago, Chicago, IL 60607, USA

Ennio Tasciotti
Center for Biomimetic Medicine, Houston Methodist Research Institute, Houston, TX 77030, USA
Department of Orthopedics & Sports Medicine, Houston Methodist Hospital, Houston, TX 77030, USA

Nemany A. Hanafy
CNR NANOTEC-Istituto di Nanotecnologia, 73100 Lecce, Italy
Department of Mathematics and Physics "E. De Giorgi", University of Salento, 73100 Lecce, Italy

Luciana Dini
Department of Biological and Environmental Sciences and Technologies (DiSTeBA), University of Salento, 73100 Lecce, Italy

Cinzia Citti
CNR NANOTEC-Istituto di Nanotecnologia, 73100 Lecce, Italy
Department of Biological and Environmental Sciences and Technologies (DiSTeBA), University of Salento, 73100 Lecce, Italy

Giuseppe Cannazza
Department of Biological and Environmental Sciences and Technologies (DiSTeBA), University of Salento, 73100 Lecce, Italy
Life Science Department, University of Modena e Reggio Emilia, 41121 Modena, Italy

Stefano Leporatti
CNR NANOTEC-Istituto di Nanotecnologia, 73100 Lecce, Italy

Yu-Jen Lu, Pei-Han Huang and Mao-Yu Chen
Department of Neurosurgery, Chang Gung Memorial Hospital Linkuo Medical Center and College of Medicine, Chang Gung University, Taoyuan 33305, Taiwan

Pin-Yi Lin, Chang-Yi Kuo and K.T. Shalumon
Department of Chemical and Materials Engineering, Chang Gung University, Taoyuan 33302, Taiwan

Jyh-Ping Chen
Department of Chemical and Materials Engineering, Chang Gung University, Taoyuan 33302, Taiwan
Department of Plastic and Reconstructive Surgery and Craniofacial Research Center, Chang Gung Memorial Hospital, Linkou, Kwei-San, Taoyuan 33305, Taiwan

Research Center for Food and Cosmetic Safety, Research Center for Chinese Herbal Medicine, College of Human Ecology, Chang Gung University of Science and Technology, Kwei-San, Taoyuan 33302, Taiwan
Department of Materials Engineering, Ming Chi University of Technology, Tai-Shan, New Taipei City 24301, Taiwan

Index

A

Anisotropy, 122, 126, 132-133, 135, 139

Antibodies, 28, 66, 88, 141, 179-182, 203, 208

Anticancer Drugs, 14, 24, 87-88, 99, 108, 111, 155-156, 166, 174, 227-228

Atomic Absorption Spectroscopy, 140, 142

Autophagy, 58-60, 65, 70-75

B

Betulinic Acid, 59-60, 62, 65, 67-72, 74

Bioavailability, 1-2, 5, 10-11, 48, 164

Biodistribution, 140, 143, 149-150, 153, 176, 193-194

Bioimaging, 76-77, 83-84, 180

Biotechnology, 155, 168, 173-174, 223

Biotoxicity, 111-112, 116, 119

Breast Cancer, 42, 47, 51, 56, 110, 139, 154-156, 165, 173-174, 176, 183, 186, 188, 190, 194, 208

Buspirone, 1-13

C

Cadmium, 76-77, 79-80, 83-84, 181

Camptothecin, 74, 88, 155, 185, 195

Cell Culture, 18, 31, 33, 47, 51, 90, 102, 108, 160, 162, 168, 170-172, 208, 213, 217-218, 222-224

Cell Lines, 16, 40, 44-47, 51, 58, 77, 90, 99-100, 102, 105, 107, 110, 131, 205

Cell Viability, 18, 23, 51, 60, 65, 76, 79, 81, 102, 113, 116-117, 141, 162-163, 172, 180, 186, 202, 217-219, 224

Chemotherapeutic Drug, 15, 154-155, 174, 225

Chemotherapy, 14-15, 24-25, 28, 41-42, 45, 56, 88, 99-100, 119, 122, 155, 174-176, 182, 184, 193, 206, 208-210, 220-221, 226-227

Cisplatin, 27-31, 33-34, 36-37, 39-42, 88, 100

Cytoplasm, 15, 81, 107, 141, 146, 161, 201-202, 216

Cytoskeleton, 78, 180, 202

Cytotoxicity, 14-15, 18, 23, 27, 29, 34, 36-37, 44, 47, 51, 65, 70, 72, 76, 82, 84, 86, 100, 107-108, 113, 116, 120, 154, 156, 158, 160-164, 172, 174, 176, 180, 188, 191, 206, 209, 216, 219-220, 222, 224-225

D

Diarrhea, 28, 41, 164

Doxorubicin, 14-16, 25-26, 28, 40-42, 60, 73-74, 99, 104, 108-112, 119-121, 154-156, 163, 168, 174-177, 181-182, 207-210, 212, 222-223, 226-228

Drug Delivery Carrier, 24, 111, 156, 184

Drug Solubility, 44, 48

E

Electron Spin Resonance, 140, 142, 144, 149, 153

Endocytosis, 38, 51, 83, 107, 141, 154-155, 160-163, 173, 182, 198, 207, 209-211, 216

Endosome, 155, 216

Ethinylestradiol, 2, 4, 8

Ethylenediaminetetraacetic Acid, 77, 171

F

Flow Cytometry, 31, 82-83, 89, 113, 117-118, 154, 163, 174

Folic Acid, 154-155, 161, 168-169, 175, 177, 197-199, 203-204

G

Gemcitabine, 45, 51, 58, 88, 110

Graphene Oxide, 154-155, 168, 174-177, 209-213, 221-222, 226-228

H

Halloysite, 76-86, 196

Hot Flushes, 1-3, 11-13

Hyaluronic Acid, 110, 154-155, 158, 168, 175-176, 186, 196

Hyperthermia, 27-29, 32, 34, 37, 39-40, 42, 59, 123, 137-138, 141, 151, 179, 181, 191, 217, 221, 225

I

Immunotherapy, 28, 208, 210, 226

Intravenous Injections, 140, 149

L

Liposomal Drugs, 87-88

Liposomes, 14, 26, 73, 87-94, 96-97, 100, 107, 109-110, 122-123, 131-137, 139, 155, 182-183, 187-188, 198, 210, 227

M

Magnetic Resonance Imaging, 32, 59, 73, 119, 123, 137, 140-141, 143, 152, 179, 190-191, 194-195, 227

Manganese Ferrite, 122-124, 127-129, 131-134, 136-138

Mass Spectrometry, 87, 89, 201-202, 205

Metal-organic Gel, 111, 119

Metastasis, 27-28, 45, 94, 97, 100, 138

Microcapsules, 140, 142-153

Mortality, 87-88, 203

Multidrug Resistance, 14, 25-26, 99-100, 108-109, 175

Multimodal Therapy, 27-28, 38, 41

N

Nanotechnology, 14, 42, 44-45, 57, 73, 88, 137, 140-141, 178, 189, 192-193, 196-197, 210

Nanovesicles, 2-3, 6, 196

Nanovesicular Delivery System, 1, 6-8, 10

Nasal Cavity, 1-2, 5
Nausea, 28, 45
Neuroblastoma, 27-32, 34-35, 37-43, 141

O
Oleic Acid, 197-201, 204, 208
Osteosarcoma, 100, 102, 106, 108, 110

P
Pancreatic Cancer, 44-46, 56-58, 87-88, 91, 93-96, 98
Pancreatic Ductal Adenocarcinoma, 87-88
Parvifloron D, 44-57
Pharmacokinetics, 12, 59, 88, 96, 108, 140, 153, 192
Phototherapy, 122, 135-136, 209
Physiological Temperature, 155, 158, 174
Plasma Proteins, 87-89, 91-92, 94-95
Plectranthus, 44-45, 56-57
Polyvinylpyrollidone, 29, 32
Protein Corona, 87-89, 96-98
Proteome, 89-90, 94

Q
Quantum Dots, 43, 76-77, 79, 82, 85-86, 168, 181, 192, 211-212, 216, 222

R
Radiation Therapy, 27-28
Radiotherapy, 28, 38, 41-42, 73
Reactive Oxygen Species, 39, 45, 180-181, 185, 198, 211

S
Serotonin, 1, 12-13
Sodium Tripolyphosphate, 100, 108
Squalene, 59-61, 65-67, 69-72, 74
Stem Cells, 141, 177, 183, 186, 196
Surface Plasmon Resonance, 123, 127, 129, 180, 192
Synuclein, 59, 72

T
Theranostics, 123, 133, 177-179, 181-182, 184, 186, 189-191, 195-196
Therapeutic Agents, 28, 32, 38, 42, 45, 56, 122-123, 178, 184, 195
Therapeutic Index, 59, 88
Thin Layer Chromatography, 60
Transition Electron Microscopy, 1, 3
Trehalose, 59-63, 65-75

Z
Zoledronic Acid, 99-100, 104, 108-109